electrical
measurement systems
for biological and
physical scientists

leonard j. weber

Oregon State University

donald l. mclean

University of California

electrical measurement systems for biological and physical scientists

▲
▼▼ **addison-wesley publishing company**

Reading, Massachusetts • Menlo Park, California
London • Amsterdam • Don Mills, Ontario • Sydney

This book is in the
ADDISON-WESLEY SERIES IN LIFE SCIENCES

Consulting Editor:
Johns Hopkins III

ISBN 0-201-04593-1
ABCDEFGHIJ-MA-798765

This book is dedicated to our families
and those who wish to learn.

preface

Nearly all scientific laboratories now contain electronic instruments or devices. These instruments or devices have become indispensable. Electronics has not only enabled scientists to obtain more accurate research data but also opened new and wider areas of research. A revolution in electronics has occurred in the laboratories of every biological discipline with the advent of such sophisticated instruments as the electron microscope, computer, gas chromatograph, spectrophotometer, instruments for measuring radio activity, and many other devices. Properly used, these instruments can yield satisfactory and accurate results even when operated by individuals who have no knowledge of electrical fundamentals or electronics. If the equipment malfunctions, it can usually be repaired by a manufacturer's representative in the area. There is no need for busy scientists to concern themselves with the electronics involved in their devices when skilled technicians are available to make adjustments and repairs.

However, not all measurements can be made with such specialized devices. It may be necessary at times to select a new instrument or device or assemble several instruments into a system. In these cases some knowledge of electrical fundamentals and electronics will be required. Scientists must be able to understand the specifications of a device such as an amplifier, power supply, or strip-chart recorder so that they can select the one that will operate more efficiently in the system. If a device or instrument is not commercially available, they must construct it by following a schematic diagram. Sometimes they may find it necessary to consult with an engineer to obtain answers to specific problems, and it may be difficult to communicate with the engineer if they are without any knowledge of electricity and electronics.

There are books on the market which will provide research scientists with a theoretical understanding of basic electronic devices and circuits. While much useful information can be obtained from these books, readers will often find difficulties in relating the theory to practical laboratory situations. This problem is especially acute for biologists since their work calls for the application of unfamiliar physical phenomena to highly variable natural phenomena.

This book is written to help biologists and other scientists bridge the gap between the familiar natural science and the unfamiliar and often "mystic" physical science. Because biologists are primarily interested in dependable electronic measuring systems, this book is designed to aid them in assembling such systems for use in the laboratory.

Two measurement systems are introduced and briefly discussed in Chapter 1. In the subsequent chapters, each device or instrument is discussed in relation to the other devices in a system. Sufficient electrical and electronic theory pertaining to the operation of these devices is presented to enable readers to understand the important factor that must be considered when setting up a measurement system. This format has the advantage of clearly relating the theory to specific situations, thereby enabling biologists to see this theory operate in an environment with which they are familiar.

Chapters 2 and 3 focus on problems which scientists can easily imagine and lay the basis for an understanding of electrical terminology used in direct-current (dc) measurement systems.

The first equations appear in Chapter 3. Equations of importance are numbered. Those of *major* importance are marked by an asterisk (*).

Chapter 4 introduces the reader to alternating-current (ac) components and their general response characteristics. The general usefulness of ac components is developed without making detailed numerical calculations. This approach will be particularly useful for readers not familiar with complex-number manipulations. Readers needing more help in circuit-analysis techniques may jump directly to Chapter 9 for this material.

Chapters 5, 6, and 7 discuss basic components and building blocks used in all electrical measuring systems. The emphasis is on the various characteristics of these components and blocks that must be considered when they are to be assembled into a complete measuring system.

Chapter 8 provides an introduction to the different types of building blocks used in biotelemetry systems.

Chapter 9 provides the important circuit-analysis laws and procedures that are needed when detailed analysis or design problems must be solved. It builds directly on the concepts introduced in Chapters 2, 3, and 4 and can be read without studying Chapters 5 through 8.

Chapters 10 and 11 deal with the ever-present noise problems that plague the experimenter, and various techniques and methods that can be used to reduce the objectionable effects of noise are discussed. Several rather sophisticated techniques are introduced in enough detail so the reader will be aware that they are available and can be useful in particularly difficult situations.

Chapter 12 covers circuits that can be used to perform mathematical operations on electrical signals as well as produce other useful functions.

A minimum of mathematical notations is used, since few biologists communicate in this language. A knowledge of basic algebra along with the meanings of slope and time-rate-of-change will enable readers to understand the principles discussed in the first ten chapters. The concepts of integration and differentiation are used briefly in Chapters 11 and 12 for those who require an introduction to the more sophisticated measurement and signal-processing problems.

Numerous examples are given throughout the book to point out how the ideas and equipment being discussed are applied to real measurement situations.

Review Questions and Problems appear at the end of each chapter except Chapter 8. These reviews are given to help the reader recall the important concepts that were stressed in the preceding chapter. These concepts should be committed to memory so that they may be used subsequently without the reader having to refer to the chapter. The idea that "I can look it up when I need it" will prove to be self-deceptive. Certain concepts are necessary tools for thinking about a subject. The Review Questions and Problems relate to such concepts.

Appendixes have been added to provide the reader with ready access to helpful information. Appendix I provides a glossary of 186 frequently used electrical terms. Every term listed in the glossary is given in *italics* the first time it appears in the text to indicate to the reader that it is defined in the glossary. Appendix 2 gives a list of symbols and subscript conventions. Appendix 3 references useful equations. These are the equations whose numbers are marked by an asterisk (*) when they first appear in the text. Appendix 4 lists books and references for those interested in further information on related subjects. Many of the references are annotated. The books and references pertinent to the various chapters are listed by numbers together with chapter numbers. Appendix 5 lists the major examples discussed in the text so that they can be readily located for reference. Appendix 6 lists basic electrical units and multiplier abbreviations. Appendix 7 provides the standard color code used on carbon-composition resistors. Answers to Selected Review Questions and Problems appear in Appendix 8.

Although the electrical theory presented in this book is relevant to devices and instruments in measuring systems, this book is also intended to provide a firm foundation for those individuals interested in acquiring a more diversified knowledge of basic electronics. Practicing biologists should find this book a good self-learning aid without the help of formal instruction. Biology students interested in learning some fundamental electronics should find this a valuable introductory classroom text.

Corvallis, Oregon   L. J. W.
Davis, California   D. L. McL.
April 1975

contents

1

the
measurement system

1.1 INTRODUCTION

The final result of almost any research investigation is an accumulation of measurement data. After compilation these data are grouped and frequently analyzed statistically. Conclusions are drawn from the analysis, and this information is then published in a scientific journal. The validity of these conclusions depends on the accurate interpretation of accurate data. The scientist must eliminate as many variables as possible from his experiments to be sure of obtaining valid data. This is especially difficult in biology since any interference by the observer with an organism's normal pattern of life will result in data that are not a true reflection of natural behavior.

The introduction of electronic measurement systems into biological research has enabled the scientist to make more precise observations and obtain data that could not have been collected by the more conventional methods. A basic measurement system is usually made up of the following: (1) a device attached to or placed near the animal which is designed to convert physiological or physical information into electrical energy (transducer); (2) a device that increases the level of the transduced signal (amplifier) so that it can be displayed on available instruments; and (3) devices to display (meter, cathode-ray oscilloscope) or permanently record (strip-chart recorder, magnetic tape recorder) the desired information. A measurement system may contain additional devices, depending on the type of measurement desired (see Fig. 1.1). To the uninitiated, an electronic measurement system may appear to be a simple array of devices or instruments, one following another in logical succession. Although it appears simple to assemble, in practice an assembled system may not adequately perform the task for which it was designed. One soon discovers that even the most modest systems can be fraught with problems. The difficulties usually involve some electrical or electronic

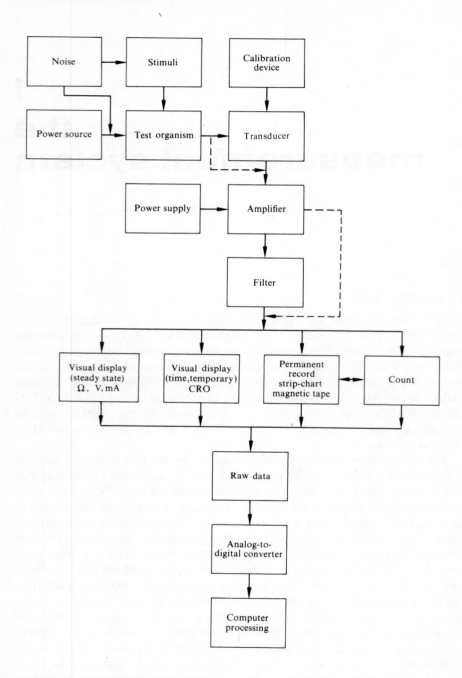

Fig. 1.1. Block diagram showing the devices that may be found in electronic measurement systems.

principles or characteristics. Lacking a knowledge of the electronics involved, the scientist may discard the system, often after having invested in it a great deal of time and money.

The most meaningful aid to attaining a full understanding of these problems and the associated electronic principles is a clear idea of their relation to an actual measurement system used in biological research. Two such systems are presented in this chapter: the *direct-coupled system* and the *biotelemetric system.* The electrical and electronic principles involved and the problems that might be encountered in the assembly and operation of such systems are discussed throughout the remainder of the book. Explanations of terms in italics used in this and subsequent chapters can be found in the glossary.

1.2 THE GENERAL BLOCK DIAGRAM

A *block diagram,* such as Fig. 1.1, is used to show the placement of instruments and other items in a system. It is a simplified means of presenting this information which does not confuse the issue by including the details of components within electronic circuits. A block diagram makes it possible to determine at a glance the position of circuits within an instrument, or instruments within a system. The *schematic diagram* is often referred to as the working diagram, since it shows all of the components within an instrument and is therefore useful as a guide for construction and repair.

For the newcomer to electronics schematic diagrams often seem complicated and confusing. While the block diagram is relatively straightforward, the schematic is often viewed as a jumble of strange symbols serving only to perplex the uninitiated.

The block diagram in Fig. 1.1 is read by following the arrows from one instrument to the next. Starting with the *power source,* we move to the *test organism,* then to or around the *transducer,* and on through the system. Items such as noise and stimuli are not instruments, but are usually present in a system used for biological measurements. *Noise* is defined as an undesirable signal, either intrinsic or extrinsic to the system, which usually masks, distorts, or destroys the display signal. This variable is very difficult to eliminate and the experimenter often must be content to have it reduced to a tolerable level. Because of its importance, noise is discussed in Chapter 10 as a separate subject.

1.3 A DIRECT-COUPLED MEASUREMENT SYSTEM

In a *direct-coupled* measurement system the transduced *signals* are transmitted by means of wire, self inductance, capacitance, or resistance to an amplifier or recorder. In some cases a transducer is not used and the signals go directly from the organism to a display device. In a *biotelemetric system,* the signals are transmitted through the air to a receiver. A direct-coupled system is depicted in block diagram form in Fig. 1.1.

The length of the wire connecting the transducer and the amplifier or recording instruments found in direct-coupled systems places restrictions on the size of the area over which the tested organism may range. Many subjects, in fact, are confined within cages in a laboratory. The organisms often tested with this system include small mammals, reptiles, arthropods, and plants. In most cases the investigations are carried out in the laboratory under programmed environmental conditions.

The classic example of the direct-coupled system in biology is the electrophysiological system used to measure nerve and muscle potentials. Since such systems have been used rather extensively for some time now, the circuitry is well established and quite dependable. In recent years additional direct-coupled systems have been developed which show much promise. The *capacitance sensing* system [18],* [31], [55] and the *insect activity sensing* system [32], [17], [40], [33] are two such systems that have become widely used. The capacitance-sensing system was developed to study locomotor activity and responsiveness to stimuli in small rodents and other animals. The insect activity sensing system is used to study locomotor, feeding, and salivation behavior in mosquitoes, aphids, and other sucking insects. This system, with aphids as the test animal, will be presented as an example of a direct-coupled measurement system.

Aphids pierce the tissues of their host plants with fine, sharp stylets in order to contact those cells preferred for the ingestion of food. Aphids have four stylets which are arranged to form a compact stylet bundle (Fig. 1.2). The bundle contains two canals, one through which the aphid secretes saliva and the other through which it aspirates the liquid food. An electrical system has been developed to measure the salivation and ingestion activities of aphids and to relate these activities to the transmission of plant viruses. Specific waveforms associated with these activities are recorded on a strip-chart recorder, enabling the investigator to determine precisely how long aphids salivate or ingest, and from which plant tissue area they obtain their food.

Figure 1.3 is a block diagram of the aphid activity measurement system. Starting with the block labeled "power source" and following the arrows, the reader can get a good picture of the system. The power source is a 120-volt alternating current (ac), which is the standard household voltage, usually called line voltage. A *voltage regulator* is the next block in the system; it is used to maintain a constant voltage in the system. Without this regulator fluctuations in line voltage, which are common in many laboratories, would affect the final recording.

Before proceeding to the next block, the reader must first understand a few basic electrical principles. It is apparent from the discussion up to this point that voltage and current are involved in the system. An analogy will aid in understand-

---

* The reference numbers are keyed to the listings in Appendix 4.

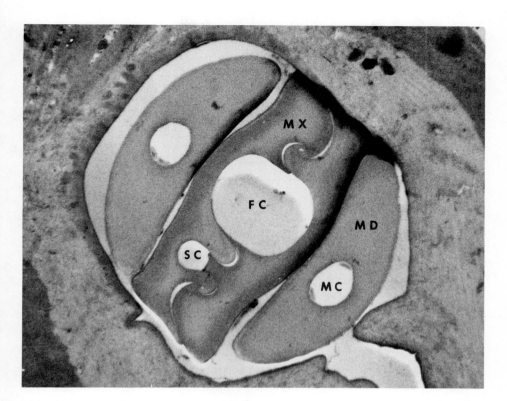

Fig. 1.2. Electron photomicrograph of the stylet bundle of a pea aphid, *Acyrthosiphon pisum* (Harris). (X16,900)

ing the meanings of some important terms. A system involving the circulation of a fluid, for example, has two major characteristics: pressure and flow. If a difference in pressure exists between two points in the system, liquid will flow, and the direction of the flow will be from the high-pressure area to the area of low pressure.

In electrical circuits a similar phenomenon exists. *Voltage* or *potential* is analogous to pressure, and *electric current* (usually called current) is analogous to flow. The concept of electric potential is related to the motion of a particle with a positive *electric charge*. If the positively charged body tends to move from one point to another, the point toward which it moves is said to be at a lower potential than the first point, or to be at a negative potential with respect to the first point. If two points are at different electric potentials, a *potential difference* is said to exist between them. If a conductive path is provided between two points having a potential difference, an electric current will flow from the point of high potential to the point of low potential.

Voltage or potential is symbolized by V, E, or *emf*. The time rate of change

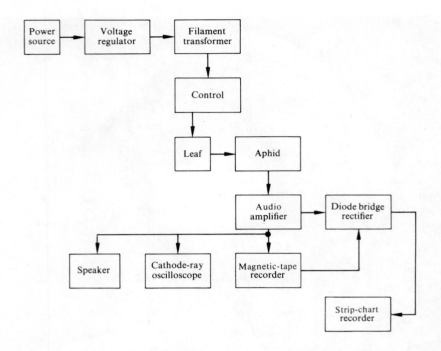

Fig. 1.3.   A block diagram of the aphid activity measurement system.

of electric charge passing through a specified area constitutes a current symbolized by I, which is measured in *amperes,* written A or amp. One-thousandth of an ampere is a milliampere, written mA. One-millionth of an ampere is a microampere, which is written μA. (Refer to Appendix 2 for more electrical symbols and their meanings.) These phenomena will be discussed more fully in Chapters 3 and 4.

If we resume our progress through the system, the next block encountered is the *transformer*. This device serves to step down the voltage from 120v ac to 6.3v ac. In thus reducing the potential, it also reduces the current. The operation of transformers will be discussed in Chapter 4.

The transformer is connected to the control unit, providing it with a fixed ac voltage of 6.3v. In this particular system it is desirable to be able to vary the amplitude of the voltage applied to the leaf. The purpose of the control is to give the experimenter a means of varying the amplitude of this ac voltage from zero to 6.3v. This can be done with a device called a *voltage divider* or *potentiometer*. The concept of a voltage divider will be discussed in Chapters 3 and 9.

The voltage available at the output of the control unit is connected to the leaf. The leaf acts as a very high resistance to current flow when there is a potential difference between two points on the leaf.

The next block in the system is the aphid, which is in contact with the leaf. A gold wire with a diameter of 15 microns is attached to the aphid's abdomen with silver conducting paint. The gold wire is fastened to another wire that goes into the input of the *audio amplifier*. When the aphid either salivates or ingests it will fill one or the other stylet canal with liquid. Then current will flow from one side of the control to the leaf, through the aphid, through the gold wire, through the amplifier, and back to the other side of the control. Saliva is secreted in spurts and solidifies almost immediately. Maximum current will flow when the saliva is in liquid form, and almost no current will flow after the solidification of the salivary material. Therefore, the salivation waveforms recorded will show sharp, narrow peaks. During ingestion, on the other hand, there will be very little fluctuation because the current will remain essentially unchanged, causing the waveform to appear as a nearly straight line (Fig. 1.4). Other waveforms will occur which reflect variations in the aphid's salivation and ingestion activities.

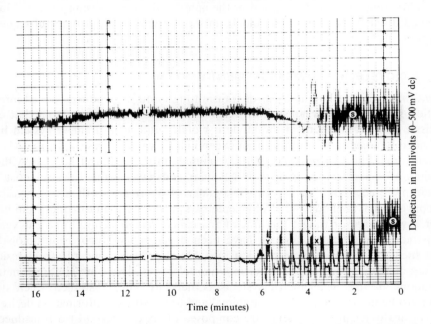

Fig. 1.4. Waveforms recorded during aphid probing of plant leaves. S is salivation, X is sieve-tube contact by stylets, I is ingestion. Strip charts are to be read from right to left.

The amplifier increases the voltage, enabling enough voltage to appear across the *diode bridge rectifier* to allow current flow through this device. The rectifier changes alternating current (ac) into direct current (dc) so that the dc chart recorder will accept the voltage. Direct and alternating currents will be discussed in Chapters 3 and 4, and rectifiers in Chapter 5.

The *strip-chart recorder* in this system records differences in potential, making it essentially a voltage recorder. Strip-chart recorders, along with other display devices, will be discussed in Chapter 7.

Another display device is also connected to the amplifier: a *cathode-ray oscilloscope* (CRO). Since this instrument will accept either alternating or direct current, there is no need to have a rectifier between it and the amplifier. The primary function of the oscilloscope is to act as a monitor for the system, detecting distortion caused by noise.

The *speaker* provides sound when the investigator is visually observing the aphid directly and not the recorder. The *magnetic-tape recorder* is another device for collecting and storing the data. The data collected on this instrument can be played back to a strip-chart recorder through the rectifier or to a cathode-ray oscilloscope. The advantage of the tape recorder is that the same data can be displayed over and over again for close study.

This completes the description of the aphid activity measuring system. More detailed discussions of the basic blocks in this system will appear in subsequent chapters.

1.4 A BIOTELEMETRIC MEASUREMENT SYSTEM

Biotelemetry is a technique used for transmitting through space transduced information from a living organism to a receiver at a remote distance from that organism. The development of the modern biotelemetric measurement system has provided biological scientists with an exceptionally valuable research tool. These systems have made it possible to study animals in their natural habitats with a minimum of interference with their behavior and have enabled the scientist to obtain more accurate data with a wider range of observations than was possible by conventional methods. Many biotelemetric systems are used to "track" animals over a wide area or range; this tracking is called *ecotelemetry*. In recent years even more sophisticated systems have been developed to record physiological data such as temperature, respiration rate, blood pressure, and pH from inside the test animals, giving rise to the term *physiotelemetry*. There are almost as many variations in types of telemetric systems as there are animals studied. Each system must be tailored to a particular animal and to the specific information desired.

Basically telemetric systems are composed of six devices: (1) a transducer, (2) a *transmitter* and its battery power, (3) a transmitting *antenna*, (4) a receiving *antenna*, (5) a *receiver* and its battery or other dc power supply, and (6) a recorder or other data-storage unit.

The measurement of internal body temperature of a ground squirrel, *Citellus beecheyi*, is representative of one kind of biotelemetry, specifically physiotelemetry. We can better understand the operation of this system by once again studying a block diagram (Fig. 1.5). In most biotelemetric systems the test organism will be the first block encountered. The test organism may be the squirrel, *C. beecheyi*.

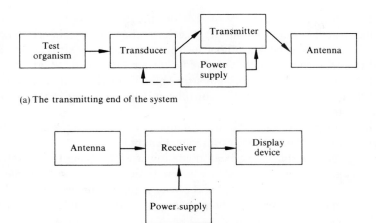

(a) The transmitting end of the system

(b) The receiving end of the system

Fig. 1.5. Block diagram of a typical telemetric system.

In this example the transducer must detect temperature and convert the information into electrical energy so that it can be transmitted to a receiver. This system uses part of the transmitter to perform this function. The circuit is called an *astable* or *free-running multivibrator*. The multivibrator functions as an electronic switch that goes on-off-on-off at programmed time intervals. When the multivibrator is connected to the transmitter through an oscillator circuit, intermittent "beats" or "pulses" are transmitted to a receiver. The multivibrator uses two transistors in its circuit which are temperature sensitive. As the ambient temperature surrounding the transistors increases, the current through them will increase and the "switch" will turn on and off faster. When the temperature decreases, the current flow will also decrease, resulting in a slower on-off activity. Therefore, if the time interval between the "pulses" is calibrated for known temperatures, any change in temperature inside the animal can be determined by timing the interval. The transmitter feeds these impulses to an antenna and the signals go off into space. The transmitter is "tuned" to a specific and constant frequency or "channel."

The transmitting antenna must also be designed to efficiently operate on this frequency. The transmitter, along with its battery power supply, is encapsulated in Saran Wrap®, beeswax, and Silastic 382 plastic. The complete unit is then surgically implanted within the peritoneal cavity of the ground squirrel. Under these conditions the transmitter has a range of 150 to 200 feet, and the batteries will last up to three months.

The transmitted impulses travel through space and eventually contact the receiving antenna, which is also designed to efficiently receive these radio waves. The impulses travel down a wire from the antenna into the receiver. The receiver is "tuned" to the exact frequency of the transmitter. The signals travel through rather complicated circuitry within the receiver and are finally changed into sound that is heard through a speaker. Other instruments, such as a strip-chart recorder, magnetic-tape recorder, oscilloscope, and a meter, may also be attached to the output of the receiver. By attaching a strip-chart recorder to the receiver output, the temperature changes within the squirrel can be permanently recorded over any given time span.

We have briefly discussed the instruments used in this example. A more thorough presentation will be found in subsequent chapters.

Although great strides have been made toward improving the versatility and dependability of biotelemetric systems, a few basic problems still plague experimenters. The size of the transmitter and power supply units are still too large for use in or on very small animals. The placement of the transmitter, power supply, and antenna on or in the animal, even though the instruments are small enough, may interfere with the animal's normal behavior. Extreme care must be taken to ensure that behavior is not influenced by these devices. The frequency of the transmitter may "drift" so that continuous adjustments must be made in the receiver to compensate for this drift. If the receiver is left unattended during a period of drift, valuable data will be lost. Drift often results from poor components within the transmitter or power supply, high temperatures, or excessively rough handling. It is very important to make the transmitter as stable as possible to minimize drift. The device should be bench tested for a period of time before being affixed to the animal. If the transmitter is surgically implanted in the animal or swallowed, it must be protected from destruction by the body fluids. This is one of the greatest problems encountered by physiotelemetrists, and an economical solution is not as yet available. If the device is to be externally attached to the animal, it must be firmly attached to prevent its removal.

Although the two measurement systems have been only briefly discussed, one can see the vast and exciting uses of these tools. The reader has probably already imagined a use for one or both of these systems in his own research. Let us become a little better acquainted with this subject by proceeding to Chapter 2.

1.5 REVIEW QUESTIONS

1.1   What are the general types of components that are commonly used in electrical measurement systems?

1.2   What type of information can a person usually expect to get from a block diagram of an electrical measurement system?

1.3   What is the distinction between a block diagram and a schematic diagram?

1.4   What are the major differences between a "direct-coupled measurement system" and a "biotelemetric system"?

1.5   What symbols are used to represent a voltage or potential difference variable? a current variable?

1.6   What are the general types of components that are commonly used in a biotele-metric system?

1.7   What is meant by the symbols "mA" and "μA"? Speculate on what the symbols "kV" or "kΩ" mean. The symbol Ω represents a unit called the ohm, which will be discussed later.

1.8   What applications can you imagine for direct-coupled electrical measurement systems needed by scientists? What inherent problems may be common for this type of system?

1.9   What applications can you imagine for biotelemetric measurement systems needed by scientists? What inherent problems may be common for this type of system?

2
coupling basic building blocks

2.1 OBJECTIVES

In this chapter we try to help the reader bridge the gap between his scientific background and an understanding of what he must look for when connecting test instruments to his electrical circuit. The chapter is written with the intention of allowing the reader to gradually work himself into the common problems and terminology associated with electrical measurements. No knowledge of electrical fundamentals is assumed. Examples of nonelectrical problems are used to introduce the concepts of potential, current flow, impedance, and resistance. The problems which often occur when test instruments are connected to an electrical circuit are discussed with examples. The use of mathematics is not required in the introduction of these concepts.

It was indicated in the previous chapter that there are many different types of measurements which you may want to make during the course of a particular experiment. Resistors, capacitors, inductors, power sources, amplifiers, and display or indicating devices are commonly used; unfortunately, they are also misused. Assembling a measuring system requires a careful selection of components so that they will perform the desired function; they must also be compatible.

The purpose of this chapter is to point out some of the pitfalls that cause difficulties and erroneous results. Any time two electrical circuits are connected together, a new circuit is formed which will not have exactly the same characteristics as the individual circuits. An electrically operated chart recorder may be operating properly before it is connected to the source of the signal which it is to record. After connection to the source, it may still record exactly the signal which is present at the input to the recorder. However, it is possible for this new recording to be in error by orders of magnitude compared to the signal generated by the source when the recorder is not connected to the source. A brief introduction to dc electrical fundamentals will make you well aware of these types of coupling problems.

2.2 THE FAULTY BATTERY PROBLEM

A scientist has been spending the past week setting up the crucial experiment in his $45,000 research project. All seems to be going properly until late in the afternoon of the sixth day. He notes that the light detector box is not giving repeatable results. This box is battery operated. "Ah," says the scientist, "I'll check this battery with my vacuum tube voltmeter." He does just this and finds that the voltage is almost at the rated value. He plugs in the battery only to find that the light detector is still erratic. This dilemma is shown in Fig. 2.1.

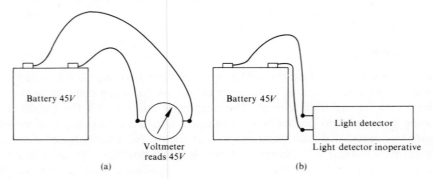

Fig. 2.1.   The dilemma!

The scientist then spends the next four hours trying to determine why he is getting erratic results. Finally he goes to the stockroom and gets a new battery even though he knows the old one passed the voltmeter test. He connects the new battery to the box and the system then functions properly. Why? The voltmeter was operating properly when the battery was measured. Indeed, the voltage measured was about right. However, if he had measured the voltage across the battery when the battery was functioning as the source of power for the light detector, he would have found the battery voltage to be only 30% of its rated value. The battery would not respond in the same way to the voltmeter alone as it would to the light detector.

Moral of this story

Any time two electrical components are connected together, a new circuit is produced which may be significantly different from the original circuits.

In this example the battery is acting as a source of energy for two different circuits or *loads*—the voltmeter and the light detector—and it responds differently to these two loads. We must, therefore, study the characteristics of sources and loads if we are to be successful in making electrical measurements.

2.3   INTERNAL CHARACTERISTICS OF SOURCES

Let us assume that a physiologist would like to open an artery of a small animal and have the animal pump its blood through a piece of test apparatus and then back into its own body (Fig. 2.2).

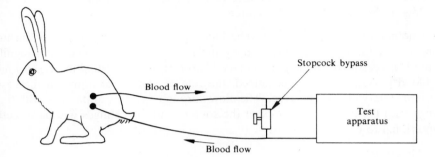

Fig. 2.2.   Blood flow experiment.

What factors are going to affect the flow of blood through the test apparatus? In this example the rate of flow of the blood may be considered the signal; it is analogous to the flow of current from the battery to the light detector in the previous example. Let us consider the animal as the source and speculate on the characteristics of this source. Blood will flow in the system when there is a complete path from one side of the pump (heart) to the other side of the pump. The amount of flow will depend on the pressure difference or *potential* difference between the two parts of the pump, the number of different blood paths through the body, the condition of these different paths, the rate at which the pump is operating, and the load which the test apparatus creates on the circulatory system of the animal. It seems reasonable to expect that as the physiological characteristics of the animal change, the blood flow through the test apparatus will change. It seems equally reasonable to expect that the blood flow through the test apparatus will change as the tubes in the apparatus change in shape.

Two things should now be apparent: we have a source whose internal characteristics can vary depending on the environment and the conditions of the animal; and we have a load external to the animal whose characteristics will affect the blood flow.

What about the source and its internal characteristics? Assume first of all that the heart produces a constant amplitude of pressure or potential regardless of the blood flow. If all of the blood passageways are to expand, the blood flow will increase and more blood will flow to the test apparatus than is possible under normal conditions. Then we can say that there is a reduction in *resistance* or *impedance* to the flow of blood when the passages expand. The opposite may occur: the blood passages leading from and to the heart may become severely constricted. Very little blood will then flow to the test apparatus. The internal resistance or impedance of the source has increased due to this constriction.

A point to remember

Even though the potential generated internally in the source is constant, changes in the internal impedance or resistance of the source will affect the flow of the signal out of the source.

Another situation may occur. The blood passages in the animal remain unchanged, but the pressure generated by the heart increases or decreases significantly. It is reasonable to assume that as this pressure or potential increases while the blood passages remain unchanged, the rate or volume of flow will increase. The converse will also be true. The flow through the test apparatus will thus change with the internal potential of the source, and the changes will be directly proportional to each other.

A point to remember

Changes in the internal potential of a source will affect the flow of a signal into a load even though the internal impedance of the source (source impedance) remains constant.

Through the physical analogy given above two very important points have been made which are directly applicable to any problem of electrical measurements. All electrical sources have an equivalent internal potential and an equivalent internal impedance. It is important to know what they are. If any load is connected to this source, the potential and the impedance of the source will affect the flow of current out of the source. You cannot expect the flow of current out of the source to be independent of the internal characteristics of the source.

2.4 CHARACTERISTICS OF LOADS

The test apparatus of the example given in the previous section serves as a load for the animal's blood system. It is not difficult to imagine some of the factors which determine its characteristics as a load. The internal works of the test apparatus may contain many different tubes of varying diameters connected one to another with many junctions. The amount of blood that can flow into this apparatus will depend on the number of tubes, the diameter of the tubes, the roughness of the interior walls of the tubes, the length of the tubes, etc. Thus the makeup of the tube network will determine how the flow of blood is impeded. The source, the blood system in this example, then works into or *drives* the load, the amount of flow depending on the impedance presented by the load.

The apparatus may have a cavity with an elastic wall, as shown in Fig. 2.3. As the pressure at the input to the cavity increases, more blood will flow into the cavity and cause the elastic wall to expand. A point will be reached when the wall will no longer expand and the pressure in the cavity will be equal to the pressure at the input to the cavity. When this occurs no more blood will flow into the cavity. Energy has been stored in the elastic wall.

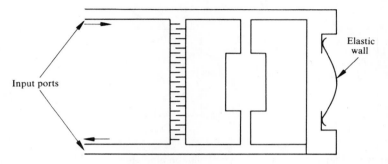

Fig. 2.3.   Interconnected tubes.

When the pressure at the input to the cavity decreases, the pressure inside the cavity will be greater than that at the input and blood will flow out of the cavity. The energy which was stored in the elastic wall when the wall was stretched is released as it drives blood out of the cavity. Again an equilibrium point will be reached when the pressure inside the cavity is no greater than the pressure at the input and there is no longer any blood flow. A cavity such as this could be used as a storage element in the test apparatus.

Points to remember

A load will present an impedance to the flow from a source.

A load may contain a storage element which will store and return flow from a source on a temporary or transient basis.

Although the discussion has been limited to the flow of blood from sources to loads, the concepts introduced here are basic to the study of electrical measurements. Terms such as resistance, impedance, source, load, signal, and drive have been introduced because they are commonly used in referring to electrical phenomena. More detailed analyses of electrical circuits will be given later.

2.5   CONSEQUENCES OF COUPLING SOURCES TO LOADS

A number of inferences have been made regarding what will happen when a source is connected to a load. It would be well at this point to relate these concepts more clearly to electrical measurement problems. Let us take the two most common electrical measurements and see what problems are involved. They are the measurement of flow or *current* and measurement of potential difference or *voltage.*

In taking the measurement of current with an *ammeter,* we find that there are three steps required (Fig. 2.4):

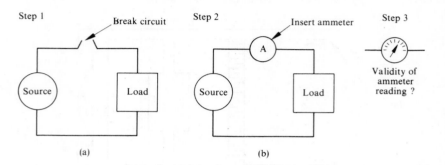

Fig. 2.4. Steps in measuring current with an ammeter.

1. Break the *circuit* at the point where current is to be measured.
2. Insert the ammeter and make the reading.
3. Determine what effect the insertion of the ammeter had on the circuit being tested. Are corrections necessary?

Step 3 is crucial. If this step is not carried out, an erroneous reading may be accepted and used as an accurate measurement of the current flow when the ammeter is not in the circuit. (Refer to the ideas introduced earlier.) When the source is connected to a load, some flow is expected. It is a measurement of this flow that is desired. Note that when the measurement is being made, the source is no longer driving the same load. Figure 2.5 helps illustrate this point.

When the ammeter is connected in the circuit, in *series* with load 1, the source is made to drive a new load, which is called load 3. Load 3 is equivalent to load 1 in series with load 2. Each load has an impedance between its two connecting terminals. Therefore, load 3 has a total impedance which is the sum of the individual impedances of loads 1 and 2. A general statement can now be made.

A point to remember

Whenever circuit element loads are connected in series, the total impedance of the combination of series circuit elements is equal to the sum of the individual circuit element impedances.

$$\text{Total series impedance} = \sum_{i=1}^{n} \text{element impedances,}$$

where n is the number of series circuit elements.

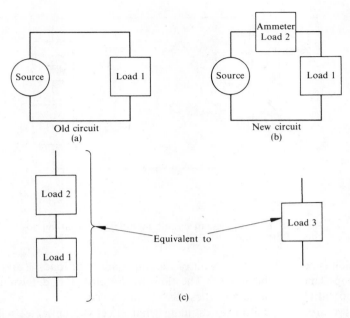

Fig. 2.5. Diagram showing change in circuit when an ammeter is inserted in the circuit.

What effect will the ammeter, the load 2 impedance, have on the current flow in the new circuit? It is fairly obvious that if the ammeter has zero impedance, often called a short circuit, the flow in the new circuit will be the same as the flow in the old circuit. No error will be introduced in the measurement other than the inherent error of the ammeter.

Let us think about what will happen if the impedance of the ammeter is the same as that of load 1. Do you think the current flow will be half what it was without the ammeter because the total series impedance is twice what it was before? Maybe yes or maybe no! It is true that the equivalent load, load 3, is twice as large as load 1. If the source voltage applied to the equivalent load remained constant while the equivalent load doubled, the current flow would indeed be half what it was without the ammeter. The important question to ask is this: will the source voltage remain constant as the load impedance is changed? At the moment we do not have enough information to answer this question.

It would be helpful to draw a more detailed picture of the new circuit to serve as an aid to answering the above question (Fig. 2.6). The new factor which has been added in the diagram is the internal impedance of the source. Unfortunately most sources do not have zero internal impedance. What effect will this internal impedance have on the current flow? This internal impedance is in series with load 1 and load 2. The constant-potential portion of the source drives

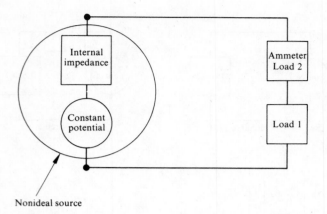

Nonideal source

Fig. 2.6. New equivalent circuit, including internal impedance of the source.

a load which is equivalent to the sum of the impedances of loads 1 and 2 and the
internal impedance of the source. The flow in the circuit is determined by the
constant potential and the sum of these three impedances.

Now we are in a position to estimate what effect the ammeter will have on
the current flow in the circuit.

1. If both the internal impedance of the source and the ammeter impedance are
   zero, the ammeter will indicate the same current as would flow in the circuit
   if the ammeter were not in the circuit.

2. If the internal impedance of the source were zero and the ammeter and load
   1 impedances were equal, the current reading on the ammeter would be half
   of what it would be if the ammeter was not in the circuit.

3. If the internal impedance is not zero and the ammeter impedance is not zero,
   the ammeter reading will be different from what it would be if the ammeter
   was not in the circuit.

A point to remember

Measured current may or may not be equal to the current which will flow
when the ammeter is not in the circuit. You must know the impedances of
the ammeter, the load, and the internal impedance of the source before you
can determine the difference.

Let us move on to the problem of measuring the potential (voltage) in a circuit and see what factors may affect the voltage reading. We will pick as our
standard of reference or comparison the voltage which appears between the two
test points in the circuit when the voltage-measuring device is not connected in the
circuit. We will compare this reference voltage with the actual voltage indicated

on the voltmeter. Indeed, errors will occur and the relative values of the source internal impedance and the load impedance are the critical factors which must be considered.

A liquid flow analogy will aid in this discussion and such a system is shown in Fig. 2.7. Assume that the pressure or potential-measuring device must have liquid flowing through it when a measurement is made. The amount of flow is directly proportional to the pressure between the two inputs to the device. This device is to be connected across the load as shown in Fig. 2.8.

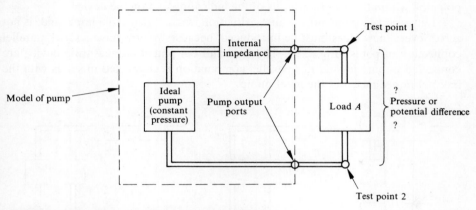

Fig. 2.7.   Liquid flow model for measuring potential.

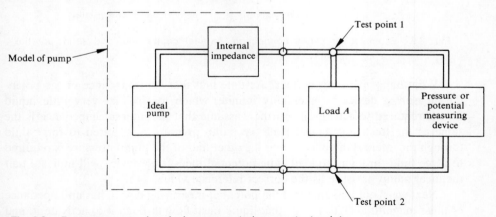

Fig. 2.8.   Pressure-measuring device connected across test points.

Different situations may occur when this measurement is made.

1. The pump may maintain a pressure difference between the two output ports which is constant regardless of the amount of liquid flow when the internal impedance of the pump is zero.

2. The pump may maintain a constant internal pressure when the internal impedance is not zero.

Let us investigate the first situation. The pressure across the output ports where the potential-measuring device is connected is equal to the constant pressure produced by the ideal pump because the internal impedance of the pump is zero. All tubes are assumed to be lossless, meaning that no pressure difference between the ends of the tubes is required to produce liquid flow. This represents an ideal situation. In this situation the potential-measuring device will read the correct potential within the accuracy limits of the indicating unit on the device.

Let us consider the more realistic situation where the internal impedance is not zero. Several new ideas must be introduced, because we now have a series-parallel connection of paths (Fig. 2.9). The load and the potential-measuring device are connected in parallel and this parallel combination is connected in series with the internal impedance and the ideal pump.

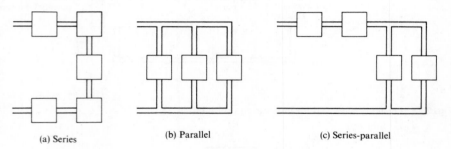

(a) Series   (b) Parallel   (c) Series-parallel

Fig. 2.9. Examples of series connection, parallel connection, and series-parallel connection.

What happens in this system? Assume first that the impedance of the potential-measuring device is essentially infinite, which means that very little liquid flow is required to activate it. Further, assume that the internal impedance is the same as the load impedance. Half the pump pressure is required to force fluid through the internal impedance and the other half of the pump pressure is required to force fluid through the load. The potential measuring device will indicate half the ideal pump pressure as the correct reference value.

Next we should assume that the potential-measuring device has an impedance of finite magnitude. This means that liquid must flow through it to activate it, and this liquid must be supplied by the pump. Thus the total flow through the pump will increase as the impedance of the potential-measuring device decreases. An increase in pressure across a fixed impedance is required if the flow through the impedance is to be increased. Therefore, when the potential-measuring device requires more flow through it on account of a decrease in its impedance, more potential must be developed across the internal impedance to sustain this higher flow. It should be apparent now that the percentage of the ideal pump's potential which appears across the output ports changes with the impedance of the potential-measuring device. The potential-measuring device will not indicate the reference potential whenever the measuring device has finite impedance and the source has internal impedance.

Now let us consider the potential-measuring problem simply as a question of connecting a source to a load (Fig. 2.10). The source has a constant internal potential with some series internal impedance. The load has two different values.

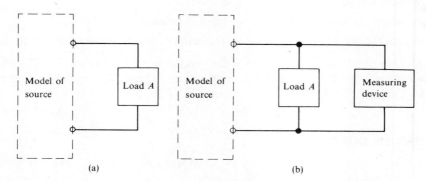

Fig. 2.10. Load conditions without and with a measuring device.

1. When the potential-measuring device is not connected, the load for the source is just load *A*.
2. When the potential-measuring device is connected across load *A,* the load for the source is the parallel combination of load *A* and the device.

If the measuring device has finite impedance, these two load conditions will differ as will the potential across load *A* under these conditions. The difference between the readings of the potential depends on the internal impedance, load *A* impedance, and the impedance of the potential-measuring device.

A point to remember

A potential-measuring device may alter a circuit significantly if its impedance is finite and the equivalent source internal impedance is nonzero. A misleading reading may therefore result.

2.6   DISCUSSION

Although we have talked primarily about fluid flow and associated measurements, all the ideas presented thus far are valid for electrical circuits. We should substitute the term "potential difference" or "voltage" for pressure and the term "current" or "amperage" for flow when talking about electrical phenomena. The term "impedance" was used because it has meaning in fluid systems and also is the correct term to use in electrical circuits. The idea that flow or current increases with pressure or potential was introduced on an intuitive basis. Similarly the idea that flow or current varies inversely with impedance was presented.

The most important piece of information that should be assimilated is the fact that three things must be considered whenever an electrical measurement is to be made.

Don't forget these questions when you make an electrical measurement!

1. What is the internal impedance of the source?
2. What are the impedances of the load and the measuring device?
3. What changes take place when the measuring device is connected to the circuit?

If these three questions are considered and answered every time an electrical measurement is made, most of the difficulties caused by misleading and erroneous readings can be alleviated.

2.7   REVIEW QUESTIONS

2.1   What important consequences can occur when an electrical measuring instrument is connected to an electric circuit?

2.2   What is meant by the term "electric potential"?

2.3   What is meant by the term "impedance"?

2.4   What is meant by the term "load"?

2.5   What are some of the general characteristics of loads?

2.6   What effect does the internal impedance of a source have on the output across a load when the load is connected to the source?

2.7   What effect does a change in the internal potential of a source have on the flow from the source?

2.8   What effect does a change in the internal impedance of a source have on the flow from the source?

2.9   What is another term used to designate an electric potential difference?

2.10   What is meant by the term "electric circuit"?

2.11   What is the term used to indicate flow in an electric circuit?

2.12   What is meant by the term "series circuit"?

2.13   What is the general equation that is used when calculating the total impedance of a series circuit?

2.14   If the impedance of one circuit element in a series circuit increases, what happens to the total impedance of the series circuit?

2.15   Is it desirable to have an ammeter of low internal impedance or of high internal impedance? Why?

2.16   What errors might occur when an ammeter is inserted in the circuit to measure current?

2.17   What might happen if an ammeter is connected directly across a voltage source?

2.18   What is meant by the term "parallel circuit"?

2.19   Is it desirable to have a voltmeter with a low internal impedance or a high internal impedance? Why?

2.20   What errors might occur when a voltmeter is connected to a circuit to measure voltage? What factors affect the magnitude of these errors?

2.21   What is meant by the term "series-parallel circuit"?

2.22   What are three important questions that should be asked whenever an electrical measurement is to be made?

3
direct-current
circuit models

3.1 OBJECTIVES

This chapter is designed to show the reader the necessity of understanding basic direct-current circuits if he is to obtain useful and accurate measurements of electrical phenomena. The idea of making a model of the circuit to be tested is introduced to illustrate how helpful it is in designing a significant experiment. The method of using these models when making calculations of voltage and current in series and parallel circuits is introduced and examples are discussed. Basic equations needed when making the calculations are given and only an elementary understanding of algebra is assumed. Three important problems are presented and solved at the end of the chapter to help the reader understand how to use the principles discussed in the chapter.

It is fairly easy to visualize fluid flow through tubes and thus gain a little insight into the factors which cause the flow to increase or decrease. What is lacking in this approach is a method to determine numerical values of current or voltage which may be needed when undertaking an experiment. Most of the analysis done with electrical circuits requires the use of a model of the circuit in question. On the basis of this model it is possible to write some simple algebraic equations which can be used to obtain specific numerical values of current or voltage. In this chapter we will restrict our thinking to *direct-current* (dc) electrical circuits. These models will also be applicable to other types of flow such as liquid or heat flow.

We will discuss the basic circuit elements used, series circuits, parallel circuits and solve some typical measurement problems for these circuits.

3.2 BASIC CIRCUIT ELEMENTS

Only three circuit elements need be considered when working with dc circuits: *resistors,* current sources, and voltage sources.

Resistance

Resistors are the elements in dc circuits which impede the flow of current and dissipate energy. They have the property of *resistance*. Resistance is a proportionality constant which relates current and voltage. This relation is stated explicitly in *Ohm's Law:*

$$\text{Voltage} = \text{Current} \times \text{Resistance} \qquad (3.0)*$$

or

$$V = IR,$$

where V is given in volts, I is given in amperes, and R is given in ohms

The relation between voltage and current may be linear or nonlinear (Fig. 3.1). Note that in the case of a *linear resistor* the ratio of voltage to current, which is resistance, is a constant regardless of the particular value of voltage applied to the resistor. In the case of a nonlinear resistor this ratio depends on the particular value of the voltage applied to the resistor.

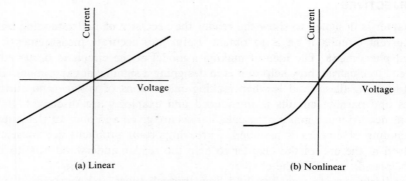

(a) Linear   (b) Nonlinear

Fig. 3.1. Possible characteristics of linear and nonlinear resistors when voltage is applied across the terminals.

A linear resistor may be some substance which does not change its physical or chemical properties with changing current. Thus any change in voltage across this substance will produce a proportional amount of current change.

A standard household 100-watt 130-volt light bulb is an example of nonlinear device. When 4 volts (V) was applied across a particular bulb, the resistance of the light filament was found to be 24 Ω (ohms). When 60 V was applied across the bulb, the resistance of the filament was found to be 117 Ω. When 120 V was applied across the bulb, the resistance of the filament became 162 Ω. The relation between voltage and current for this light bulb is nonlinear.

---

* The asterisk is used to indicate equations of major importance.

There is also the possibility that the resistance of a particular material will change in an irreversible way. For example, a small piece of animal tissue may be subjected to an electrical potential in an experiment. Current will flow through the tissue and produce heating in the tissue which will tend to dry it and make it become a poorer conductor of electric current. This change is probably irreversible. Recall the aphid experiment discussed in Chapter 1. How much current can flow through the aphid before it affects the aphid's habits or alters its physiology? This is an important question.

The less complicated of the two types of resistors is obviously the linear resistor, because only a minimum of effort is required to establish a mathematical model for it. For this reason we will assume in this section that all the resistors discussed are linear. However, when making actual measurements, you should always determine whether or not the resistors involved are linear.

A point to remember

Is the resistance of the test specimen linear or nonlinear and will its value change during the experiment?

More information about resistors will be presented in Chapter 4.

Ideal Voltage Source

An *ideal voltage source* is one that will produce a constant voltage across its output terminals regardless of the current flow. Actual sources only approximate this ideal. Mercury batteries, for example, have characteristics similar to those of an ideal voltage source, but they cannot supply excessively high currents. Manufacturer's ratings must be observed. The characteristics of an ideal voltage source are shown in Fig. 3.2(a) and those of a nonideal voltage source are shown in Fig. 3.2(b).

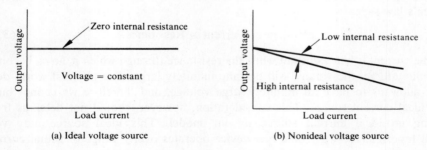

(a) Ideal voltage source   (b) Nonideal voltage source

Fig. 3.2. Characteristics of ideal and nonideal voltage sources.

The actual or nonideal voltage source of Fig. 3.2(b) has some internal resistance which causes the terminal voltage to drop as the current flow is increased. Recall that just such a difficulty was encountered in the battery problem discussed in Chapter 2. The amount of voltage drop per unit change in current depends on the magnitude of the internal resistance.

We will use the ideal voltage source when we make our models of dc circuits. Nonideal voltage sources exist and may be modeled as a combination of an ideal voltage source and a resistor. There are many interesting and important characteristics of voltage sources or *power supplies,* as they are commonly called, but we will leave those details for later discussion.

Ideal Current Source

The last circuit element which is required is the current source. Again we will use only an *ideal current source* when we make our models of dc circuits. They will prove useful in circuit analysis and can be approximated by some existing devices. The characteristics of an ideal current source are shown in Fig. 3.3.

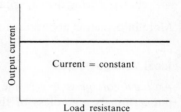

Fig. 3.3. Characteristics of an ideal current source.

An ideal current source will supply a constant current to a load regardless of the value of the impedance or resistance of the load. A little reflection may lead you to suspect that an ideal current source is impossible to build. For example, Ohm's law says:

$$\text{Voltage} = \text{Current} \times \text{Resistance}. \tag{3.0}$$

If the current is held constant while the resistance through which it flows becomes infinitely large, the voltage will become infinitely large. The physical world does not allow us to have an infinitely large voltage, and therefore we cannot build an ideal current source. This consideration, however, should not deter us from using an ideal current source in our model. This ideal source may very well represent the way some real device operates over a range of actual current values.

Now we have the three basic circuit elements required to set up a model of the dc circuits we need to study. The following is a list of the symbols used to represent them.

1. Linear resistor, whose basic unit of measurement is the ohm (Ω):

2. Ideal voltage source, whose basic unit of measurement is the volt (V):

3. Ideal current source, whose basic unit of measurement is the ampere (A):

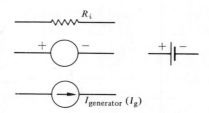

3.3 SERIES-CIRCUIT MODEL

The *series-circuit* model is shown schematically in Fig. 3.4. In this example four circuit elements are connected in series, which means that they are connected end to end. The lines connecting the element symbols represent a short circuit or a zero-resistance wire. This model will prove to be very useful.

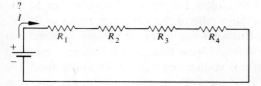

Fig. 3.4. Series connection of circuit elements.

An example at this point will show how such a model may be used to aid the scientist. We would like to make an electrical model of an experiment that a biologist wishes to perform. He wants to know how a certain biological specimen functions when it is illuminated with various intensities of light while being maintained in an environment of constant atmospheric pressure, temperature, and humidity. Very little is known about this specimen other than the fact that it is capable of generating a small measurable voltage at its surface. This voltage is said to vary with the light intensity. Let us see what the model might look like and how the specimen might be tested.

If the specimen does generate a voltage, we may consider it to be a nonideal voltage source. Recall that sources have both voltage and internal impedance. It seems reasonable to set up a model of the specimen as an ideal voltage source in series with a resistor that represents the internal impedance of the specimen. This model is just a guess at this point, but it is the best we can do with the information available. The model may give us some clue as to how we should perform the experiment.

The biologist wants to use a dc voltmeter to measure the voltage. The voltmeter will draw current from the source when the meter is connected to an illuminated specimen. The amount of current drawn by the voltmeter depends on its *input resistance*. This model is shown in Fig. 3.5.

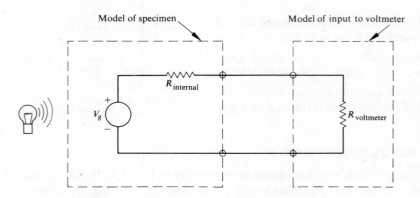

Fig. 3.5. Electrical model of the experiment.

The experiment is performed. The biologist connects the voltmeter to the specimen, turns on the light, and sees the needle of the voltmeter move to 0.3 V. Eureka! The experiment is a success. But what has he learned about the specimen other than the fact that it produced a voltage? Very little as yet, though something did happen. Before the significance of this voltage reading can be understood it is necessary to consider the three crucial questions emphasized in the previous chapter:

1. What is the internal impedance of the source?
2. What is the impedance of the measuring device?
3. What changes take place when the measuring device is connected to the source?

Questions 1 and 3 cannot be answered yet. The instruction manual for the voltmeter should give its input resistance. The biologist must then ask the following:

1. How should the experiment be performed, and why is one procedure better than another?
2. What characteristics should he look for when choosing the voltmeter?

These are difficult questions to answer, and we should spend some time introducing some of the possible implications.

The biologist now begins to apply some of the basic concepts discussed earlier. The voltmeter resistance is constant. There are two unknowns in our series-circuit model: V_g and R_{int} ("int" for "internal"). Let him vary the light intensity and get a second reading of voltage. With two unknowns and two data points should he be able to determine the two unknowns?

He increases the light intensity linearly and finds that the voltage increases linearly. The data are given in Table 3.1.

TABLE 3.1
Data from the experiment

Light intensity (lumens)	Voltage (V)	Calculated current (μA)
0.0	0.0	0.0
0.1	0.2	0.2
0.2	0.4	0.4
0.3	0.6	0.6
0.4	0.8	0.8

Sample calculation:

$$I = \frac{V_{vm}}{R_{vm}}$$
$$R_{vm} = 10^6 \ \Omega$$
$$I = 0.2 \times 10^{-6} \ A$$
$$= 0.2 \ \mu A$$

It may appear that this linear relation between light intensity and measured voltage is an obvious way for the specimen to function. Further discussion will show that there are many other possibilities. Reference to the hypothetical model and Ohm's law leads us to conclude that if V_g increases linearly, the results will be as observed if R_{int} is constant. Would it be possible for the observed results to occur if R_{int} decreased linearly when V_g was constant? These two effects might indicate two entirely different mechanisms in the specimen reacting to increases in light intensity. Thus the answer to the stated question could give a significant clue about the functioning of the specimen under varying light conditions.

Let us speculate about our model. If R_{int} is very small compared to R_{vm} ("vm" for "voltmeter"), variations in R_{int} will have essentially no effect on the voltmeter reading. Hence if this is true, we would suspect that V_g is varying significantly. *What chemical action in the specimen could cause V_g to vary?* If R_{int} is about the same as R_{vm}, it is possible that all the variations in voltage measured are caused by variations in R_{int} alone. *What chemical action in the specimen could cause R_{int} to vary?* It is also possible that both V_g and R_{int} vary together to produce the observed results. This possibility leaves us in a dilemma. What is the fact of the case? It may have been difficult to follow the word description of these various possibilities. This is where simple mathematics becomes very helpful.

We must resort to applying Ohm's law to gain further information. Recall that

$$\text{Voltage} = \text{Current} \times \text{Resistance} \tag{3.0}$$

The total resistance in a series circuit is the sum of all of the resistances of the individual resistors.

$$R_{\text{Total(series)}} = \sum_{i=1}^{n} R_i,$$
(3.1)*

where i is the index number of the resistance and n is total number of resistors.

In this example of a series circuit

$$V_g = I\,(R_{\text{int}} + R_{\text{vm}}),$$
(3.2)

where $I =$ current flowing in the series circuit. The voltage across the voltmeter is

$$V_{\text{vm}} = I\,R_{\text{vm}}.$$
(3.3)

We can rearrange these two equations to show the relations among V_{vm}, R_{int}, and V_g:

$$I = \frac{V_g}{R_{\text{int}} + R_{\text{vm}}},$$
(3.4)

$$V_{\text{vm}} = I\,R_{\text{vm}} = \left(\frac{V_g}{R_{\text{int}} + R_{\text{vm}}}\right)\left(R_{\text{vm}}\right).$$
(3.5)

An inspection of the last equation will disclose that all three of the possibilities offered above may exist. In fact, R_{int} may have any finite constant value and the voltage measured is linearly related to V_g.

Let us rearrange the terms in the last equation to see if it will help:

$$V_{\text{vm}} = \frac{V_g}{R_{\text{int}}/R_{\text{vm}} + 1}.$$
(3.6)

Choose a voltmeter with a very high input resistance. Assume that

$$R_{\text{vm}} \gg R_{\text{int}}.$$

Then

$$V_{\text{vm}} \cong V_g.$$

Under this condition the voltmeter essentially measures V_g.

As a second possibility choose a voltmeter with a very low input resistance. Assume that

$$R_{\text{vm}} \ll R_{\text{int}}.$$

Then

$$V_{\text{vm}} \cong \frac{V_g R_{\text{vm}}}{R_{\text{int}}}.$$
(3.7)

In the study of Eq. (3.6) we found that we could determine V_g if we made our measurement with a high-resistance voltmeter. Values of voltmeter resistance can be found in the instruction manuals for the voltmeters. We now need to determine R_{int} by means of Eq. (3.7). Rearranging Eq. (3.7), we get

$$R_{int} = \frac{V_g R_{vm}}{V_{vm}} \qquad (3.8)$$

We have now determined all of the values for our model of the specimen. Whether or not these values are correct depends on whether or not the assumptions that in the first measurement

$$R_{vm} >> R_{int}$$

and in the second measurement

$$R_{vm} << R_{int}$$

were valid. Also we must determine whether or not the current flow during the second measurement was large enough to damage or temporarily alter the specimen.

These arguments have been brought up to point out how the simple series circuit model can be used to aid the scientist in designing his experiment and picking the proper voltmeter. The previous example was not intended to provide you with all of the answers, but the importance of certain factors should have begun to emerge:

1. Models can be made to represent physical phenomena in terms of electrical circuits.

2. The elements which are used in dc circuit models are resistors, constant voltage sources, and constant current sources.

3. The determination of the actual values of the resistances and sources may be difficult, but a model may give some clues as to how an experiment should be performed.

4. Relatively simple equations may be used to help determine how the model circuit operates under varying conditions. These equations are an essential part of the analysis of the circuit.

5. Measurement of the circuit with meters having different input resistances can yield useful information about the circuit.

3.4   PARALLEL-CIRCUIT MODEL

The *parallel-circuit* model is widely used in measurement problems and must be understood if the experimenter is to obtain valid data. Like the series-circuit model, it is not difficult to understand. Let us first consider an experiment which uses an ideal voltage source, to determine the basic relations of parallel circuits. Then, for comparison, let us consider an experiment which uses an ideal current source to find out what differences may result from the same parallel load being driven by these two basic sources.

The experiment consists of connecting an ideal voltage source to a test specimen and then monitoring the voltage across the specimen (Fig. 3.6). Part (a) of the figure shows the specimen to be connected to the source. Since it is a simple series circuit, I_{Ta}, the total current from the source in circuit (a) is equal to the current I_1 flowing through R_1:

$$I_{Ta} = I_1 = \frac{V_b}{R_1}. \tag{3.9}$$

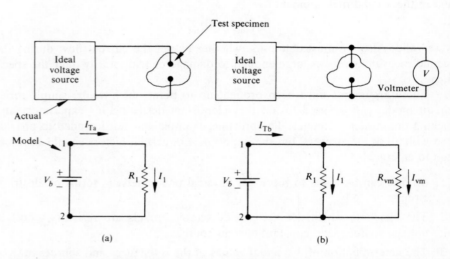

Fig. 3.6. Test specimen connected to ideal voltage source for voltage measurement.

Part (b) of the figure shows the voltmeter to be connected across the resistor so that the experimenter may observe both the voltage across the specimen and the action of the specimen resulting from the applied voltage. The voltmeter is represented by a resistor whose value is equal to that of the input resistance to the voltmeter. This is a simple but accurate model of the voltmeter's input characteristics. What changes take place in the circuit when the voltmeter is connected across the test specimen? The voltmeter is connected directly across points 1 and 2, as is R_1. When they are connected in this way, the voltmeter is said to be in parallel with the resistor R_1. Since they are connected to the same points in the circuit, the voltage across the voltmeter and across R_1 must be the same.

The current flow from the ideal voltage source is made up of two parts: I_1 and I_{vm}. I_1 must be the same as it had been before the voltmeter was connected, because the voltage across R_1 has not changed. The current through the voltmeter is given by the following equation:

$$I_{\text{vm}} = \frac{V_b}{R_{\text{vm}}}. \tag{3.10}$$

The total current flowing from the ideal voltage source is the sum of these individual currents:

$$I_{\text{Tb}} = I_1 + I_{\text{vm}} \tag{3.11}$$

$$= \frac{V_b}{R_1} + \frac{V_b}{R_{\text{vm}}}. \tag{3.12}$$

An important fact to note at this point is that the addition of the voltmeter to the circuit does not change the current flow through the specimen. This is true when an ideal voltage source is used. We shall see later whether or not this is true when an ideal current source is used.

Suppose that the experimenter wants to vary the voltage across the specimen and photograph the specimen's behavior in response to this variation. To correlate the photographs and the voltage, he will need a record of the voltage. He may choose to manually record the voltage at specified times or connect a chart recorder to read the voltage across the specimen. The latter will make a permanent and continuous recording for future reference. Assume both the voltmeter and the chart recorder to be connected to points 1 and 2 so that the accuracy of the readings can be checked (Fig. 3.7). Note that the chart recorder is modeled as a resistor, as is the voltmeter. This resistance R_{cr} is the input resistance to the chart recorder. Again this is a simple yet valid model for the chart recorder. What changes will occur because of the addition of the chart recorder?

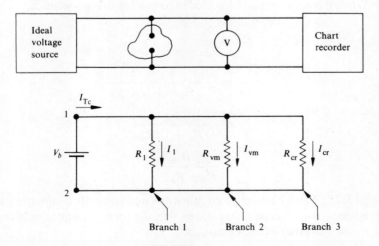

Fig. 3.7. Voltmeter and chart recorder connected across the specimen.

The currents I_1 and I_{vm} do not change because the voltage across R_1 and R_{vm} do not change. The current through the chart recorder is given by the following equation:

$$I_{cr} = \frac{V_b}{R_{cr}}. \tag{3.13}$$

The total current flow from the ideal voltage source is the sum of the three branch currents:

$$I_{Tc} = I_1 + I_{vm} + I_{cr} \tag{3.14}$$

$$= \frac{V_b}{R_1} + \frac{V_b}{R_{vm}} + \frac{V_b}{R_{cr}}. \tag{3.15}$$

The addition of the chart recorder has no effect on the voltage across and the current through the specimen when the ideal voltage source is driving the test specimen.

Another point of interest is the determination of the total resistance between points 1 and 2. This resistance can be determined by dividing the ideal source voltage by the total current flow from the source—another application of Ohm's law.

a) For the specimen alone

$$R_T = \frac{V_b}{I_{Ta}} \tag{3.16}$$

$$= R_1. \tag{3.17}$$

b) When the voltmeter is connected in parallel with the specimen,

$$R_T = \frac{V_b}{I_{Tb}} \tag{3.18}$$

$$= \frac{V_b}{V_b/R_1 + V_b/R_{vm}} \tag{3.19}$$

$$= \frac{1}{1/R_1 + 1/R_{vm}} \tag{3.20}$$

$$= \frac{R_1 R_{vm}}{R_1 + R_{vm}}. \tag{3.21}*$$

Equation (3.21) is very useful in circuit work and is worth committing to memory. An inspection of this equation shows that the total resistance between points 1 and 2 is less than that of either resistor.

c) When the chart recorder and the voltmeter are connected in parallel with the specimen,

$$R_{\mathrm{T}} = \frac{V_b}{I_{\mathrm{Tc}}} \qquad (3.22)$$

$$= \frac{V_b}{V_b/R_1 + V_b/R_{\mathrm{vm}} + V_b/R_{\mathrm{cr}}} \qquad (3.23)$$

$$= \frac{1}{1/R_1 + 1/R_{\mathrm{vm}} + 1/R_{\mathrm{cr}}}. \qquad (3.24)$$

Equations (3.20) and (3.24) are very similar in form. You will note that with each additional parallel branch in the circuit, a term of the form

$$\frac{1}{R_i}, \qquad \text{where } i \text{ represents an index number,}$$

is added to the denominator. The total resistance of a parallel combination of resistors is less than the resistance of any one of the individual resistors.

Important points to remember for parallel circuits driven by an ideal voltage source

1. The current in branch i is

$$I_i = \frac{V_b}{R_i}, \qquad (3.25)$$

where i is an index number for branch.

2. Total current flow from an ideal voltage source is

$$I_{\mathrm{T}} = \sum_{i=1}^{n} I_i, \qquad (3.26)*$$

where i is an index number for branch, n is the total number of branches.

3. The total resistance across parallel resistors is

$$R_{\mathrm{Tp}} = \frac{1}{\sum_{i=1}^{n} (1/R_i)}. \qquad (3.27)*$$

As the number of parallel branches increases, the resistance R_{Tp} decreases.

4. The voltage across a parallel circuit is the same for all branches.

Another test may be made on the specimen when it is driven by a constant current source. The experimenter may again want to use a voltmeter and a chart recorder to measure the voltage across the specimen. We will assume that an ideal current source is to be used. Figure 3.8 shows the circuit when the voltmeter is connected in parallel with the specimen.

In Fig. 3.8(a) the current from the source is defined as I_s, which is equal to I_1, since the current is a simple series circuit. When the voltmeter is connected to points 1 and 2, some very interesting things begin to happen as compared to the results obtained when the voltmeter was connected in parallel with the constant voltage source. Since the ideal current source drives the load with a fixed current, this current is divided between the resistor branch and the voltmeter branch. Therefore, the current through the specimen will now be smaller than it had been before the voltmeter was connected in the circuit. It follows from Ohm's law that the voltage applied to the specimen will decrease when the voltmeter is in the circuit. In this situation the voltmeter is said to load down the circuit, because it causes the voltage at the test point to drop.

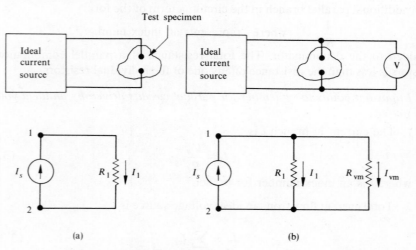

Fig. 3.8. Test specimen connected to ideal current source for voltage measurement.

How much of the source current is flowing in the specimen compared to what is flowing through the voltmeter? Let us start with the fact that the total current flow in a parallel circuit is the sum of the individual branch currents:

$$I_s = I_1 + I_{vm} \tag{3.28}$$

$$= \frac{V_{12}}{R_1} + \frac{V_{12}}{R_{vm}}, \tag{3.29}$$

where V_{12} is the voltage between points 1 and 2. Therefore,

$$I_s = V_{12}\left(\frac{1}{R_1} + \frac{1}{R_{vm}}\right) \tag{3.30}$$

$$= V_{12}\left(\frac{R_1 + R_{vm}}{R_1 R_{vm}}\right). \tag{3.31}$$

Note that the term in parentheses in Eq. (3.31) is the inverse of the total resistance of the parallel combination of R_1 and R_{vm} obtained in Eq. (3.21). The voltage across points 1 and 2 is simply the product of the current flowing into the parallel combination times the resistance of the parallel combination:

$$V_{12} = \left(\frac{R_1 R_{vm}}{R_1 + R_{vm}} \right) I_s. \tag{3.32}$$

Now we can easily calculate the current flow through the specimen:

$$I_1 = \frac{V_{12}}{R_1} \tag{3.33}$$

$$= \frac{R_1 R_{vm}}{R_1 + R_{vm}} \frac{I_s}{R_1} \tag{3.34}$$

$$= \frac{I_s}{R_1/R_{vm} + 1} \tag{3.35}$$

An important revelation of Eq. (3.35) is that, as the resistance of the voltmeter increases, the current flow through the specimen increases. In other words, *the current shunted by the voltmeter* decreases as the voltmeter resistance increases. If the input resistance to the voltmeter R_{vm} becomes infinite, the current through the specimen becomes equal to the source current, and the circuit diagram becomes the same as that in Fig. 3.8(a).

The other extreme value of the voltmeter resistance will occur when the instrument is damaged. If R_{vm} becomes zero—a short circuit—then Eq. (3.35) indicates that the current flow through the specimen will be zero, so that all of the current will be shunted through the voltmeter short circuit.

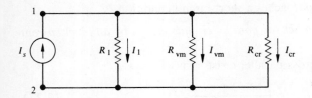

Fig. 3.9. Voltmeter and chart recorder connected across the specimen.

Assume now that the experimenter wants to have a permanent recording of the voltage across the specimen. So he connects the chart recorder between points 1 and 2 in addition to the voltmeter (Fig. 3.9). Will the addition of the chart recorder affect the voltage across and the current through the specimen? We can answer this question by following the procedure given in the last example: Solve for the voltage between points 1 and 2, divide the voltage between points 1 and 2 by the specimen resistance R_1:

$$I_s = I_1 + I_{vm} + I_{cr} \tag{3.36}$$

$$= \frac{V_{12}}{R_1} + \frac{V_{12}}{R_{vm}} + \frac{V_{12}}{R_{cr}} \tag{3.37}$$

$$= V_{12} \left(\frac{1}{R_1} + \frac{1}{R_{vm}} + \frac{1}{R_{cr}} \right), \tag{3.38}$$

$$V_{12} = \left(\frac{1}{1/R_1 + 1/R_{vm} + 1/R_{cr}} \right) I_s. \tag{3.39}$$

Note that the term in parentheses is the total resistance between points 1 and 2 as given by Eq. (3.24). Also

$$I_1 = \frac{V_{12}}{R_1} \tag{3.40}$$

$$= \left(\frac{1}{1/R_1 + 1/R_{vm} + 1/R_{cr}} \right) \frac{I_s}{R_1}. \tag{3.41}$$

The form of Eq. (3.41) is identical to that of Eq. (3.34). As the resistance of the chart recorder decreases, the current flow through the test specimen decreases. Since the chart recorder usually has a finite resistance, we can say that the chart recorder will *load down* the circuit and cause the voltage across the specimen to be lower than it would be without the chart recorder.

We can now make a general observation as a result of the study of the last two circuits. The current flow through one of the branches of a parallel circuit is directly proportional to the total resistance of the parallel combination and inversely proportional to the resistance of the branch carrying the current when the combination is driven by an ideal current source. It seems reasonable to expect the current flow in a particular branch to increase as the resistance of that branch becomes smaller and approaches a short-circuit condition.

Important points to remember for parallel circuits driven by an ideal current source

1. The total resistance across parallel resistors is

$$R_{Tp} = \frac{1}{\sum_{i=1}^{n} (1/R_i)}. \tag{3.27}$$

2. The voltage across the branches of a parallel circuit is the same and depends on the number of parallel branches and the resistance of the individual branches:

$$V_{12} = I_s R_{Tp}, \tag{3.42}$$

where I_s is the source current.

3. The current flow in each branch depends on the number of parallel branches and the resistance of the individual branches:

$$I_1 = \frac{V_{12}}{R_i}. \qquad (3.43)$$

4. The sum of the branch currents must be equal to the source current:

$$I_s = \sum_{i=1}^{n} \frac{I_i}{I_i}. \qquad (3.44)$$

Refer to the previous list of important points to remember for parallel circuits driven by an ideal voltage source and compare it with this list. You will note that there are some similarities. The voltage across the branches of a parallel circuit is the same for all branches. The current through each branch may be calculated by dividing the voltage across the parallel combination by the branch resistance. The total resistance across the parallel combination is given by Eq. (3.27).

There are some differences in the characteristics of driving a parallel circuit with an ideal current source and driving it with an ideal voltage source. When using an ideal current source, the voltage across the parallel combination is dependent on the branch resistances. When driven by an ideal voltage source, the voltage across the parallel combination is independent of the branch resistances. When using an ideal current source, the current through a particular branch is affected by the resistance of the other branches. When using an ideal voltage source, the current through a particular branch is independent of the other branch resistances.

We have spoken only of driving the parallel circuit with an ideal current source or an ideal voltage source. In most circuits which you will have to analyze, your circuit will probably be somewhat different from these ideal cases. Actually they can be considered as combinations of series and parallel circuits. Examples of these are shown in Fig. 3.10.

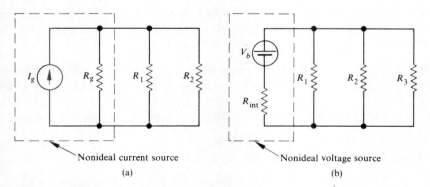

Nonideal current source

(a)

Nonideal voltage source

(b)

Fig. 3.10.   Models of realistic measurement problems.

3.5 CONCLUSIONS

The discussion in this chapter has shown that relatively few circuit elements and equations are required in making models of and analyzing simple series or parallel dc circuits. To summarize, they are as follows.

1. Circuit elements
   a) Ideal voltage source, constant voltage
   b) Ideal current source, constant current
   c) Resistor
2. Equations
   a) Ohm's law:
$$V = IR. \tag{3.0}*$$
   b) Series circuit total resistance:
$$R_{Ts} = \sum_{i=1}^{n} R_i \tag{3.1}*$$
   c) Parallel circuit total resistance:
$$R_{Ts} = \frac{1}{\sum_{i=1}^{n} (1/R_i).} \tag{3.27}*$$
   d) Special case of two resistors in parallel:
$$R_{Tp} = \frac{R_1 R_2}{R_1 + R_2}. \tag{3.21}*$$

All the characteristics of series and parallel circuits which have been obtained are derived from Ohm's law. A good understanding of the application of this law is essential when setting up measurements of electrical circuits.

3.6 PROBLEMS WITH SOLUTIONS

The material which has been presented in this chapter will assume more relevance if we look at some typical problems with appropriate numerical values for the instruments.

Problem 3.1 A measurement of voltage is to be made between two electrodes inserted in an electrolyte. A theoretical study indicates that the chemical action should produce 1.3V in the absence of current flow. The internal resistance of the solution should be 1,000 Ω. Three instruments are available to measure voltage:

1. Panel type voltmeter 0-5 V (1,000 Ω/V)
2. Multimeter (VOM) 0-3 V (20,000 Ω/V)
3. Vacuum tube voltmeter (VTVM) 0-5 V (10^6-Ω input resistance)

What readings could be expected from these three voltmeters if the values obtained by the theoretical study are valid?

Solution   The first step in the solution is to draw the equivalent circuit for the problem (Fig. P3.1). Given this circuit, which is an equivalent electrical model of the physical problem, we can calculate the expected voltmeter readings and determine what effect the different types of voltmeters have on the readings.

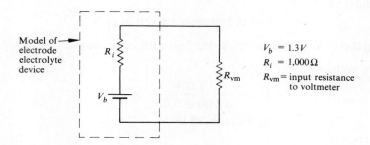

Fig. P3.1.   Equivalent circuit for electrode-electrolyte voltage measurement problem.

As the second step, we should write the equation that describes the circuit in mathematical form:

$$V_b = IR_i + IR_{vm},$$
$$V_b = I\,(R_i + R_{vm}). \tag{3.2}$$

The internal voltage V_b must be equal to the sum of the voltages across the resistors in series with this voltage. The voltage across the voltmeter will be given by the equation:

$$V_{vm} = I\,R_{vm}. \tag{3.3}$$

If we solve for the current flow in the circuit, we will be able to calculate the required readings:

$$I = \frac{V_b}{R_i + R_{vm}}, \tag{3.4}$$

$$V_{vm} = \frac{R_{vm}}{R_i + R_{vm}}\,V_b. \tag{3.5}$$

The resistance of voltmeters is quite often given in ohms per volt. This provides a standard for comparison. Improved performance is usually obtained as the ohms-per-volt rating increases. The total resistance of the voltmeter is calculated by multiplying the ohms-per-volt rating by the full-scale reading of the voltmeter.

Panel type voltmeter:

$$R_T = \left(\frac{1{,}000\ \Omega}{V}\right)(5\ V) = 5{,}000\ \Omega.$$

Multimeter:

$$R_T = \left(\frac{20{,}000\ \Omega}{V}\right)(3\ V) = 60{,}000\ \Omega.$$

Vacuum tube voltmeter:

$$R_T = 10^6\ \Omega \ \text{(rating not given in } \Omega/V).$$

Using these values, we can make the following calculations.*

Panel type voltmeter:

$$V_{vm} = \frac{5{,}000}{1{,}000 + 5{,}000} \times 1.3$$
$$= 1.0833\ V.$$

Multimeter:

$$V_{vm} = \frac{60{,}000}{1{,}000 + 60{,}000} \times 1.3$$
$$= 1.2787\ V.$$

Vacuum tube voltmeter:

$$V_{vm} = \frac{10^6}{1{,}000 + 10^6} \times 1.3$$
$$= 1.2987\ V.$$

The statement of the problem did not give the percentage deviation we can expect from the correct voltage applied to the voltmeters. Plus or minus 3% of full-scale reading is a fairly standard tolerance for voltmeters. If we include this fact in our study, then the final results will be as follows.

Panel type voltmeter: $1.0833 \pm 0.15 = 1.2333$ to 0.9333 V.
Multimeter: $1.2787 \pm 0.09 = 1.3687$ to 1.1887 V.
Vacuum tube voltmeter: $1.2987 \pm 0.15 = 1.4487$ to 1.1487 V.

These results may appear very discouraging if you need an accurate value for the internal voltage V_b. However, they are valid and are what you should expect with instruments of this quality. Which meter would you recommend using?

We may need to know how much current is flowing through each of the voltmeters. We can find this value by dividing V_b by the total series resistance (Eq. 3.4).

---

* The voltages calculated in this section carry more decimal places than is reasonable. Meters can usually be read only to three digits unless a digital meter is used.

Panel type voltmeter:

$$I = \frac{1.3}{1{,}000 + 5{,}000} = 217 \times 10^{-6} \text{ A.}$$

Multimeter:

$$I = \frac{1.3}{1{,}000 + 60{,}000} = 21.3 \times 10^{-6} \text{ A.}$$

Vacuum tube voltmeter:

$$I = \frac{1.3}{1{,}000 + 10^{6}} = 1.3 \times 10^{-6} \text{ A.}$$

The panel type voltmeter draws the most current and thus loads down the circuit, causing the voltage reading to be much less than V_b. The vacuum tube voltmeter draws the least current and gives the highest nominal voltage reading.

Problem 3.2   A chemist has developed a solution that produces a desired chemical reaction when 10 mA of current flows through the solution. The solution presents a constant resistance of 5,000 Ω to the external circuit. The chemist has on hand a regulated power supply. This voltage source maintains an output voltage of 200 $\pm$ 0.2. He connects a resistor in series with the solution and power supply, as shown in Fig. P3.2. This series resistor limits the current to 10 mA. After noting the chemical reaction which occurs when the current is passed through the solution, the chemist decides that he needs to record the voltage across the solution. He has two chart recorders with appropriate voltage ranges:

1. Recorder model A (3,000-Ω input resistance)
2. Recorder model B (10,000-Ω input resistance)

What will happen to the current flow when one or the other of these recorders is connected across the solution? What can be done to maintain the desired current through the solution?

Solution   This problem involves a series-parallel circuit, so material from both major sections of this chapter must be used.

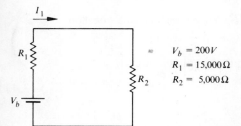

$V_b = 200V$
$R_1 = 15{,}000\,\Omega$
$R_2 = 5{,}000\,\Omega$

Fig. P3.2.   Circuit for chemical-reaction experiment.

Step 1. Draw the circuit which is the electrical equivalent of the physical problem (Fig. P3.2s1). The chart recorder is connected in parallel with the solution resistance, and this combination is in series with the power supply and the 15,000-Ω resistor.

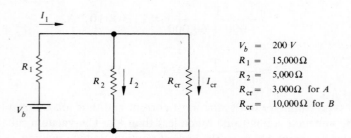

$$
\begin{aligned}
V_b &= 200\ V \\
R_1 &= 15,000\,\Omega \\
R_2 &= 5,000\,\Omega \\
R_{cr} &= 3,000\,\Omega \ \text{ for } A \\
R_{cr} &= 10,000\,\Omega \ \text{ for } B
\end{aligned}
$$

Fig. P3.2s1. Equivalent circuit for chemical-reaction problem.

Let us consider the case of recorder model A.

Step 2. Determine the total resistance across the parallel combination:

$$
R_{Tp} = \frac{R_2 R_{cr}}{R_2 + R_{cr}} \tag{3.21}
$$

$$
= \frac{(5,000)\,(3,000)}{5,000 + 3,000} = 1,875\ \Omega.
$$

Step 3. Draw the new equivalent circuit, reducing the series-parallel circuit to a series circuit (Fig. P3.2s2).

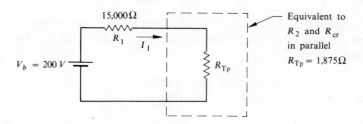

Fig. P3.2s2. Simplified equivalent circuit for chemical-reaction problem.

Step 4. Calculate the current flow in the simplified circuit:

$$
I_1 = \frac{V_b}{R_1 + R_{Tp}} \tag{3.4}
$$

$$
= \frac{200}{15,000 + 1,875} = 0.01185\ A = 11.85\ mA.
$$

Step 5. Calculate the voltage across the resistor which is equivalent to the parallel resistors:

$$V_{R_{\text{Tp}}} = I\,R_{\text{Tp}}$$
$$= (11.85 \times 10^{-3})\,(1.875 \times 10^{3}) \qquad\qquad (3.3)$$
$$= 22.25 \text{ V.}$$

We have found that when the chart recorder is connected across the solution, the voltage across the solution drops to 22.25 V. The current flow through the solution is given by Ohm's law:

$$I_1 = \frac{\text{Voltage across solution}}{\text{Resistance of solution}}$$
$$= \frac{22.25}{5,000} = 4.45 \text{ mA.}$$

This current is much too low to effect the desired chemical reaction. If this chart recorder is to be used, how can the circuit be changed to raise the current through the solution to the required 10 mA?

Step 6. Referring to Fig. P3.2s2, we see that we can increase the current flow in the circuit if we lower the resistance R_1. We have no control over R_{Tp} with this solution and recorder A. We must find the current flow from the power supply when 10 mA flows through the solution. The current flow from the power supply through R_1 is the sum of the currents through all the branches of the parallel combination:

$$I_1 = I_2 + I_{\text{cr}} = I_2 + \frac{V_{R_{\text{Tp}}}}{R_{\text{cr}}}$$

$$= 10 \times 10^{-3} + \frac{50}{3 \times 10^{3}} = 10 \times 10^{-3} + 16.667 \times 10^{-3}$$

$$= 26.667 \text{ mA.}$$

The voltage across R_1 must be the difference between the supply voltage and the voltage required across the solution:

$$V_b = V_{R_1} + V_{R_{\text{Tp}}},$$
$$V_{R_1} = V_b - V_{R_{\text{Tp}}} = 200 - 50 = 150 \text{ V.}$$

Knowing the voltage across the resistor, R_1, and the current through R_1, we can calculate R_1:

$$R_1 = \frac{V_{R_1}}{I_1} = \frac{150}{26.667 \times 10^{-3}} = 5.62 \times 10^{3} \ \Omega.$$

If a resistor of this size is used in the circuit, 10 mA will flow through the solution when chart recorder A is connected across the solution.

Now we turn to the case of recorder model B. What change can we expect if recorder B is used in place of recorder A? We will follow the same steps as before, but in an abbreviated fashion.

Step 1. Refer to Fig. P3.2s1 and note that we should use the 10,000-Ω value for R_{cr}.

Step 2. Determine the total resistance across the parallel combination:

$$R_{Tp} = \frac{(5,000)\ (10,000)}{5,000 + 10,000} = 3,333\ \Omega.$$

Step 3. Draw the new simplified equivalent circuit (Fig. P3.2s3).

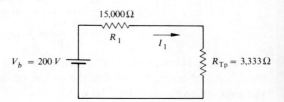

Fig. P3.2s3. New simplified equivalent circuit when recorder *B* is used.

Step 4. Calculate the current flow in the simplified circuit:

$$I_1 = \frac{200}{15,000 + 3,333} = 10.9\ \text{mA.}$$

Step 5. Calculate the voltage across the resistor which is equivalent to the parallel resistors:

$$V_{R_{Tp}} = (10.9 \times 10^{-3})\ (3,333) = 36.3\ \text{V.}$$

Calculate the current flow through the solution:

$$I_2 = \frac{36.3}{5 \times 10^3} = 7.27\ \text{mA.}$$

Step 6. Determine the current flow from the power supply when 10 mA of current flows through the solution:

$$I_1 = I_2 + I_{cr} = 10 \times 10^{-3} + \frac{50}{10 \times 10^3} = 15\ \text{mA.}$$

Calculate the value of resistance for R_1 when 10 mA of current flows through the solution:

$$R_1 = \frac{150}{15 \times 10^{-3}} = 10,000\ \Omega.$$

The following table of values will help us compare the results of using these two recorders.

TABLE P3.2
Summary of results of Problem 3.2

	Current through solution, I_1	Value of R_1 required to make $I_1 = 10$ mA	Total current, I_1
Recorder A in circuit	4.45 mA	5.62×10^3 Ω	11.85 mA
Recorder B in circuit	7.27 mA	10.0×10^3 Ω	10.9 mA
No recorder in circuit	10.0 mA	15.0×10^3 Ω	10.0 mA

Recorder A has a lower input resistance than recorder B. Thus recorder A shunts more of the current away from the solution than does recorder B. Note also that the total current flow from the power supply is dependent on the recorder resistance.

Problem 3.3 A very common problem of obtaining a specific voltage is the following situation. A voltage source is on hand with an output voltage of 200 V. The experimenter needs a voltage of 125 V to drive a load with an input resistance of 1 MΩ (megohm). How can he use this voltage source to produce the desired voltage?

Solution Since the source produces more than the required amount of voltage, it is possible to build a circuit that taps off the percentage of the total voltage required to drive the load. Such a circuit is shown in Fig. P3.3s1. An exact solution for the load voltage V_L can be readily obtained given the equivalent circuit. Equation (3.21) is used to determine the equivalent resistance of the parallel combination of R_2 and R_L:

$$R_p = \frac{R_2 R_L}{R_2 + R_L}.$$

The current I can be determined:

$$I = \frac{V_b}{R_1 + R_p}.$$

The voltage across the load V_L can be determined:

$$V_L = I\,R_p = \frac{V_b}{R_1 + R_p}\,R_p,$$

$$V_L = \frac{R_p}{R_1 + R_p}\,V_b. \tag{3.45}*$$

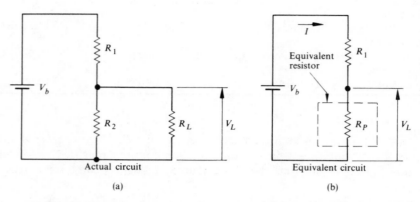

Fig. P3.3s1.   Circuit used to tap off a given percentage of a source voltage.

Note that V_L is determined by the ratio of R_p to the total resistance across the source. Thus the resistance across the terminals where the voltage is to be measured or used is a certain percentage of the total resistance across the source. This type of circuit is usually called a *voltage divider*, because the voltage that is used is less than the source voltage.

The final step in the solution of this problem is to determine the resistances R_1 and R_2. If the load resistance R_L is much larger than R_2, the equation for the load voltage V_L can be simplified: For $R_L \gg R_2$,

$$R_p = \frac{R_2\,R_L}{R_2 + R_L} = R_2 \left(\frac{1}{1 + R_2/R_L} \right) \cong R_2,$$

$$I = \frac{V_b}{R_1 + R_p} \cong \frac{V_b}{R_1 + R_2},$$

$$V_L = \frac{R_p}{R_1 + R_p}\,V_b \cong \frac{R_2}{R_1 + R_2}\,V_b.$$

With the assumption that R_L is much greater than R_2, R_1 and R_2 make a simple divider network to reduce the voltage V_b to the desired V_L. The resistance of R_1

plus R_2 can be any amount so long as the current I is not too large for the source to deliver.

Now we are able to specify the resistor values. Let R_L be 100 times larger than R_2. Let $R_2 = 10,000\ \Omega$. We can now solve for R_1 (Fig. P3.3s2):

$$R_L \gg R_2, \quad V_L \cong \frac{R_2}{R_1 + R_2}\ V_b,$$

$$\frac{R_2}{R_1 + R_2} \cong \frac{V_L}{V_b},$$

$$\frac{10^4}{R_1 + 10^4} \cong \frac{125}{200},$$

$$R_1 + 10^4 = 1.6 \times 10^4$$

$$R_1 = 6 \times 10^3\ \Omega.$$

Fig. P3.3s2.

Essentially the same results could be obtained if $R_1 = 600\ \Omega$ and $R_2 = 1000\ \Omega$. The only major difference would be the increase in current flow from the source. The following table shows the effect of varying R_1 and R_2 on V_L and I when $R_L = 10^6\ \Omega$.

TABLE P3.3

R_1 (kΩ)	R_2 (kΩ)	V_L (V)	I (mA)
0.6	1	125	125
6	10	124.5	12.5
60	100	120.5	1.3
600	1000	90.9	0.18

Note the loading effect that occurs when R_L and R_2 are nearly equal. The load voltage V_L begins to drop below the desired value of 125 V.

3.7 REVIEW QUESTIONS AND PROBLEMS

3.1   What is a resistor and what properties might it have?

3.2   What is the difference between a linear and a nonlinear resistor?

3.3   Give the mathematical expression defining Ohm's law.

3.4   What is an ideal voltage source? What are its characteristics?

3.5   What is an ideal current source? What are its characteristics?

3.6   Two voltmeters (a and b) are available to measure the voltage of a source. They have internal resistances of 10 kΩ and 100 kΩ, respectively. (The letter k represents "kilo" or a factor of 1000.) The source is known to have an internal resistance of 50 kΩ. Assume that the source has an internal voltage of 75 V. What will each of the voltmeters read if they are individually connected across the source? Next, assume the internal resistance of a source is 75 kΩ. If the two above specified voltmeters are connected across the source individually, and if the 10 kΩ voltmeter reads 11.76 V and the 100 kΩ voltmeter reads 57.2 V, what is the internal voltage of the source?

3.7 A number of circuit elements are connected in parallel with an ideal voltage source. How can the total current flowing from the source be calculated?

3.8 When resistors are connected in parallel, how can the total resistance of the parallel combination of resistors be calculated?

3.9 A current source is designed to drive a desired amount of current through a test specimen. What will happen in the circuit if a voltmeter is connected across the test specimen when the current source is also connected to the specimen?

3.10 What is meant by the expression, "The measuring instrument loads down the circuit"? Is this a desirable or an undesirable action to occur? What causes it to occur?

3.11 A chart recorder is to be used to measure the variations in voltage that may occur in an experiment. The input resistance for the chart recorder is 100 kΩ. The circuit to be tested can be modeled as shown in Fig. R3.1. The voltage across R_1 is to be measured. What voltage variations will be read across R_1 if V_s varies from 10 to 20 V? What voltage variation will occur across R_1 if the chart recorder is not connected to R_1?

Fig. R3.1

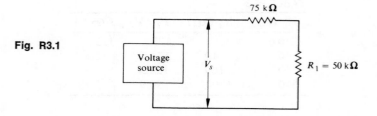

3.12 Determine the current I_s that will flow from the source in Fig. R3.2. Determine the voltage V_{12}.

Fig. R3.2

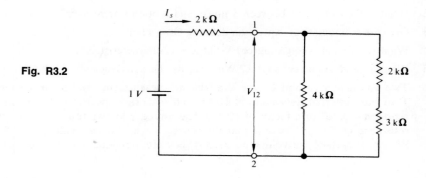

3.13   Determine the current I_a that will flow in the circuit of Fig. R3.3. [*Note:* This can be solved without the use of the network analysis laws given in Chapter 9.]

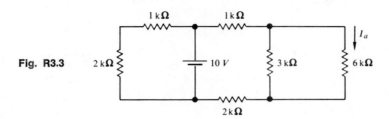

Fig. R3.3

3.14   A voltmeter (a) and an ammeter (b) have been placed in the circuits of Fig. R3.4. Each of these meters has an internal resistance, R_A or R_V, as given. What resistance is given by the ratio of the voltage and current reading on these meters? What is the actual resistance of R_1? Why are these two values different?

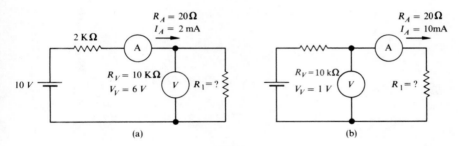

Fig. R3.4

3.15   A current source is to be produced so that a 1-mA current will flow through a test specimen. Two proposals have been made and the diagrams are shown in Fig. R3.5. The specimen has a resistance that will probably vary from 1k to

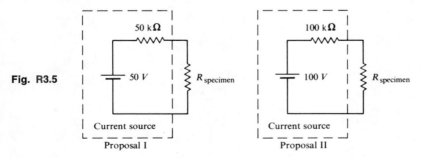

Fig. R3.5

10 kΩ. What variation in current will flow through each of the sources as the specimen resistance changes? Is one source better than the other? What generalizations can be made about this method of producing a current source?

4
alternating-
current circuit models

4.1 OBJECTIVES

This chapter builds on the concepts introduced in the previous chapters. Emphasis is given to the fundamental ideas about dc circuits that can also be used in the study of ac circuits. The terminology that is used in specifying the value of an alternating current or voltage is given so that the reader will understand what the test instrument values mean.

The *capacitor* and the *inductor* are introduced in a way that will enable the reader to understand why these elements have useful characteristics. Basic definitions and waveforms are used as aids in the development of the impedance relations for the inductor and the capacitor. The influence of element size and source frequency on impedance is given. Applications of these devices in low-pass and high-pass filters are discussed in the examples. The mathematical models of these circuits are given to show the usefulness of these models even though no numerical calculations are required.

The basic voltage and impedance transformation characteristics of a transformer are introduced to show that it is a useful and needed element in ac circuits. Problems with solutions are given to help the reader learn how to use the basic models for the circuit elements used in ac circuits.

The intent of the discussions in this chapter is to aid the reader in developing an intuitive feeling of the characteristics and operation of these circuit elements. A number of equations is given, but actual numerical calculations are not required. Insight to the circuits discussed can be gained by considering only what happens when the several variables become large or small.

Many times the current that flows in a circuit during an experiment is not constant in direction and magnitude, as is the case in dc circuits. Current flow may change in magnitude or direction depending on the circuit and its power source. In this chapter we shall discuss the fundamentals relating to circuits driven by alternating-current or voltage sources. We shall define an *alternating current* (ac) or voltage as one that changes direction rhythmically. It rises from zero to a maximum value in one direction, returns to zero, rises to the same value in the opposite direction, and returns to zero, etc. The values form a periodic wave and are specified mathematically as follows:

$$v\,(t) = V_{\max} \sin\,(2\pi f t + \theta), \tag{4.1}$$

where t is time, $V_{\max}$ is the maximum or peak value, f is frequency at which the reversals take place (in cycles per second or *hertz,* abbreviated Hz), T is the period of the wave and equals $1/f$, and θ is an angle displacing the wave along the t-axis.

This type of current or voltage can be graphically shown as a function of time (Fig. 4.1). Since this current or voltage varies as a function of time, as do water waves, this picture in Fig. 4.1 is often called a *waveform*. Note that this voltage or current is periodic for all values of time t. There are other types of voltage or current variations occurring in some experiments that are not periodic. The analysis methods presented in this chapter are not applicable to those types of voltage or current. Only alternating currents as defined above will be considered.

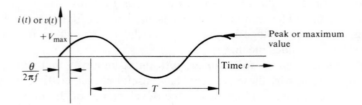

Fig. 4.1. Waveform of an alternating voltage or current. Example of a periodic wave.

A number of important questions come to mind as we recall the material presented in the previous chapter.

1. How must the circuit model be changed when the experiment involves ac rather than dc signals?
2. Is Ohm's law valid when the source of power or signal is ac rather than dc?
3. What new circuit elements do we have available for use in ac circuits?
4. How can we develop an intuitive feeling for the responses that these new circuit elements will have in ac circuits?
5. What types of things can be done with these new circuit elements in ac circuits that could not be done with dc sources and resistors?

In the following sections in this chapter we shall pursue answers to these questions so as to enhance the readers capability to effectively perform experiments involving alternating currents. The discussion in this chapter will serve as an introduction to the concept of alternating currents while leaving the study of the more detailed mathematical operations for Chapter 9.

4.2   SERIES-CIRCUIT MODEL

The models that were used in the discussion of dc circuits involved only dc voltage or current sources and resistors. In Chapter 2 we used the terms "resistance" and "impedance" interchangeably, whereas in Chapter 3 the term "resistance" was used and "impedance" was dropped. This was done because only one circuit element, the resistor, besides the power or signal sources was used in the discussion of dc circuits. Two additional circuit elements may be used in ac circuits; the capacitor and the inductor. These elements also can impede the flow of current in ac circuits, so we use the term "impedance" for the opposition to current flow which may be caused by a resistor, a capacitor, an inductor, or any combination of these three circuit elements.

General Form of Series-circuit Model

The series-circuit model for ac circuits is a very simple extension of the series-circuit model for dc circuits. In its most general form the model can show an impedance in place of a resistor, as in Fig. 4.2. The symbol Z_i is used to represent the impedance of each block in the diagram. The symbol $i_g(t)$ or $i_s(t)$ is used to represent an ideal current generator or source, while the symbol $v_g(t)$ or $v_s(t)$ is used to represent an ideal voltage generator or source. These are time-varying sources; hence t is included in the symbol.

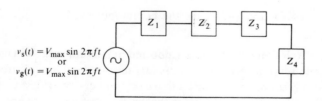

Fig. 4.2.   Block diagram for series ac circuits.

Total Impedance of Series Circuit

The total impedance across the source is equal to the sum of the individual impedances. This law is the direct counterpart of Eq. (3.1) used in dc-circuit analysis.

$$Z_{\text{Total}} = \sum_{i=1}^{n} Z_{i,}$$ (4.2)*

where Z_i represents the individual impedances, whose values may be complex numbers, † and n is the total number of series impedances.

AC Current and Voltage Terminology

The current flow in the circuit is determined by dividing the source voltage by the total impedance:

$$i_{\text{Total}}(t) = \frac{v_g(t)}{Z_{\text{Total}}} \tag{4.3}$$

where $v_g(t) = V_{\max} \sin 2\pi ft$.

Equation (4.3) is one form, though not a particularly good one, of Ohm's law. Most of the time we do not need to know the particular value of current at any one instant in time, but would rather have a number or symbol that would describe a *sine wave* of the current. This number should be the one that could be read on an ac voltmeter or ammeter commonly found in laboratories. The appropriate number is defined as the maximum value of the sine wave divided by the square root of two and is known by several names: *effective value, root-mean-square value, rms value of the sine wave*. When rms values are used, the symbols for current and voltage are I and V, respectively. Ohm's law for ac circuits takes on the following form:

$$I = \frac{V}{Z}, \tag{4.4}$$

$$V = IZ, \tag{4.5}*$$

where V is an rms voltage value, and I is an rms current value.

Equations (4.4) and (4.5) are the commonly used relations for ac-circuit calculations.

Example 4.1   Relation between rms value and maximum value of voltage.   Some examples should serve to bring this confusing terminology into clearer focus. The 60–Hz ac power supplied to most laboratory outlets provides voltages in the range of 110 to 120 V rms. Usually the term "root-mean-square" is dropped when referring to power line voltage, but the number stated is an rms voltage. Assume that the voltage in a particular laboratory is 115 V rms as measured on an rms-reading voltmeter. If you were able to look at the waveform of the sinusoidal voltage at the power line outlet, you would see a curve such as shown in Fig. 4.3. The maximum or peak value of the voltage is $115 \times \sqrt{2}$ or 162 V. The peak-to-peak voltage is twice the maximum value or 324 V. Thus, if someone says

---

† Complex numbers must be treated differently from real numbers. No numerical calculations are required in this chapter. Complex-number operations are introduced with examples in Chapter 9 when they are needed to get numerical results.

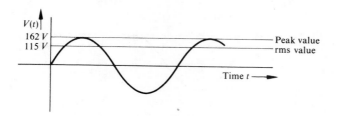

Fig. 4.3. Waveform of a 115-V rms voltage.

that a sinusoidal voltage of 115 V is available in the laboratory, he is referring to an ac voltage that swings from zero to plus 162 V, back to zero, to minus 162 V, back to zero, and so forth, as shown in Fig. 4.3. The polarity of the voltage reverses every half cycle.

Example 4.2   Relation between rms value and maximum value of current.   A second example of applying Ohm's law is in order. Suppose the manufacturer of a piece of laboratory equipment states that the impedance of this equipment is 50 Ω when the power line frequency is 60 Hz. How much current will flow into the equipment when the power line voltage is 115 V rms and the frequency is 60 Hz? What will the waveform of the current look like? Solving for current, we have

$$I = \frac{V}{Z}$$ (4.4)

$$= \frac{115 \text{ v rms}}{50 \text{ }\Omega} = 2.3 \text{ A rms}$$

To draw the current waveform we must convert the rms current value to an equivalent sinusoidal current maximum or peak value. Recall that

$$\text{rms value} = \frac{\text{maximum value}}{\sqrt{2}}.$$ (4.6)*

Therefore:

$$\text{maximum or peak value} = \text{rms value} \times \sqrt{2}$$ (4.7)*

$$I_{\text{peak}} = 2.3 \sqrt{2}$$
$$= 3.25 \text{ A.}$$

This waveform is shown in Fig. 4.4.

Example 4.3   Frequency-selective circuit.   The third example will illustrate a major application of ac circuits in many experiments. Assume that a study is to be made involving an experiment to find a signal of a particular frequency that might be generated by a source which also generates many other undesired frequencies of no particular importance. The investigator would like to be able to

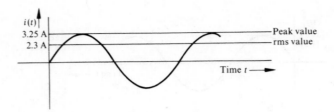

Fig. 4.4. Waveform for an ac current of 2.3 A rms.

reject or block out all the undesired frequencies and retain or pass only the wanted frequency. A frequency-selective circuit is required to solve this experimental problem. A simple series circuit can be developed to accomplish this. Let us look at the series-circuit model to see what characteristics might be needed for the individual impedances.

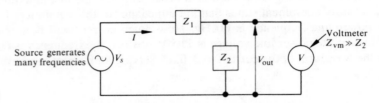

Fig. 4.5. Block diagram for frequency-selective circuit.

Figure 4.5 shows the general block diagram. Assume that the voltage-sensing device used to measure this desired frequency voltage has a very high input impedance and does not act as a *shunt* on Z_2. The voltage generated by the source must equal the sum of the voltages across the individual impedances. In general we can state the following for series circuits:

$$Z_{total} = \sum_{i=1}^{n} Z_i, \tag{4.2}*$$

$$V = IZ, \tag{4.5}*$$

$$V_{total} = IZ_{total} \quad \text{for series circuit} \tag{4.8}$$

$$= I(Z_1 + Z_2 + \cdots + Z_n) \tag{4.9}$$

$$= IZ_1 + IZ_2 + \cdots + IZ_n \tag{4.10}$$

$$= V_1 + V_2 + \cdots + V_n \tag{4.11}$$

$$= \sum_{i=1}^{n} V_i. \tag{4.12}*$$

In this example $n = 2$. If two of the impedances were made up of circuit elements that did not change their characteristics with frequency, this circuit would be a simple voltage divider and would not be frequency-selective. (Refer to problem 3.3 for the analysis of a voltage divider.) We conclude that we need an impedance that varies as a function of frequency if a frequency-selective circuit is to be produced.

We would like the voltage across the output to be high when the desired frequency is present and to be low when the unimportant or undesired frequencies are present. There are two possible solutions to this problem:

1. Make Z_1 a fixed impedance regardless of the frequency. Let Z_2 have a high impedance at the desired frequency and a low impedance at all other frequencies.

2. Make Z_2 a fixed impedance regardless of the frequency. Let Z_1 have a low impedance at the desired frequency and a high impedance at all other frequencies.

Let us look at the first solution. If Z_2 has a high impedance relative to Z_1 at the desired frequency, most of the source voltage at that frequency will appear across Z_2 and very little will appear across Z_1. Therefore the output voltage will be high as is required. This can be shown mathematically. The current through Z_1 = current through $Z_2 = I$. The voltage across Z_1 is

$$V_{Z_1} = I\,Z_1.$$

The voltage across Z_2 is

$$V_{Z_2} = I\,Z_2.$$

If $Z_2 > Z_1$, $V_{Z_2} > V_{Z_1}$, then

$$I = \frac{V_{Z_1}}{Z_1} = \frac{V_{Z_2}}{Z_2},$$

$$\frac{Z_2}{Z_1} = \frac{V_{Z_2}}{V_{Z_1}}.$$

If Z_2 has a low impedance relative to Z_1 at all other frequencies, most of the source voltage will appear across Z_1 and very little will appear across the output. This is the desired response for the circuit. This action can also be shown as follows:

$$I = \frac{V_s}{Z_1 + Z_2}, \tag{4.13}$$

$$V_{out} = I\,Z_2 \tag{4.14}$$

$$= \frac{Z_2}{Z_1 + Z_2}\,V_s \tag{4.15}$$

$$= \frac{1}{1 + Z_1/Z_2}\,V_s. \tag{4.16}*$$

Compare Eq. (4.16) with Eq. (3.45).

The characteristic curve for Z_2 vs. frequency could be as shown in Fig. 4.6. In this figure the desired frequency could be f_0, and the undesired frequencies could be f_1, f_2, f_3, f_4.

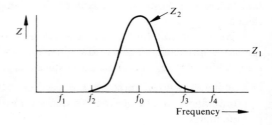

Fig. 4.6. Characteristic curve for the frequency-selective impedance Z_2 (first solution); Z_1 is constant.

The second solution can be analyzed in the same way. When Z_1 has a low impedance relative to Z_2, most of the source voltage will appear across Z_2 and very little will appear across Z_1. This is the desired response. When Z_1 is a large impedance compared to Z_2, most of the source voltage will appear across Z_1 and very little will appear across the output. Thus the undesired frequencies would be blocked by Z_1, as is required. The mathematics necessary to validate this line of reasoning has already been developed. A reference to Eq. (4.16) for V_{out} will verify that this is another solution to the problem. The characteristics required for Z_1 in this case are shown in Fig. 4.7.

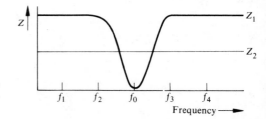

Fig. 4.7. Characteristic curve for frequency-selective impedance Z_1 (second solution); Z_2 is constant.

Note that very little new information was required to develop a feel for the operation of a very important ac circuit that finds almost universal application in laboratory equipment. The fundamentals required to develop this "feel" should be thoroughly understood.

The discussion above reveals that the major difference between the analyses of ac and dc series circuits is terminology. The total impedance of an ac series circuit is the sum of the individual impedances. The general form of Ohm's law for ac circuits is the same as for dc circuits, except that impedance is used instead of resistance. The method of determining the individual impedances will be discussed in Sections 4.5, 4.6, and in Chapter 9.

4.3 PARALLEL-CIRCUIT MODEL

General Form of Parallel-Circuit Model

The most general form of the parallel-circuit model for ac circuits is a minor variation of the parallel-circuit model for dc circuits. The terminology introduced in the previous section is also standard for parallel circuits. I and V represent the rms values of current and voltage, respectively. Figure 4.8 shows the general form of the parallel circuit with impedances in every branch.

The total current that flows from the source is equal to the sum of the individual currents in the several branches:

$$I_{total} = \sum_{i=1}^{n} I_i, \tag{4.17}*$$

where I_i represents the individual branch currents and n is the total number of parallel branches. The current flow in the individual branches is determined by Ohm's law:

$$I_i = \frac{V_s}{Z_i}. \tag{4.18}$$

Equivalent Impedance of a Parallel Circuit

The equivalent impedance driven by the source can be readily determined by means of Ohm's law and the equations above:

$$Z_{eq} = \frac{V_s}{I_{total}} = \frac{V_s}{\sum_{i=1}^{n} I_i},$$

$$= \frac{V_s}{V_s/Z_1 + V_s/Z_2 + \cdots + V_s/Z_n} = \frac{1}{\sum_{i=1}^{n} (1/Z_i)}. \tag{4.19}*$$

Note that the equation for the total or equivalent impedance Z_{eq} of parallel branches has the same form as Eq. (3.27) for the parallel combination of resistors.

Fortunately, these simple equations are all that are necessary to describe the general operation of ac circuits. The dc problems discussed in Section 3.4 have

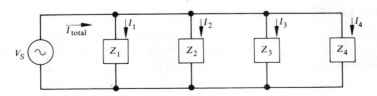

Fig. 4.8. Block diagram for a parallel ac circuit.

their exact analogies in ac problems, where every resistor in the diagrams is replaced by an impedance block and every R in the equations are replaced by a Z. Therefore, the experimenter can easily discover trends in his experiment as the various impedances in the circuit increase or decrease. However, it would be misleading to say that the calculation of the individual impedances and combined impedances is as simple as it is for dc circuits. Methods of making numerical calculations of these impedances will be deferred until Chapter 9.

4.4 ac POWER AND SIGNAL SOURCES

Both ac current and voltage sources will be used in the models of ac circuits. They will be ideal sources as in the dc circuit models. An *ideal ac voltage source* is one that will produce a sinusoidal voltage of constant maximum or peak value across its output terminals regardless of the current flow. The internal impedance of an ideal ac voltage source must therefore be zero. If the actual voltage source does not have zero internal impedance, an impedance can be placed in series with an ideal voltage source to make a model of the actual voltage source.

An *ideal ac current source* is one that will supply a sinusoidal current of constant maximum or peak value to a load regardless of the impedance of the load. A nonideal current source can be considered as an impedance placed in parallel with an ideal current source.

Sources of ac *power* differ from sources of ac *signals* in that the former can deliver a large amount of power to a load while maintaining a sinusoidal waveform with constant peak value.

ac power = rms voltage × rms current × cosine of the phase angle.† (4.20)*

dc power = dc voltage × dc current. (4.21)*

If a source can deliver a large amount of power, it is usually called a power source. If it can produce any reasonable peak value of sinusoidal voltage while delivering a relatively small current, it may be called a signal source. Similarly, if the source will deliver any reasonable peak value of sinusoidal current to a load while producing a limited voltage, it may be called a signal source. In general the term "signal" is used when the voltage or current represents some information about an experiment.

4.5 THE RESISTOR MODEL

The *resistor* in an electrical circuit is the element that can dissipate energy and give off heat. It impedes the flow of current in the circuit in conformity with Ohm's law. The actual device used as a resistor in a circuit may be fabricated in a num-

---

† Phase angle will be defined in Section 4.6.

ber of ways. It may be a solid cylinder of carbon with wires attached to each end. It may be a thin layer of resistive material coating an insulated cylinder. It may be a coil of wire that has a high resistance per length of wire.

These differences explain the fact that some resistors have other properties besides resistance. Some have the characteristics of a capacitor or an inductor in addition to being resistors. In a dc circuit the inductive or capacitive characteristics of a resistor have no importance. As will be shown in later sections, however, when the frequency of ac signals varies, the responses of inductors and capacitors also vary, thus complicating the analysis of resistor circuits when the frequency is in the order of megahertz or higher.

Ideal resistors will be used as models in this study. An ideal resistor is one that has only the property of resistance, and the symbol for it is the same as that used in Chapter 3. If in fact the resistor used has some properties of an inductor or a capacitor, it is possible to add the appropriate inductor or capacitor model to the ideal resistor model for purposes of analysis.

4.6   THE CAPACITOR MODEL

In the discussion thus far we have indicated only that there is a circuit element called a *capacitor* and implied that it has some desirable characteristics. In fact, it is the most widely used circuit element after the resistor. It is very important that the reader develop an intuitive understanding of the characteristics of the capacitor and its uses in experimental work, even though he may not have to make any detailed numerical calculations. This will enable him to understand the general characteristics of ac circuits which he may find useful in his work. For example, the capacitor is one of the essential elements in the impedance used in the frequency-selective network discussed in Section 4.2.

Unique Property of a Capacitor

One of the interesting properties of the capacitor is that it will prevent the flow of direct current but not the flow of alternating currents. This is a very useful characteristic which explains the wide application of capacitors in experimental work. Imagine, for example, that an experiment requires that a dc voltage be applied across a specimen and the specimen responds by generating a rapidly fluctuating, measurable voltage. This rapidly fluctuating voltage is of primary interest to the experimenter. Unfortunately, at the point where the measurement is to be made, both the fluctuating ac and the dc voltages are present. Some means must be found to remove the dc voltage while retaining the ac voltage. The capacitor is the logical element to use since it will let pass only ac signals and will reject or block dc signals. To understand this property we must visualize the physical structure of a capacitor.

Let us look at the circuit in Fig. 4.9 and see how we might obtain the desired property of a capacitor. Note that in (a) a resistor is connected across a battery and thus current will flow. In (b) the wire to the resistor has been broken so that air occupies the gap between the ends of the wire. Since air will not conduct electrical charges across the gap unless it is ionized, direct current will not flow in this circuit.

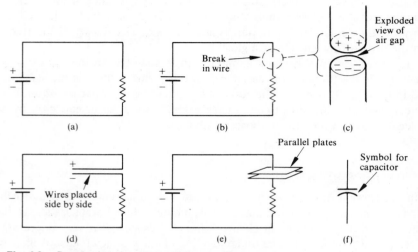

Fig. 4.9. Developing the concept of capacitance.

An interesting phenomenon occurs at the ends of the wires. Positive charge will appear on the top wire, because it is connected to the positive terminal of the battery and the mobile electrons in the wire are attracted to the battery, leaving only positive charges at the end. Negative charges will appear on the bottom wire, because it is connected to the negative terminal, and the mobile electrons in the wire are repelled from the negative terminal, thus forcing an excess of negative charge on the bottom end of the wire. This is shown in (c). These negative charges cannot move across the gap because the air is not ionized. Thus an *electric field* is set up in the gap between the positive and negative charges. If an electric field exists, there must be a potential difference between the ends of the wires. The voltage across the gap is equal to the battery voltage. So long as the battery voltage does not change, the charges on the ends of the wire will not change and there will be no current flow. We recall that electric current is defined to be the time rate of change of electric charge passing through a specified area. There must have been charge flow initially to charge the ends of the wires.

It is possible to change the physical configuration of the wires, as shown in (d), where the wires are bent so that the two ends are side by side but not touching. The area of exposure of the wire ends to each other is now much greater than in (b). Charges will once again accumulate along the wires; only this time more positive charges will be near the negative charges, and vice versa. Hence there must have been more charge flow initially to build up this charge from the situation in (c). We can connect large plates to the wire ends and place them very close together as in (e), to get still more charges close together.

Thus each of the situations (b) through (e) will initiate a charge flow until the voltage across the ends of the wire or across the plates has become equal to the source voltage, and the flow will cease. This current flow takes only a very short time and is called a transient current.

Capacitance

The device we have described as adjacent wires or metal plates is able to obtain and store charge when a voltage is applied across the device. The capacity to store charge depends on the mutually exposed surface area and the spacing between them. This device is called a *capacitor* because it has the capacity to hold or store charge. The capacity or *capacitance* is defined by the following equation:

$$C = \frac{q}{v},$$
(4.22)*

where q is the charge in coulombs, $+q$ on one plate and $-q$ on the other plate, v is the voltage in volts, and C is the capacitance in farads. Thus the voltage across the capacitor is directly proportional to the charge that is accumulated on the capacitor and inversely proportional to the value of capacitance.

ac Current and Voltage Relation

We have seen that a capacitor can act as an open circuit to dc and still allow charge to flow on a short-term or transient basis. How will it respond when a sinusoidal current flows in the circuit? How will it respond when the voltage applied across it is sinusoidal? How can we make a model for this circuit element to predict how the circuit will operate under ac voltages? The waveforms shown in Fig. 4.10 will be helpful when answering these questions.

Assume that a sinusoidal voltage appears across the capacitor. By our defining equation (4.22), if the capacitance is constant, the charge q must also vary sinusoidally. The time rates of change of the voltage and charge across the capacitor are shown in (a) and (b). Again referring to the definition of current in Chapter 1, we can write a current equation in terms of charge and time:

$$
\begin{aligned}
i(t) &= \text{time rate of change of charge} \\
&= \frac{\text{incremental change of charge}}{\text{incremental change of time}} = \frac{dq}{dt} \\
&\cong \frac{\Delta q}{\Delta t}.
\end{aligned}
$$
(4.23)*

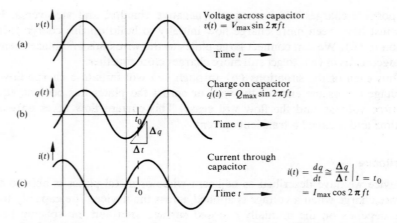

Fig. 4.10.   Waveforms of v(t), q(t), and i(t) for a circuit with only a capacitor and an ac power source.

(Refer to Fig. 4.10 for Δq and Δt.) Note that the time rate of change of the charge wave form (b) is simply the slope of this wave at any point of time. The maximum slope occurs when q is zero, and zero slope occurs when q is at its maximum positive or negative values. On the basis of this information we can construct the waveform for i(t) as shown in (c). A more mathematical treatment of this phenomenon will prove that the current waveform is a cosine wave when the voltage wave is a sine wave. The current through the capacitor reaches its peak one quarter of a cycle (90°) before the voltage across the capacitor reaches its peak. A common way of describing this difference between the times when the voltage and the current peak is to say that the *current leads the voltage by 90° or the voltage lags the current by 90°*. Either statement is correct. The current and voltage are *out of phase* with each other, and the *phase angle* is 90°.

A point to remember

When a sinusoidal voltage is applied across a capacitor, the sinusoidal current through the capacitor will lead the voltage by 90°. They are out of phase by 90°. The phase angle between voltage and current is 90°.

The Impedance of a Capacitor

Now that we know how the capacitor responds to a sinusoidal current or voltage, how can we make a model for it that will enable us to write some simple equations that can be used to predict the performance of circuits with capacitors? Let us rearrange Eq. (4.22) as shown in Eq. (4.24) and look at the waveforms again:

$$v = \frac{q}{C}.$$ (4.24)

If v is held constant while C is increased, the charge q must increase proportionally. This is shown for the time-varying waveforms in Fig. 4.11 (a) and (b). When the value of capacitance doubles at any instant, the value of charge must also double in order to maintain constant voltage across the capacitor ($v = q/C$). The current flow at any instant of time is equal to the slope dq/dt of the $q(t)$ wave. When the capacitance is C_1, the slope at the zero crossing points is one-half the slope at the zero crossing points when the capacitance is $2C_1$. This can be proved mathematically, but the proof will be omitted at this time. Therefore, the current flowing through the larger capacitor is twice as great as the current flowing through the smaller capacitor as shown in Fig. 4.11(c). We can say that the larger capacitor does not impede the current flow as much as does the smaller capacitor.

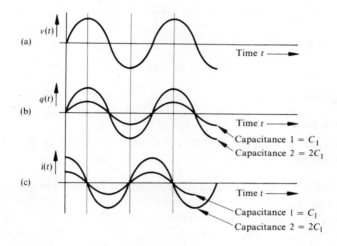

Fig. 4.11. Effect of varying capacitance on current flow in a capacitor.

In this example we are solving for the current flow for two different values of capacitance. Recalling that

$$I = \frac{V}{Z},\qquad(4.4)$$

we let Z_1 be the impedance offered by capacitor 1 and Z_2 be the impedance offered by capacitor 2. The currents are then given by the following equations:

$$I_1 = \frac{V}{Z_1},\qquad(4.25)$$

$$I_2 = \frac{V}{Z_2}.\qquad(4.26)$$

We found earlier that the current through capacitor 2 is twice as great as the current through capacitor 1 when V is held constant.

$$I_2 = 2I_1.$$

Using Eqs. (4.25) and (4.26), we find that the impedance of the larger capacitor, capacitor 2, is half the impedance of capacitor 1.

V is held to a fixed peak value of the waveform for each case.

$$V = I_1 Z_1 = I_2 Z_2.$$

Since $I_2 = 2I_1$,

$$I_1 Z_1 = 2I_1 Z_2 \quad \text{and} \quad Z_2 = \frac{Z_1}{2}.$$

We are now able to observe that

$$Z_2 \text{ is less than } Z_1$$

when C_2 is greater than C_1.

A point to remember

The impedance of a capacitor at a particular frequency is inversely proportional to the value of capacitance.

Thus the model for a capacitor must be described by an equation that accounts for this observation. Recall also that the model must account for the fact that the current through a capacitor and the voltage across the capacitor are one quarter of a cycle or 90° out of phase with each other. The equation below incorporates these considerations:

$$Z = -j \left(\frac{1}{kC} \right),$$

where j indicates a 90° phase angle between current and voltage, k is a proportionality constant, C is the capacitance.

Next we must determine the effect produced by varying the voltage frequency across the capacitor (Fig. 4.12). Note that in (b) when the frequency doubles, the slope at the zero crossing points increases. A mathematical analysis will show that the slope doubles when the frequency doubles. Therefore, the current flow doubles when the frequency doubles, because the current at any instant is equal to the slope of $q(t)$ at that time. See Fig. 4.12 (c). When the peak value of the sine wave of voltage is held constant and the frequency doubles, the current doubles or we can say that the impedance of the capacitor must have halved.

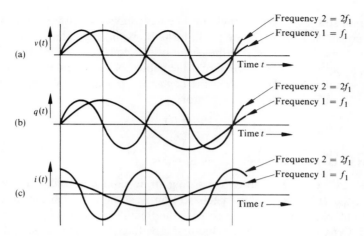

Fig. 4.12. Effect of varying frequency on current flow in a capacitor.

Let Z_1 be the impedance offered by a capacitor when the frequency is f_1 and Z_2 be the impedance offered by the same capacitor when the frequency is $2f_1$. The currents are then given by the following equations:

$$I_1 = \frac{V}{Z_1},\tag{4.25}$$

$$I_2 = \frac{V}{Z_2}.\tag{4.26}$$

We found earlier that the current for frequency 1 is half as large as for frequency 2:

$$I_1 = \frac{I_2}{2}.\tag{4.27}$$

$$\frac{V}{Z_1} = \frac{V}{2\,Z_2}\tag{4.28}$$

Therefore,

$$Z_1 = 2\,Z_2\tag{4.29}$$

when frequency $1 = \frac{1}{2}$ (frequency 2).

A point to remember

The impedance of a capacitor is inversely proportional to the frequency of the ac voltage applied across the capacitor.

With this new information we are now able to understand the form of the general equation for the impedance offered by a capacitor when a sinusoidal voltage is applied across the capacitor:

$$Z = -j\left(\frac{1}{2\pi f C}\right),\tag{4.30}*$$

where j indicates a 90° phase angle between current and voltage, 2π is a proportionality constant, f is the frequency in hertz, C is the capacitance in farads, and Z is the impedance in ohms. Another form of this equation is often used when the phase angle between the voltage across the capacitor and the current through the capacitor is not needed. It is called the *capacitive reactance, X_c,* and is the magnitude of the impedance of the capacitor:

$$X_c = \left(\frac{1}{2\pi fC}\right) \qquad (4.31)*$$

where f is in Hz, C is in farads, X_c is in ohms.

Example 4.4   High-pass filter consisting of a capacitor and a resistor. The example cited at the beginning of this section was one in which the experimenter wanted to block the dc voltage and pass the fluctuating voltage generated by the specimen. Let us assume that the fluctuating voltage is sinusoidal so that we may use the information discussed thus far. A relatively simple circuit, such as shown in Fig. 4.13(a), may be used to block or filter out the dc voltage while passing the ac voltage. This circuit consists of a resistor and a capacitor connected in series across the specimen with the output taken across the resistor. An ac voltmeter could be used to measure this output voltage.

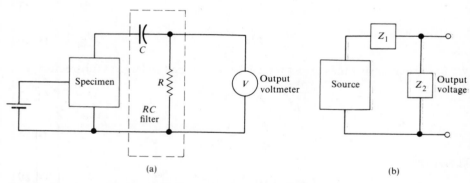

(a)   (b)

Fig. 4.13.   Circuit for filtering out dc voltage while passing ac voltage.

The capacitor will block the dc voltage as required, but it will also present an impedance to the flow of ac current. How will this impedance affect the amplitude of the ac signal that is developed across the resistor? To answer this question we examine the simplified block diagram shown in Fig. 4.13(b). Z_1 represents the impedance of the capacitor at any particular frequency. Z_2 represents the resistor whose resistance does not change with frequency.

We recall from our arguments and Eq. (4.30) that the impedance Z_1 offered by the capacitor decreases as frequency increases. The value of Z_2 is equal to the parallel combination of the resistor R and the input resistance of the voltmeter.

This block diagram is of the same form as that of the voltage divider studied in problem 3.3 and in Section 4.1. Part of the ac voltage generated by the specimen will appear across Z_1 and part of it will appear across Z_2. If Z_1 is large compared with Z_2, most of the ac voltage will appear across Z_1 and very little will appear across Z_2 at the output. If Z_1 is small compared with Z_2, most of the ac voltage will appear across Z_2 at the output and very little will appear across Z_1. This may be shown mathematically by substituting the equation for the impedance of a capacitor, for Z_1 in Eq. (4.15):

$$V_{\text{out}} = \frac{Z_2}{Z_1 + Z_2} V_s, \qquad\qquad (4.15)$$

where $Z_1 = -j/2\pi f C$, $Z_2 = R \, R_{\text{vm}}/(R + R_{\text{vm}})$, and R_{vm} is the voltmeter input resistance. For the moment let us speak in generalities and ignore the phase-angle term that appears in the equation for the impedance of the capacitor. We can discover trends following this path even though we cannot calculate specific numerical values of the output voltage.

With the aid of Eq. (4.15) the experimenter should be able to determine whether he should have a large or small capacitance C when the frequency f is at a specific value, f_1.

Let the resistance of the voltmeter be large compared to R. We have

$$Z_2 = \frac{R \, R_{\text{vm}}}{R + R_{\text{vm}}}.$$

Since $R_{\text{vm}} >> R$,

$$Z_2 \cong R.$$

Rearranging Eq. (4.16), we obtain

$$V_{\text{out}} = \left(\frac{1}{Z_1/Z_2 + 1} \right) V_s, \qquad\qquad (4.16)$$

where $Z_1 = -j/2\pi f C$, $Z_2 \cong R$. When f equals f_1, C can be made large enough so that Z_1 is much less than Z_2 and the output voltage is almost equal to the source voltage. As C becomes smaller Z_1 increases and the denominator of Eq. (4.16) becomes larger, causing the output voltage to decrease. Thus the amplitude of the output voltage is dependent on the size of the capacitor and Z_2. These equations verify the fact that the dc output voltage is zero because the amplitude of Z_1 is infinite when f is zero.

The specimen may generate a frequency which changes with the applied dc voltage. How will the filter output change as the frequency changes? If frequency increases, Z_1 decreases, making the denominator of Eq. (4.16) decrease. The output voltage then increases toward the source voltage. If the frequency is very high, the output voltage is almost equal to the source voltage. As the frequency decreases, the output voltage approaches zero. Variations of C or f produce the same results in the output voltage. The reader should verify this line of reasoning while looking at Fig. 4.13 (a), because it will prove very valuable when analyzing instrumentation circuits. This discussion can be summarized pictorially by Fig. 4.14, which shows a typical frequency-response curve of a high-pass *RC* filter. This type of filter is called a high-pass filter because it passes high frequencies while attenuating low frequencies.

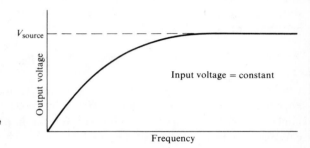

Fig. 4.14. Frequency response curve for a simple *RC* filter.

A point to remember

A capacitor may be used with a resistor to produce a filter that will let pass high frequencies while attenuating low frequencies.

In the study of problem 4.2 in Section 4.10 we will find that a simple capacitor-resistor combination can be used to pass low frequencies while attenuating high frequencies.

The example we have just studied reveals the importance of understanding the model for a capacitor in an ac circuit. An intuitive feeling of how a capacitor will affect signals will be helpful, even though we have made no numerical calculations.

4.7 THE INDUCTOR MODEL

The capacitor was found to have an impedance that varies inversely with frequency. In a dc circuit the capacitor acts as an open circuit and at very high frequencies it acts as a short circuit. It is desirable to have an element with characteristics that are the opposite of those of the capacitor. Such an element will act as a short circuit in a dc circuit and as an open circuit at very high frequencies. The *inductor* is such an element. Later it will be shown that combinations of these two circuit elements can be produced that have high impedances at certain frequencies and low impedances at all other frequencies. These devices are required to produce the characteristics pictured in Figs. 4.6 and 4.7. Before proceeding to combinations of capacitors, resistors, and inductors, it would be well to develop a good understanding of the characteristics of the inductor.

To understand the characteristics of an inductor, we must first look at what happens when current flows in an electric conductor. Whenever a current flows, a magnetic field is produced around the current which changes proportionally with the current flow. The term *magnetic flux* is used in describing this field. If this field has a high density (strength), it is said to have a large amount of flux per unit area.

Induced Voltage

If a magnetic field around a conductor varies in strength, a voltage will be induced in the conductor and this voltage will produce current flow in a complete circuit. Two effects may occur simultaneously: a varying current through the conductor producing a varying magnetic field and a varying magnetic field around the conductor inducing a voltage in the conductor. The polarity of the voltage induced in this situation is such as to tend to oppose the flow of the current that produced the varying magnetic field. The magnitude of this *induced voltage* is directly proportional to the time rate of change of the magnetic field around the conductor. That is, the more rapidly the strength of the magnetic field around the conductor changes, the greater is the voltage induced in the conductor. Since this voltage opposes the flow of current in the conductor, the impedance of the conductor increases when there is an increase in the rate at which the magnetic field strength varies.

Consider Fig. 4.15. In (a) a small area in the center of the cross section of a conductor is shown to be carrying a small portion of the current flowing through the conductor. The magnetic field due to this current is indicated by the circle with the arrowhead. The arrowhead indicates the direction of the field. In (b) a larger current is flowing through the same square cross section of the conductor, and the circle around the square is thicker indicating that the magnetic field is stronger due to the larger current flow than in (a).

In (c) a portion of a complete circuit with current flowing in it is shown. If the conductor is driven by an ac voltage source with a small peak value, a current will flow which produces a magnetic field. This magnetic field around the square section of the conductor will vary by a small amount, inducing a small voltage across this section of the conductor with the polarities as shown. The voltage of this polarity will oppose the flow of the current that produced the magnetic field in the first place. The net result is that the current flow in the circuit will be less than it would have been if this induced voltage was not produced.

In (d) we see that a much higher peak value of current is flowing in the circuit than in (c). Let us assume that the circuit is driven by an ac voltage source with a large peak value. This means that there will be large current variations, which will produce large variations in the magnetic field strength, which in turn will induce a large voltage along this section of the conductor. This induced voltage will oppose the flow of current from the source. The net result in both cases (c) and (d) is that the induced voltage impedes the flow of current in the circuit.

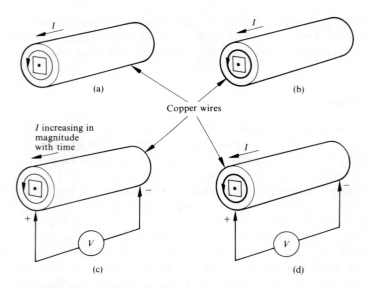

Fig. 4.15. Developing the concept of inductance.

A physical change in the configuration of the conductor can change the magnitude of the induced voltage. This is shown in Fig. 4.16. The wire has now been turned into a coil. The magnetic fields due to the current flowing in the adjacent turns of the coil will add together to produce a much stronger field than is possible with a straight conductor. If we drive this new circuit with the same current source that was used in the example of Fig. 4.15(c), larger variations in the magnetic field about the conductor will result, and the voltage induced across the turns will be larger than it was for the short section of a straight wire. As the number of turns of the coil increases, the voltage induced in the coil will increase if the ac current flow is held constant.

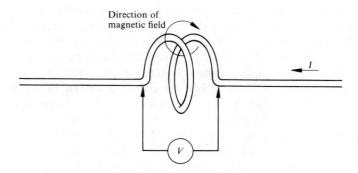

Fig. 4.16. The inductor as a coil of wire.

Inductance

It was stated in the above discussion that the voltage induced in the circuit is proportional to the rate of change of the magnetic field, which is in turn proportional to the rate of change of current flow. These relations can be written in the form of an equation:

Induced voltage = Time rate of change of current × Proportionality constant

where the proportionality constant indicates the ease with which the magnetic field around the conductor is established. This constant is called the *inductance* and given the symbol L. Thus the induced voltage is

$$V_{\text{ind}} = L \left(\frac{\text{Incremental change in current}}{\text{Incremental change in time}} \right) \tag{4.32}$$

$$= L \frac{di}{dt}. \tag{4.33}*$$

The proportionality constant L is based on the physical make-up of the device which we shall now call an *inductor*. The number of turns, the closeness of the turns to one another, the diameter of the turns, and the magnetic material that may be near the turns all have an effect on the magnitude of the magnetic field that may develop around the turns of the inductor.

The Impedance of an Inductor

The factors that influence the impedance of the inductor may be determined by means of Eq. (4.33). Assume that a current source of sinusoidal waveform is used to drive the inductor. Figure 4.17(a) shows the waveform of the current flowing through the inductor. By Eq. (4.33) the voltage induced across the inductor is directly proportional to the rate of change of current for a given inductance L (Figure 4.17(b)). If the inductance is increased, the voltage will increase.

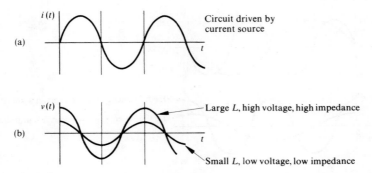

Fig. 4.17. Waveforms of $i(t)$ and $v(t)$ for a circuit with only an inductor and a current source.

When the voltage across a device increases while the current is held constant, the impedance of the device must have increased:

$$V = Z I. \tag{4.5}$$

Note also that in Fig. 4.17(b) the current peaks lag behind the voltage peaks by 90°. This angle is derived from the fact that the voltage wave is proportional to the slope of the current wave. Our model for the inductor impedance must include the following factors:

$$Z = j k L, \tag{4.34}$$

where j indicates the $+90°$ phase angle between current and voltage, k is a proportionality constant, and L is the inductance. The basic unit of inductance is the *henry*.

Figure 4.18 shows the effects of varying the frequency of the applied sinusoidal current. At the higher frequency the slopes at the zero crossings are larger in magnitude than at the lower frequency. Therefore, Eq. (4.33) indicates that the voltage across the inductor is higher at these points. The conclusion is that the rms voltage across the inductor increases when the frequency increases. Again using Eq. (4.5), we find that the impedance of the inductor increases when the frequency increases:

$$V = Z I. \tag{4.5}$$

Combining these various observations, we obtain an equation for the impedance of an inductor:

$$Z_\mathrm{L} = j2\pi f L, \tag{4.35}*$$

where j indicates the $+ 90°$ phase angle between current and voltage, 2π is a proportionality constant, f is the frequency of the voltage across the inductor, and L is the inductance of the inductor.

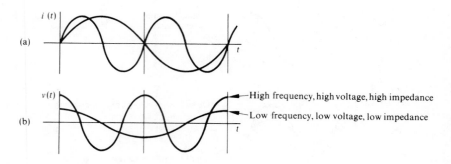

Fig. 4.18. Effect of varying the frequency of current flowing through an inductance (I_{max} = constant).

Another form of this equation is often used when the phase angle between the current through the inductor and the voltage across the inductor is omitted. We then have the *inductive reactance*.

$$X_L = 2\pi f L. \tag{4.36}*$$

A point to remember

The impedance of an inductor is directly proportional to the inductance and to the frequency of the signal across the inductor. The current through an inductor lags behind the voltage across the inductor by 90°.

Example 4.5 Low-pass filter composed of an inductor and a resistor. In the beginning of this section it was said that the inductor's characteristics are the opposite of those of the capacitor. In this example let us investigate an application of inductors and resistors which substantiates this statement. A circuit with a resistor and a capacitor was shown in Figs. 4.13 and 4.14 to be a filter that passed high frequencies and attenuates low frequencies. In a similar way we can show how an inductor may be used with a resistor to make a filter that will pass low frequencies and attenuate high frequencies. This circuit is shown in Fig. 4.19(a). In Fig. 4.19(b) is the generalized form of this circuit showing that this filter is just a voltage divider. Equation (4.16) is again applicable:

$$V_{out} = \left(\frac{1}{1 + Z_1/Z_2} \right) V_s. \tag{4.16}$$

In this example Z_1 is an inductor whose impedance is given by Eq. (4.35), Z_2 is a resistor whose characteristics do not vary with frequency. Substituting these expressions into Eq. (4.16) gives the following:

$$V_{out} = \frac{1}{1 + j2\pi f L/R} V_s. \tag{4.37}$$

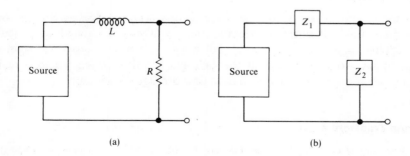

(a)   (b)

Fig. 4.19. Circuit for filtering out high frequencies while passing low frequencies.

From Eq. (4.37) we can see that when the frequency is very large, the denominator becomes very large and the output voltage approaches zero. As the frequency becomes very small, the denominator approaches 1 and the output voltage is essentially equal to the input voltage. The frequency-response characteristic of this circuit is given in Fig. 4.20.

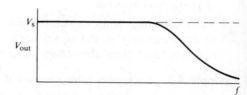

Fig. 4.20. Frequency response characteristic of a low-pass *RL* filter.

4.8 THE TRANSFORMER MODEL

In addition to the resistor, the capacitor, and the inductor, there remains one more component that is commonly used in ac circuits. This component is the *transformer,* and its principle of operation is similar to that of the inductor. In Fig. 4.21 two coils of wire are shown interleaved.

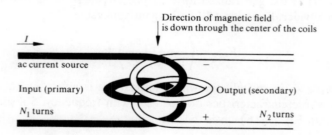

Fig. 4.21. Transformer made by interleaving two wire coils.

Magnetic Coupling

Assume that the coil on the left-hand side is driven by an ideal ac current source. A magnetic field will enclose both coils and it will vary in strength as the current varies. This varying magnetic field will induce a voltage across the right-hand coil with polarities as shown. If the right-hand coil is connected to a resistor, the induced voltage will cause current to flow through the resistor.

Voltage Transformation

The side that is driven by the ac current source is called the *primary* side of the transformer. The other side is called the *secondary* side of the transformer. The voltage induced in the secondary is dependent on the magnetic field strength established by the current in the primary circuit and the number of turns of the secondary encompassed by this magnetic field. The general relation between the input and the output voltages is given in terms of a turns ratio:

$$\frac{\text{Output voltage}}{\text{Input voltage}} = \frac{\text{Number of turns in the secondary, } N_2}{\text{Number of turns in the primary, } N_1}$$

or

$$\frac{V_{out}}{V_{in}} = \frac{N_2}{N_1}. \tag{4.38}*$$

This relation between the voltages and the turns is valid only over a limited range of frequencies. V_{out}/V_{in} will be zero for dc and will approach zero at high frequencies.

If there are more turns on the secondary side than on the primary side, the output voltage will be greater than the input voltage. This type of transformer is called a *step-up transformer*. If there are fewer turns on the secondary side than on the primary side, then the output voltage will be lower than the input voltage and the transformer is called a *step-down transformer*. Thus it is possible to use a transformer to increase or decrease the amplitude of an ac voltage.

Impedance Transformation

A transformer is used for one other important purpose: to transform the magnitude of an impedance. Consider a transformer that is designed to have an output voltage of 10 v when the input voltage is 100 v. The turns ratio in this case is 0.1:

$$\frac{N_2}{N_1} = \frac{V_{out}}{V_{in}} = \frac{10}{100} = 0.1.$$

We want to know the input impedance of the transformer when the secondary is connected to a load resistance of 10 Ω. Figure 4.22 shows the circuit for this example. Several steps are required to determine this impedance. The following questions must be asked:

1. What is the input power to the transformer compared to the output power delivered to the resistor?
2. What is the output voltage at the load?
3. What is the output current at the load?
4. What is the input current to the transformer?
5. What is the input voltage to the transformer?

If we work through the answers to these questions, we will arrive at a general relation between impedances and turns ratios. Starting with the first question, the

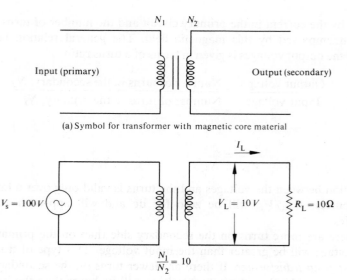

(a) Symbol for transformer with magnetic core material

(b) Circuit diagram for impedance transformation problem

Fig. 4.22.   Transformer used for impedance transformation.

total power output of the transformer can be no more than the power put into the transformer. Actually the output power will be somewhat less than the input power, about 80% to 99%. Recall from Eq. (4.20) that ac power is the rms voltage times the rms current times the cosine of the phase angle. The phase angle between the current through the resistor and the voltage across the resistor is zero. The cosine of zero is 1. Therefore, the power at the secondary is given by Eq. (4.39):

$$\text{Power delivered to the load} = V_{\text{load}} \, I_{\text{load}} \qquad (4.39)$$
$$= (10 \text{ V}) \, (1 \text{ A})$$
$$= 10 \text{ V-A}$$
$$= 10 \text{ W}.$$

If we assume the input power to the transformer to be equal to the output power delivered to the load resistor, the input power is also 10 W (watts). The input power of the transformer is equal to the voltage across the transformer times the current flowing in the primary circuit:

$$\text{Input power of transformer} = V_{\text{primary}} \, I_{\text{primary}}, \qquad (4.40)$$
$$10 \text{ W} = (100 \text{ V}) \, (I_{\text{primary}})$$
$$I_{\text{primary}} = \frac{10 \text{ W}}{100 \text{ V}}$$
$$= 0.1 \text{ A}.$$

Now we can determine the impedance which the ac source drives: the imped-ance of the primary of the transformer is

$$\text{Primary impedance} = \frac{\text{Primary voltage}}{\text{Primary current}} \qquad (4.41)$$
$$= \frac{100 \text{ V}}{0.1 \text{ A}}$$
$$= 1,000 \ \Omega.$$

This is a very significant result. The resistance connected to the secondary is $10 \ \Omega$ but the impedance of the primary of the transformer is $1000 \ \Omega$. Therefore, it is possible not only to vary the voltage with a transformer, but also to vary the impedance that the source may drive. This principle finds wide application when sources of one internal impedance must be connected to loads of vastly different impedances. An example of this application will be given in the problems with solutions at the end of this chapter (problem 4.4).

The relation between the input and the output load impedance is given by Eq. (4.42):

$$\frac{Z_{in}}{Z_{out}} = \frac{V_{in}/I_{in}}{V_{out}/I_{out}}. \qquad (4.42)$$

If the power into the transformer equals the power delivered to the load, then

$$V_{in}I_{in} = V_{out}I_{out}. \qquad (4.43)$$

Equation (4.42) says

$$\frac{Z_{in}}{Z_{out}} = \frac{V_{in}}{V_{out}}\frac{I_{out}}{I_{in}}. \qquad (4.44)$$

Substituting (4.43) into Eq. (4.44) gives

$$\frac{Z_{in}}{Z_{out}} = \frac{V_{in}}{V_{out}}\frac{V_{in}}{V_{out}}. \qquad (4.45)$$

Substituting (4.38) into Eq. (4.45) gives

$$Z_{in} = \left(\frac{N_1}{N_2}\right)^2 Z_{out}. \qquad (4.46)^*$$

This last equation indicates that the input impedance is proportional to the square of the turns ratio. If you know the voltage ratio for the transformer, you can determine the impedance ratio by determining the turns ratio and using Eq. (4.46).

A point to remember

A transformer can be used to step up or step down an ac voltage and it can be used to change the impedance of a load. Its characteristics depend on the frequency of the signals applied at the primary side of the transformer.

4.9 CONCLUSIONS

The questions that were asked at the beginning of this chapter may now be answered in summary form.

1. The rules given for the solution of simple series and parallel dc circuits are directly applicable to ac circuits once the resistance elements in all parts of the circuits have been replaced by impedance elements. Ideal resistors are assumed to be the same in both the ac and the dc circuits.

2. Ohm's law is valid for ac circuits if impedance replaces the resistance used in dc circuits:

$$V = I R \quad \text{for dc circuits,}$$
$$V = I Z \quad \text{for ac circuits.}$$

3. Circuit elements used in ac circuits:

   a) resistors

   b) capacitors

   1. The impedance of the capacitor is inversely proportional to both the capacitance and the frequency.

   2. The phase angle between the current flow through the capacitor and the voltage across the capacitor is 90°. The current peaks lead the voltage peaks by 90°.

   c) Inductors

   1. The impedance of the inductor is directly proportional to both the inductance and the frequency.

   2. The phase angle between the voltage across the inductor and the current flow through the inductor is 90°. The voltage peaks lead the current peaks by 90°.

   d) Transformers

   1. Transformers may be used to increase (step up) or decrease (step down) ac voltages.

   2. Transformers may be used to transform the value of impedances. A given impedance can be increased or decreased by the appropriate choice of turns ratio.

4. Ohm's law for ac circuits and the voltage-divider equation are useful in analyzing the operation of circuits composed of a signal source and a load.

5. The addition of the capacitor and the inductor along with the resistor allows the possibility of developing circuits that are frequency sensitive. Low-pass and high-pass filters may be constructed with these components.

There has been no attempt in this chapter to provide all of the mathematical tools required for numerical solutions for ac circuits. Instead, the approach has been to try to develop an intuitive feeling for the general characteristics of simple ac circuits. An understanding of these concepts is essential if the experimenter is to begin to effectively plan studies involving electrical measurements.

4.10 PROBLEMS WITH SOLUTIONS

The ac concepts discussed in this chapter can be applied to many different experimental situations. The following problems will serve to show how these concepts may be used.

Problem 4.1   A scientist would like to apply a voltage to a douglas fir sapling to learn something about the conduction properties of the sapling. He would like to use both ac voltage and dc voltage not exceeding 60 V. He has a dc-reading voltmeter and an rms-reading voltmeter. What readings should he look for to ensure that the voltage never exceeds 60 V?

The dc voltmeter will give the correct dc voltage but it will not read accurately when the voltage is ac. Since the ac voltmeter will read only the rms value of the voltage, we must convert the maximum value to root-mean-square. Using Eq. (4.6), we get the following:

$$V_{rms} = \frac{\text{maximum value of voltage}}{\sqrt{2}}$$

$$= \frac{60}{\sqrt{2}} = 42.4 \text{ V}. \tag{4.6}$$

This is the largest value of voltage that should be allowed to register on the ac voltmeter when the ac voltage applied to the sapling is measured.

Problem 4.2   In a certain experiment a filter is needed to pass low frequencies and reject or attenuate high frequencies. Only resistors and capacitors are available in the laboratory. What type of circuit could be used?

Recall the circuit shown in Fig 4.13: a high-pass filter made with a resistor and a capacitor. If we refer to Eq. (4.16), we will get a clue:

$$V_{out} = \frac{1}{1 + Z_1/Z_2} V_s. \tag{4.16}$$

At low frequencies we want Z_1/Z_2 to be very small. At high frequencies we want Z_1/Z_2 to be very large, so that V_{out} will be large for low frequencies and small for high frequencies (Fig P4.2s1). With the resistor and the capacitor so located the desired results can be obtained. Substitution of Eq. (4.30) into Eq. (4.16) shows the final result:

$$\frac{V_{out}}{V_{in}} = \frac{1}{1 + R/(-j/2\pi f C)} = \frac{1}{1 - 2\pi f C R/j}.$$

The frequency response for this low-pass filter is shown in Fig. P4.2s2.

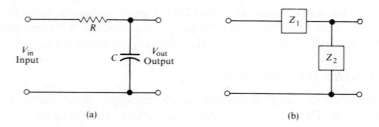

(a)   (b)

Fig. P4.2s1.   Low-pass *RC* filter.

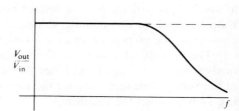

Fig. P4.2s2.   Frequency response curve for low-pass *RC* filter.

Problem 4.3   An experiment requires the use of a high-pass filter. Resistors and inductors are available for use in constructing this filter. What circuit configuration could be used with these components?

Again it will be helpful to refer to Eq. (4.16). At low frequencies we want Z_1/Z_2 to be very large. At high frequencies we want Z_1/Z_2 to be very small. This will result in V_{out} being small for low frequencies and large for high frequencies (Fig. P4.3s1). With the resistor and the inductor in these locations, the desired results can be obtained. Substitution of Eq. (4.35) into Eq. (4.16) shows the final results:

$$\frac{V_{out}}{V_{in}} = \frac{1}{1 + R/j2\pi fL}.$$

The frequency response for this high-pass filter is shown in Fig. P4.3s2.

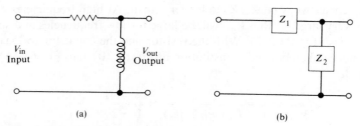

(a)   (b)

Fig. P4.3s1.   High-pass *RL* filter.

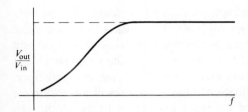

Fig. P4.3s2. Frequency response curve for high-pass *RL* filter.

Problem 4.4 An entomologist wants to record the chirps of crickets. He buys a microphone and an amplifier to drive the recorder. Much to his dismay, his recordings are very unsatisfactory. He tests the individual components and finds them to be operating according to manufacturer's specifications. What may be wrong and what can he do about it?

We must refer to Section 2.5. The microphone can be considered as the source and the amplifier as the load on the microphone. We must know something about the characteristics of the microphone and the amplifier. The microphone is a crystal microphone with an internal impedance of 100 000 Ω. The amplifier has an input impedance of 1000 Ω. The two are connected together as shown in Fig. P4.4s1. This problem is now similar to the voltage-divider problem discussed in Chapter 3 (problem 3.3). Equation (3.45) is now applicable if $R_p = R_A$, $R_1 = R_M$, $V_L = V_{out}$, and $V_b = V_M$:

$$V_L = \frac{R_p}{R_1 + R_p}\, V_b, \tag{3.45}$$

$$V_{out} = \frac{R_A}{R_M + R_A}\, V_M.$$

Substituting the appropriate values into this equation yields the following:

$$V_{out} = \frac{10^3}{10^5 + 10^3}\, V_M = \frac{1}{101}\, V_M.$$

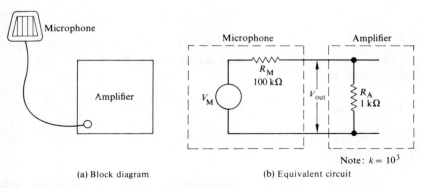

(a) Block diagram   (b) Equivalent circuit

Fig. P4.4s1. Equivalent circuit for the microphone-amplifier problem.

Note that the voltage out of the microphone is approximately one one-hundredth of the voltage generated in the microphone. The cricket does not make a very loud chirp, so the voltage generated in the microphone is very small and when that small voltage is divided by 101 the signal level into the amplifier (V_{out}) is very small indeed. This may be the reason why his recordings are unsatisfactory.

What can be done to improve the situation? One of the uses of a transformer is to transform impedances. The ratio of the input impedance to the output impedance for a transformer is given by Eq. (4.46):

$$Z_{in} = \left(\frac{N_1}{N_2}\right)^2 Z_{out}. \tag{4.46}$$

Maybe we can increase the voltage into the amplifier by using this impedance-transforming characteristic. Let $N_1/N_2 = 10$. Connect a transformer with this turns ratio between the microphone and the amplifier input as shown in Fig. P4.4s2.

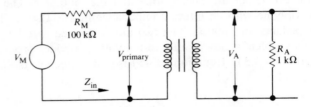

Fig. P4.4s2. Transformer coupling the microphone to the amplifier.

By Eq. (4.46) we find that the impedance into the primary of the transformer is 100 000 Ω:

$$Z_{in} = (10^2)(10^3) = 10^5 \ \Omega.$$

Now,

$$V_L = \frac{R_p}{R_1 + R_p} V_b, \tag{3.45}$$

where $R_p = Z_{in} = 10^5 \ \Omega$, $R_1 = R_M = 10^5 \ \Omega$, $V_b = V_M$. Referring once again to Eq. (3.45) for a voltage divider, we can determine that the voltage at the primary of the transformer is now $V_M/2$:

$$V_{primary} = \frac{Z_{in}}{R_M + Z_{in}} V_M = \frac{10^5}{10^5 + 10^5} V_M = \frac{V_M}{2}.$$

Using Eq. (4.38), we find that the output voltage of the transformer is one-tenth the input voltage to the transformer:

$$\frac{V_{out}}{V_{in}} = \frac{N_2}{N_1}, \tag{4.38}$$

where $V_{out} = V_A$, $V_{in} = V_{primary}$. Combining the last two results shows that the voltage into the amplifier will be

$$V_A = \frac{1}{10}\left(\frac{V_M}{2}\right) = \frac{V_M}{20}$$

when the transformer is placed in the circuit. This represents an increase in voltage delivered to the amplifier by a factor of 5.

We have assumed in the above solution that the transformer is capable of passing the frequencies generated by the cricket. It is possible that the transformer will not pass all of the frequencies of the signal picked up by the microphone. Would it be possible to use a transformer with a different turns ratio to make the voltage delivered to the amplifier even larger?

4.11 REVIEW QUESTIONS AND PROBLEMS

4.1 A waveform of voltage is observed on a display device. It shows that the voltage being measured is a periodic sinusoidal wave with a peak-to-peak voltage of 15 V. Its period is 0.7 sec. What is the rms value of this voltage? What is the frequency of this voltage waveform?

4.2 A periodic sine wave of current has been measured by an rms-reading ammeter. The value read is 4 mA. What is the peak value of the wave?

4.3 A frequency-selective circuit has been designed so it has the characteristics shown in Fig. R4.1. Sketch an approximate shape of the curve of the output voltage V_{out} as a function of frequency.

Fig. R4.1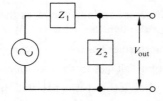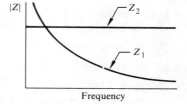

4.4 An ideal ac current source causes a 10-mA rms current to flow through an impedance that varies as Z_1 does in Fig. R4.1. Sketch the approximate shape of the curve of the voltage that will be produced across this impedance as a function of frequency.

4.5 What type of component could have an impedance characteristic similar to that of Z_1 in Fig. R4.1?

4.6 What type of component could have an impedance characteristic similar to that of Z_2 in Fig. R4.1?

4.7 What is the general form of the equation used to determine the total impedance of a series connection of capacitors? of inductors? of a combination of resistors, capacitors, and inductors?

4.8   What is the general form of the equation used to determine the total impedance of a parallel connection of capacitors? of inductors? of a combination of resistors, capacitors, and inductors?

4.9   What is meant by the term "phase angle"?

4.10   In a laboratory, the power line voltage was measured to be 125 V rms and the power line current was measured to be 9 A rms. The phase angle between the current and voltage was measured to be 20°. What is the ac power being delivered by this power line?

4.11   How is electric current related to electric charge?

4.12   Does the ac current flowing through a capacitor lead or lag the voltage across the capacitor? What is the angle between this current and voltage?

4.13   What is the general equation for determining the impedance of a capacitor? Define each of the terms in the equation.

4.14   Sketch a general curve of the amplitude of the impedance of a capacitor as a function of frequency.

4.15   If the ac voltage across a capacitor is held constant, how will the current through the capacitor vary as frequency increases?

4.16   What is the symbol j used for in electric circuit analysis problems?

4.17   What is the equation used to define the impedance of an inductor?

4.18   How is the ac current flowing through an inductor related to the ac voltage across the inductor?

4.19   What is the difference between the terms "impedance" and "reactance"?

4.20   Does the impedance of an inductor increase linearly or nonlinearly as the frequency increases? (If the frequency doubles, does the impedance double?)

4.21   If an ideal ac current is connected across an inductor, does the voltage across the inductor lead or lag the current through the inductor? By what angle?

4.22   Describe in words what action a transformer has in a dc circuit: in an ac circuit.

4.23   In what way are the input and output voltages in a transformer related?

4.24   How is the impedance seen looking into a transformer related to the impedance connected across the output of the transformer? Assume a simplified model of the transformer.

4.25   An ideal voltage source is connected across a series combination of resistors as shown in Fig. R4.2. Calculate the value of power delivered to R_2 as a function of the ratio R_1/R_2. Plot a curve of the results. Is there an optimum value of R_2 for a given value of R_1 if the maximum possible power is to be delivered to R_1 for a given value of source voltage V_s?

4.26   Think of the 10 V battery and the resistor R_1 in Fig. R4.2 as being the source of a voltage signal. This source has an internal resistance R_1. Is there an optimum value of R_2 for any particular value of R_1 that will maximize the power delivered to R_2?

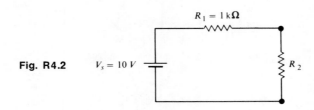

$R_1 = 1 \text{k}\Omega$

Fig. R4.2 $V_s = 10\ V$ R_2

4.27   An ac source has an internal resistance of $2\ \text{k}\Omega$. It is to deliver the maximum power possible to a load resistance of $100\ \Omega$. Assuming that the internal voltage of the source is 20 V, how much power would be delivered to the load if it is connected to the output terminals of the source? What characteristics should a transformer have if it is to be connected between the source and the load so as to maximize the power delivered to the load? Assume a simplified model of the transformer.

5
characteristics of
basic building blocks

5.1 OBJECTIVES

The measurement of electrical signals often requires the use of circuits that will take the signal from the transducer (a component to be discussed in Chapter 6) and perform operations on it so that it can be utilized by display and storage units (to be discussed in Chapter 7). In some cases dc voltages are needed and the signal must be amplified so that it will be large enough to display. In other cases there may be noise present along with the signal and this noise must be filtered out. If the signal is to be transmitted to a distant location, a transmitter must be used. There are electric circuits that are designed to perform these operations and they may be called the basic building blocks for electronic equipment and systems. These building blocks are power supplies, amplifiers, filters, oscillators, and modulators. In a particular application any one of these blocks may be used separately or all of them may be used together.

The discussion that follows will provide an introduction to these widely used building blocks. The intent of the discussion is to alert you to the characteristics that must be considered when setting up a system to measure a particular signal. How specific blocks operate will be briefly discussed, but no attempt will be made to introduce the fundamentals needed to design the circuits. Equipment that will perform these functions may be on hand in the scientist's laboratory and, if not, is available on the market from a large number of suppliers. This chapter should help the readers who need to use these blocks by themselves as well as those who need to understand the operations of the equipment that utilizes all of these blocks.

5.2 POWER SUPPLIES

Electrical instruments require either an ac or a dc source of power. This power may be supplied by the ac power line available in most laboratories, chemical batteries, or some type of solar cell. Regardless of the source of energy to be used by the instrument or system, there are certain characteristics which are desired of a source of power.

1. Capability to adjust the amplitude of the voltage to the value desired.
2. Capability to maintain a specific amplitude of voltage regardless of the current flow from the source (voltage regulation).
3. Capability to maintain a purity of waveform desired whether it be a sine wave or direct current.
4. Capability to protect the power source against short circuits (current limiting).

In many laboratories it is convenient to have power sources that will supply a range of output voltages depending on the particular application. Thus it is necessary to have a control that may be adjusted to set the voltage to the desired value. Once the voltage is set to the desired value, the experimenter does not want it to vary even though the current flowing in the load circuit changes. The figure of merit for this characteristic of maintaining a fixed voltage is defined as

$$\text{Voltage regulation} = \frac{V_{\text{no load}} - V_{\text{rated load}}}{V_{\text{rated load}}} \times 100\%. \qquad (5.1)*$$

The voltage regulation should be as low as possible. Usually it ranges from a high of 50%, which is very poor, to a low of 0.0005%, which is very good.

The power line usually supplies a 60-Hz sine wave voltage. There are times when this waveform may become distorted. The distorted wave is periodic in that its waveshape repeats every cycle of the wave. Such a wave is found to be the sum of a 60-Hz sine wave component plus other sine wave components that are harmonics of the 60-Hz fundamental component. A harmonic of a particular frequency is an integral multiple of the frequency of the fundamental component. The amplitudes of particular harmonics depend on the amount of distortion. For example, in Fig. 5.1 wave 3, which is the distorted periodic wave, is the sum of a 60-Hz wave of peak value 1 and a third-harmonic wave, 180 Hz, of peak value 0.1. Other distorted periodic waves may contain different harmonic components. This distortion may or may not cause problems in the operation of the particular equipment used.

Constant-voltage dc power supplies obtain their energy from ac power sources if they are not powered by batteries. This means that a conversion must be made from a sinusoidal voltage waveform to a constant voltage. This conversion cannot be done perfectly so that the output voltage of the dc power supply will always have some fluctuations, however minor. In Fig. 5.2 the output voltage of the power supply varies by ±0.1 V about an average value of 10 V. There is a 0.2-V fluctuation instead of a constant 10-V output of an ideal dc power supply. The amplitude of these fluctuations in part determines the quality of the power

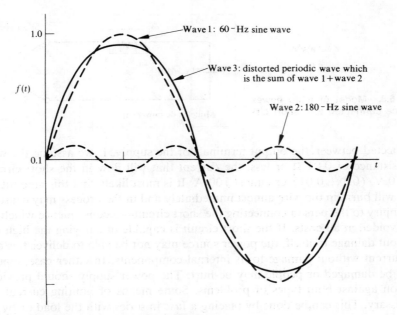

Fig. 5.1. A distorted periodic wave and its components.

supply. These fluctuations are called ripple and may range from 3 V peak to peak for a 300-V dc power supply to 100 μV peak to peak for a precision 100-V dc power supply. In most applications the peak-to-peak fluctuations of the output voltage of the power supply must be kept as small as possible.

All power sources are subject to being *short-circuited*. A short circuit may be defined as a path of almost zero resistance through which current can flow. Since the resistance is almost zero, essentially no voltage can be developed across this short circuit. An *open circuit* is the opposite of a short circuit. The open circuit defines an infinite-resistance path and thus no current can flow through it even though a potential exists across the path. If the internal resistance of the power source is very small, the current that is delivered to the short circuit can be tens or hundreds of amperes for a short period of time. Figure 5.3 shows a 10-V power supply with an internal resistance of 0.1 Ω short-circuited by a wire

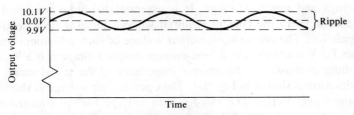

Fig. 5.2. A possible dc power supply output voltage.

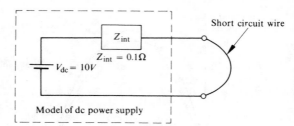

Fig. 5.3. Model of a dc power source connected to a short circuit.

connected between the output terminals of the supply. If we assume the wire has a resistance of 0.01 Ω or less, the current that will flow in the short circuit will be 10 V/(0.1 + 0.01) or almost 100 A. It is most likely that this amount of current will burn up the wire almost immediately and in the process may cause physical injury to the person connecting the short circuit—a consequence which should be avoided at all costs. If the short circuit is capable of carrying the high current without damage to itself, the power source may not be able to deliver this amount of current without damage to its internal components. In either case, equipment may be damaged or people may be hurt. The power supply should provide protection against both types of problems. Some means of limiting current flow is necessary. This can be done by placing a *fuse* in series with the load or by having an internal regulating circuit in the power supply.

ac Power Sources

The 60-Hz ac power line voltage usually ranges from 110 V to 120 V rms. If the regulation of this voltage is not good, it may drop to as low as 90 V or rise to 135 V. Either extreme is not desirable for the proper operation of electrical equipment. Some equipment is designed to perform within specified limits, such as $\pm 10\%$ of 115 V. Other equipment is designed to operate satisfactorily for input voltages of 90 V to 136 V. Still other pieces of equipment have provisions to accommodate several specific input voltages by adjustable taps built into the equipment.

A transformer can be used to change the 60-Hz power line voltage to the value needed by the load. For example, many electron tube heaters require a 6.3-V power source. Standard transformers called filament transformers are available to step the voltage down from 115 V to 6.3 V. Such transformers have voltage ratings and current ratings. It is essential to make sure that a transformer is able to carry the current required without burning up or causing poor voltage regulation. The open-circuit output voltage of such a filament transformer may be 7 to 7.5 V while the rated-load-current output voltage is 6.3 V. This variation in voltage is caused by the internal impedance of the transformer. A model of such a situation is shown in Fig. 5.4. The open-circuit voltage is shown to have a 60-Hz sine wave source. The rated output voltage for the transformer is 6.3 V when the output current is 2 A. In this example the load resistance is 3.15 Ω.

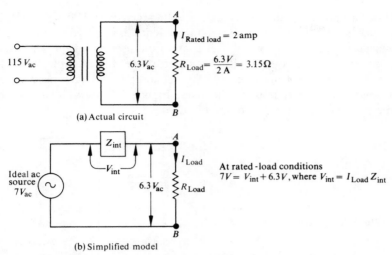

(a) Actual circuit

(b) Simplified model

Fig. 5.4. Model of a nonideal transformer connected to a load.

The voltage across the ideal ac source is 7 V and must equal the voltage across the internal impedance V_{int} plus the voltage across the load. If a load resistance of more than the rated value of 3.15 Ω is connected between points A and B, the current in the circuit will be less than 2 A. Thus the value of V_{int} will decrease, because $V_{int} = I_L Z_{int}$ and Z_{int} is a constant. When V_{int} decreases, a higher percentage of the source voltage appears across the load. [Refer to Eq. (3.45) for the mathematical explanation of this situation.] The important thing to note is the fact that the output voltage across a transformer is dependent on the particular load resistance connected across its output terminals. An ideal transformer is one with zero internal impedance so that its voltage regulation would be zero. There is a wide variety of step-up and step-down transformers that can be purchased to provide the proper voltage for a particular job.

The physical location of a power transformer may be critical in a measuring system used to detect very small voltages. If the transformer does not have a good magnetic shield, and many do not, it is possible to have the magnetic field produced by the current flowing through the transformer couple into the circuit being tested. This means that a 60-Hz related noise will be induced into the measuring system by the magnetic field that is varying at a 60-Hz rate. It is possible for the induced noise to be larger than the signal, thus causing the experiment to fail. This possibility can be reduced by placing the transformer as far away from the detecting circuit as possible and by shielding the transformer from the detecting circuit. (Refer to Chapter 11 for more information on noise problems.)

Some measurement systems require that there be a variable ac power source. This capability can be provided by an *autotransformer.* The autotransformer is made with either a set of taps to be connected to the load or a sliding tap connection.

The set of taps provides specific secondary voltages, such as 100 V, 110 V, 120 V, 130 V, etc., when the primary-side voltage is constant at 115 V ac. The sliding tap connection provides a control that enables the user to set the secondary-side voltage to any desired voltage within a stated range, for example 90 to 130 V. These autotransformers are specified by the output voltages needed and the current that will be required by the load. Figure 5.5 shows diagrams for the two types of autotransformers commonly used.

Fig. 5.5. Autotransformers.

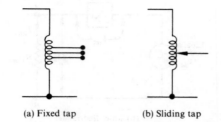

(a) Fixed tap   (b) Sliding tap

dc Power Supplies

The major source of dc voltages are dc power supplies. They differ from batteries in that they obtain energy from an ac power source. The conversion of ac into dc can be accomplished in several different ways depending on the requirements for dc power. Half-wave *rectifiers,* full-wave rectifiers, filtered power supplies, and regulated power supplies are used.

Half-wave rectifier. There are applications where all that is needed is a voltage that is always of one polarity with respect to a reference terminal. Variations in this voltage may not be important. In such applications the half-wave rectifier can be used to provide a fluctuating, unidirectional voltage. The circuit for such a supply is given in Fig. 5.6. The ideal *diode* is a device that acts like a short circuit when the voltage polarity is positive on the left (as shown in the figure) and negative on the right side. It is said to be forward biased with this set of polarities. It will act as an open circuit when it is negative on the left-hand side (as shown in this figure) and positive on the right-hand side. It is said to be reverse biased with this set of polarities. Thus it acts as a switch that opens and closes the path from the transformer to the load resistor.

The characteristic curve for a typical diode is shown in Fig. 5.6(c). The voltage across the diode in the forward biased condition is usually a few tenths of a volt. In the reverse biased condition the current through the diode will be in microampere range. Thus a typical diode only approximates the ideal diode conditions stated above.

Referring to the waveform for $v_s(t)$, we note that when $v_s(t)$ is positive, the diode conducts and current can flow through R_L which produces a $v_L(t)$ voltage that follows the shape of $v_s(t)$. When $v_s(t)$ is negative, the diode is reverse biased

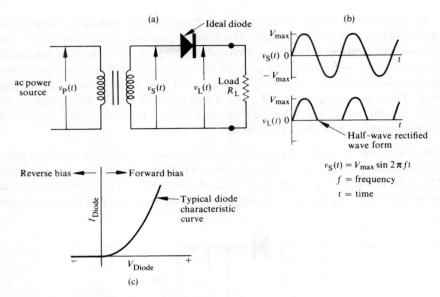

Fig. 5.6. Half-wave rectifier power supply.

and acts like an open circuit. No current can flow and thus no voltage is produced across R_L during this interval of time. This cycle repeats itself during every period of the $v_s(t)$ wave. This particular waveshape across R_L is called a half-wave rectified sine wave. Note that it is a severely distorted sine wave and thus must contain harmonics of the single-frequency $v_s(t)$ wave. This half-wave rectified sine wave contains an average or dc component in addition to the harmonics. The dc component has a value of V_{max}/π. This wave can be represented by the following equation:

$$v_L(t) = V_{max} \left[\frac{1}{\pi} + \frac{1}{2} \sin (2\pi)ft - \frac{2}{3\pi} \cos (2\pi)(2f)t \right.$$

$$\left. - \frac{2}{15\pi} \cos (2\pi)(4f)t - \cdots \right], \tag{5.2}$$

where f is the line frequency, and $2f$ and $4f$ are the second and fourth harmonics, respectively. Thus this wave contains a strong line frequency component plus harmonics of this frequency.

The half-wave rectified sine wave across a load resistor always has the same polarity but varies in amplitude. A pulsating current results in the load resistor. The average value of voltage can be varied by changing the peak or maximum value of voltage V_{max} at the transformer secondary. This may be accomplished by changing the primary-side voltage or by picking a transformer with a different voltage ratio.

In practice an actual diode does not have infinite resistance between its terminals when it is reverse biased. The reverse resistance may range from several thousand ohms to several megohms, depending on the quality of the diode. The transformer will have some internal resistance due to the windings of wire and the diode will have a varying resistance of low value when it is forward biased. These two resistances will cause a voltage drop that is dependent on the current flowing in the secondary circuit: the larger the current, the smaller the voltage available across the load resistor.

Full-wave rectifier.   A full-wave rectifier can be used if half-wave rectifiers prove to be unsatisfactory because there are times when no current flows. Two diodes act as switches which are turned on and off alternately. This operation can be explained by referring to Fig. 5.7. The center of the secondary of the transformer

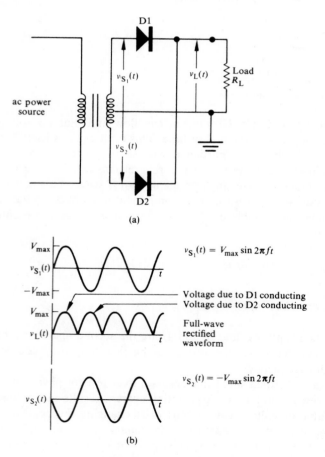

Fig. 5.7.   Full-wave rectifier power supply.

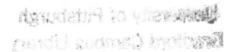

is taken as the reference point for $v_{s_1}(t)$ and $v_{s_2}(t)$. Note that these two waves are the negatives of each other. When $v_{s_1}(t)$ is positive, $v_{s_2}(t)$ is negative, and vice versa. Thus when $v_{s_1}(t)$ is positive, diode D1 is forward biased and acts like a short circuit. During this interval the voltage across the load resistor follows that of $v_{s_1}(t)$. While this is occurring $v_{s_2}(t)$ is negative and is reverse biasing diode D2. This diode thus acts as an open circuit and no current flows through it.

During the next half cycle $v_{s_1}(t)$ is negative and diode D1 is biased to produce an open circuit, while $v_{s_2}(t)$ is positive and diode D2 is forward biased. The voltage across the load resistor follows $v_{s_2}(t)$ during this half cycle. This action causes a positive-going varying voltage every half cycle. This type of *rectification* is called full-wave rectification. The full-wave rectifier output can be described by the following equation. Note that the load voltage does not contain the fundamental frequency component from the source:

$$v_L(t) = V_{max} \left[\frac{2}{\pi} - \frac{4}{3\pi} \cos(2\pi)(2f)t - \frac{4}{15\pi} \cos(2\pi)(4f)t - \cdots \right]. \quad (5.3)$$

The waveform of the load voltage $v_L(t)$ has an average voltage that is twice the half-wave rectifier output. The load voltage does not have a line frequency component if the diodes are identical and the secondary voltages are of the same peak value. However, there is a strong second harmonic of the line frequency in the load voltage. Higher harmonics are also present at the load resistor. These may be objectionable.

Filtered dc power supply. Most measurement applications require a dc power source that does not have the pulsating voltages that the half-wave or full-wave rectifiers produce. These fluctuations of voltage must be filtered out to leave an almost constant voltage. The filter may be relatively simple or it may be complicated and involve electronic control circuits. A simple filtered dc power supply is shown in Fig. 5.8. The filter consists of an inductor and two capacitors. An inductor is a device that opposes rapid change in the current flowing through it. A characteristic of a capacitor is that the voltage across the capacitor cannot change unless the electric charge stored on the capacitor changes. It takes time for this charge to accumulate and to discharge from the capacitor. A combination of these two types of components results in a filtering action that provides a voltage at the output terminals similar to that shown in the figure. This ripple-like voltage is predominately a second harmonic of the power line frequency. This fluctuation in voltage is commonly called the ripple voltage and may be specified by its peak-to-peak value or the rms value of this fluctuation.

The dc component of the output voltage from this power supply will decrease as the load current increases. This decrease is caused by a combination of things, including the transformer resistance, the diode forward resistance, the resistance in the windings of the inductor, and the discharging action of the capacitors. A V_{dc}-vs.-I_L curve is easy to obtain by connecting a dc ammeter and a dc volt-

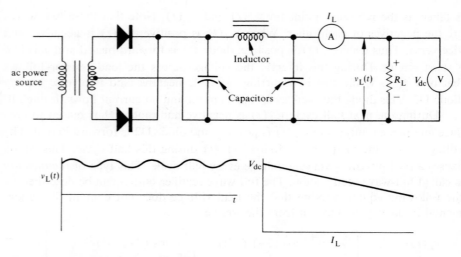

Fig. 5.8.   Filtered full-wave rectifier dc power supply.

meter as shown in Fig. 5.8 and then making measurements as R_L is varied. Once you have this curve, you know how the power supply will perform for any value of dc load current within the ratings of the power supply. Of course, any variation of the power line voltage will cause the dc load voltage to vary. The voltage regulation for this type of dc power supply is not particularly good compared with that of a regulated dc power supply.

Regulated dc power supplies.   The most versatile and stable dc power source is the regulated dc power supply, which can maintain an almost constant output voltage (or current) amid changes in the power line voltage, output load resistance, ambient temperature or time. The block diagram in Fig. 5.9(a) shows the major components of a regulated dc power supply. The voltage is stepped up or stepped down as needed by a transformer. The secondary voltage is rectified and filtered. A variable resistance is placed in series with the load. The resistance of this component in the circuit is increased or decreased depending on the variation of the load voltage. A reference potential is established and the load voltage is compared to this reference. A model for this system of regulation is shown in Fig. 5.9(b) in which a dc circuit consisting of V_b and R_{int} represent the action of the power line, transformer, rectifier, and the filter circuit. As the current I_L drawn from the source increases, the voltage drop across the internal resistance R_{int} increases. This means that there is a lower voltage available at points 1 and 2 than before. If the R_{var} resistance is lowered by an appropriate amount, the voltage across R_{var} will drop. This action counteracts the increase in voltage across R_{int}. Thus the voltage V_L across the load can be maintained almost constant. Of course there must be a slight voltage change across the load so the comparator

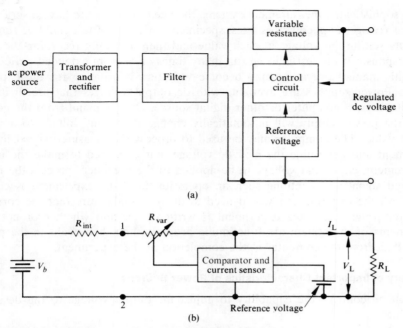

Fig. 5.9. Block diagram of a regulated dc power supply.

circuit can sense the change and control the value of the variable resistance. The opposite action will take place if I_L decreases. This dc load voltage variation may be a few millivolts or a fraction of a millivolt, depending on the quality of the power supply. The regulation circuit also produces filtering action to help reduce the ripple to a peak-to-peak value of approximately $100\mu V$ for precision power supplies.

In many of these dc regulated power supplies there is a current-limiting control that can be set to the maximum amount of current that you want the power supply to deliver to a load regardless of the resistance of the load. In effect, the regulating circuit senses the load current, so that if the current rises above the set limit, the circuit will increase the variable resistor R_{var}. When the load current tries to exceed this maximum allowable current, the output voltage will begin to drop. If a short circuit is connected across the output terminals, the variable resistor will be so set that the voltage across R_{int} and R_{var} equals V_b when the current flow is at maximum allowable value. Thus in the current-limiting mode of operation, the voltage-regulation circuit no longer functions to maintain a constant output voltage.

The control of R_{var} in all of the cases described above is done electronically. This current-limiting feature of the power supply is especially good because it not only protects the circuit connected to the supply but also prevents the possibility of damaging the power supply by exceeding its current delivery capability.

In sophisticated measurement systems the need may arise to have a series of different voltages applied across a test specimen. This type of test could be run by manually setting the voltage at each value and then manually recording the desired response. If the test is to be run many times or over an extended period of time, this manual operation may become very time-consuming for the experimenter. Power supplies are available with dc output voltages that are digitally controllable by a computer or other digital source. On command from the computer, the power supply will automatically change its output voltage to a prescribed value. The computer may be used to process the measured signal in an experiment and determine the next dc voltage that is needed to make the next measurement, cause that voltage to be applied to the specimen, process the new measured signal and continue such an operation until the experiment is completed. All the experimenter would need to do is to make sure that the correct computer program for the experiment is written, ascertain whether or not all components of the system are functioning properly, and then evaluate the processed data from the computer at the completion of the experiment.

Summary of Important Characteristics of Power Sources

1. Voltage control: the capability to adjust the output voltage to the desired value.

2. Voltage regulation: The variation in output voltage with the load current; the numerical value is given by the equation

$$\text{Voltage Regulation} = \frac{V_{\text{no load}} - V_{\text{rated load}}}{V_{\text{rated load}}} \times 100\%.$$

3. ac voltage waveform distortion: the waveshape of the single-frequency ac power source should contain a minimum of harmonic frequency components.

4. dc power supply ripple: ripple is the variation of the output voltage when the load resistance is constant; in most applications this variation should be a small percentage of the dc output voltage.

5. Limitation of current: a capability designed into the power supply so that a specified maximum output current cannot be exceeded when a low load resistance is connected across the power supply output terminals; it is especially convenient if the maximum allowable current can be varied by the operator.

5.3 AMPLIFIERS

An electronic *amplifier* is one of the most important building blocks used in measurement systems. The amplifier is a device that enables an input signal to control power from a source independent of the signal and thus be able to deliver an output that bears some relationship to, and is generally greater than, the input signal. An amplifier may be designed to increase the voltage, current, or the power level of the signal to be amplified. It may include circuits to enhance or minimize certain frequency components in the signal and there may be filters to reduce the noise that combines with the signal.

Amplifiers may be linear or nonlinear. A linear amplifier is one in which the output signal waveshape is exactly the same as the waveshape of the input signal except that it has a larger amplitude. A nonlinear amplifier is one that changes the shape of the signal so that the output signal no longer looks like the input signal, although there may be some relationship between them.

These characteristics are shown in Fig. 5.10. One characteristic of an amplifier can be specified by a curve showing the relation between the input signal voltage and the output signal voltage. The points at which these voltages are measured are shown in part (a). Part (b) shows a specific curve for an amplifier that is operating linearly. The input signal waveform in this example is a sawtooth-shaped wave. When $t = 0$, the input voltage is 0 and thus the output voltage is 0. When $t = 1$, the input voltage is 1 V and the output voltage is 10 V. When the input voltage is 2 V, the output voltage is 20 V. Note the linear relationship between the input and output voltage waves. The output wave is of the same shape as the input wave but is ten times larger in amplitude at corresponding instants of time.

In (c) the curve relating the input voltage and the output voltage is nonlinear. Once again a sawtooth wave is assumed for the input signal voltage. Tracing along point by point through the waveform, we note that the output waveform is of a different shape than the input waveform. Thus distortion of the wave is produced. Usually this distortion is not desirable.

Simplified Model of an Amplifier

The heart of an amplifier is the *vacuum tube* or *transistor,* which controls the flow of current from a power source. A simple model of a one-transistor or one-vacuum-tube amplifier is shown in Fig. 5.11. The transistor or vacuum tube can be thought of as a *control device.* The function of this device is to control the flow of current from the power supply in a way that is related to the input signal. In effect, the control device acts like a variable resistor whose resistance is changed by the amplitude of the input signal current or voltage.

A transistor control device may be described by a set of curves, as in Fig. 5.12(a). In this case the input signal is a current I_{in}. When this current is held constant and the voltage V_{out} across the transistor is varied, the output current I_{out} varies as shown. If the input current is changed to another value and then held constant while V_{out} is varied, a new curve of I_{out} will result. A family of such curves is shown in Fig. 5.12(b). Note that the input current I_{in_1} is less than I_{in_4}. In the case of a transistor the control variable is the input current.

It is possible to show that the resistance of the control device changes de-

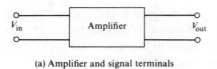

(a) Amplifier and signal terminals

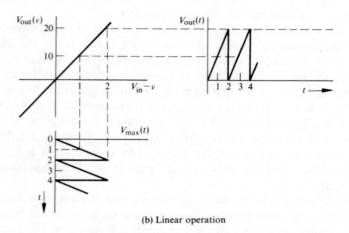

(b) Linear operation

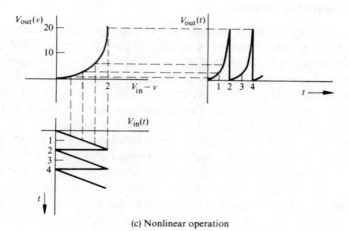

(c) Nonlinear operation

Fig. 5.10. Effects of a linear and a nonlinear amplifier on an input signal.

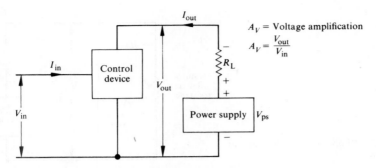

Fig. 5.11.   Simplified model of a single-stage amplifier.

pending on how the device is operated. This resistance equals V_{out}/I_{out}. At point 1 the voltage across the device is large while the current through the device is small. The ratio V_{out}/I_{out} is equal to V_1/I_1 and is relatively large. At point 2 the voltage is low and the current is high. The ratio V_{out}/I_{out} is equal to V_2/I_2 and is relatively small. This means that the resistance of the control device can be changed by changing the input control signal.

The control device is connected in series with the power supply and R_L, as shown in the simplified model of Fig. 5.13. As the resistance of the control device changes, the current flow in this series circuit changes. The smallest value of resistance the control device can have is zero and the largest value it can have is

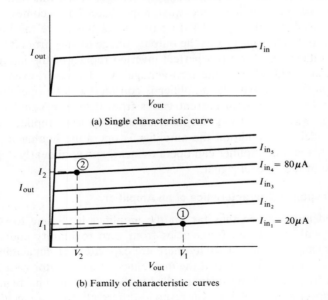

Fig. 5.12.   Output characteristic curves for a transistor.

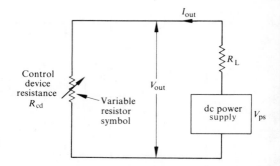

Fig. 5.13. Simplified model of an amplifier.

infinity. Knowing these two limits, we can analyze the series circuit to determine the maximum variation of V_{out} that can be expected. Note that this is just a voltage-divider circuit as was discussed in Section 3.6, where

$$V_{out} = \frac{R_{cd}}{R_L + R_{cd}} V_{ps}. \qquad (3.45)$$

When R_{cd} is zero, the output voltage V_{out} is zero. When R_{cd} is infinite, the output voltage is equal to V_{ps}. Thus there are limits to the output voltage that can be obtained from this circuit. If the control device ranges over these two extremes, the output voltage change is equal to the dc power supply voltage value.

The input signal, no matter how large it is, cannot cause the output voltage variation to be larger than the power supply voltage. When this limit is reached, the amplifier becomes nonlinear and waveshape distortion becomes severe. This type of effect is shown in Fig. 5.14. In part (a) of the figure the input current varies from 0 to 2 mA. This causes the output voltage to vary from 20 V to 10 V. The output voltage waveform is a perfect inverted replica of the input waveform which has been displaced from the zero-voltage axis. However, even though it is displaced from the zero axis, the amplifier is considered to be operating linearly.

In Fig. 5.14(b) the input current varies from 0 to 6 mA and produces an output voltage waveform that is an inverted and distorted replica of the input waveform. Under this condition the amplifier is operating nonlinearly. It is important to note that an amplifier can operate linearly or nonlinearly depending on the amplitude of the control signal.

Frequency Response Characteristics of an Amplifier

The simplified model given thus far for the amplifier leads one to suspect that the amplifier will amplify all frequencies from zero to infinity equally well. A real amplifier cannot do this. Usually there are capacitors or capacitance properties in amplifier circuits. Recall that the impedance of a capacitor is dependent on the particular frequency of the signal applied to the capacitor. This being the case, we should suspect that amplifiers will respond differently to frequencies in widely different ranges.

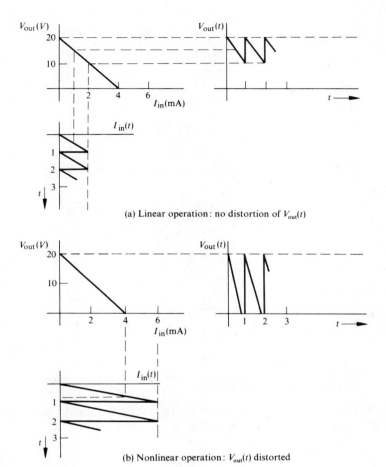

(a) Linear operation: no distortion of $V_{\text{out}}(t)$

(b) Nonlinear operation: $V_{\text{out}}(t)$ distorted

Fig. 5.14.   Linear and nonlinear operations of an amplifier.

A modification to the simplified amplifier model will show how the capacitive effect can affect the operation of an amplifier. Such a modification is shown in Fig. 5.15(a), where a capacitor and resistor are connected in series and placed across the control device. If the input control signal is sinusoidal and the amplifier is operating linearly, V_{cd} will be a sinusoidal wave. In effect, the resistance R_{cd} of the control device is varied sinusoidally by the input control signal. This voltage is directly across the two terminals 1 and 2, where the series combination of C and R is connected. Once again we have a voltage-divider problem. V_{output} is now taken across R and is given by

$$V_{\text{output}}(f) = \frac{R}{Z_c + R}\, V_{\text{cd}}(f),$$

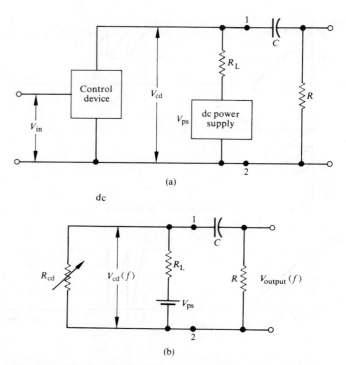

Fig. 5.15. Simplified amplifier model with an *RC* circuit connected across terminals 1 and 2.

where $V_{cd}(f)$ is a varying voltage that is dependent on the input signal and on all of the components in the circuit. Substituting

$$Z_c = \frac{-j}{2\pi fC} \tag{4.30}$$

into the above equation, we get

$$V_{output}(f) = \frac{R}{-j/2\pi fC + R} V_{cd}(f).$$

If the frequency of the signal V_{cd} is zero, that is if there is only a dc voltage, the capacitor has an infinite impedance and V_{output} is zero. As the frequency increases, the impedance of the capacitor decreases and the value of V_{output} increases. The voltage amplification of this amplifier will have a response that depends on the input control signal frequency. Its frequency-response characteristic curve is shown in Fig. 5.16.

An amplifier with a different circuit containing resistors and capacitors could have a frequency-response characteristic curve as shown in Fig. 5.17. At low and high frequencies the amplification of voltage, $A_v = V_{out}/V_{in}$, drops off. This

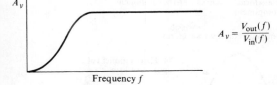

$$A_v = \frac{V_{out}(f)}{V_{in}(f)}$$

Fig. 5.16. Amplifier frequency response characteristic curve.

means that a sinusoidal wave of frequency f_1 will be amplified more than a sinusoidal wave of frequency f_3.

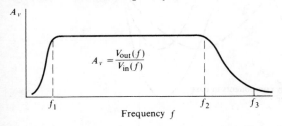

$$A_v = \frac{V_{out}(f)}{V_{in}(f)}$$

Fig. 5.17. Amplifier frequency response characteristic curve.

Often an input signal is the sum of two or more waves. In these cases each frequency component will be amplified and the sum of all of the components will be the output wave. For example, in Fig. 5.18 the input signal is assumed to be a wave which is the sum of a sine wave of peak value 2 V and a second-harmonic component of peak value 2 V. This input waveform is significantly different in shape from a sine wave. Assume that this is the input signal for an amplifier with a characteristic as shown in Fig. 5.17 and that 100 Hz and 200 Hz are both in the range between f_1 and f_2. Each frequency component would be amplified by an equal amount and the waveform of the signal at the output of the amplifier would have exactly the same shape as the input waveform.

Now consider a second case where the input signal waveform of Fig. 5.18(a) is amplified by an amplifier with a different characteristic than that discussed in the previous paragraph. Assume that the 200-Hz component is at f_3 in Fig. 5.17 and the 100-Hz component falls between f_1 and f_2. In this case the 200-Hz signal will receive very little amplification compared to the 100-Hz signal. Figure 5.18(b) shows a possible output waveshape for this condition. Note that the output signal is almost a sinusoidally shaped wave.

If the amplifier is designed to amplify current, it has a current-amplification factor $A_i = I_{out}/I_{in}$ as a function of frequency. The frequency response curve of A_i will give another indication of the performance of the amplifier.

Amplifier Drift and Feedback

The components in an amplifier may change their characteristic with age or be affected by temperature and humidity. As component values change, the amplification may be altered significantly. Such alteration is very undesirable especially in an experiment requiring constant amplification. The amplifier is said to

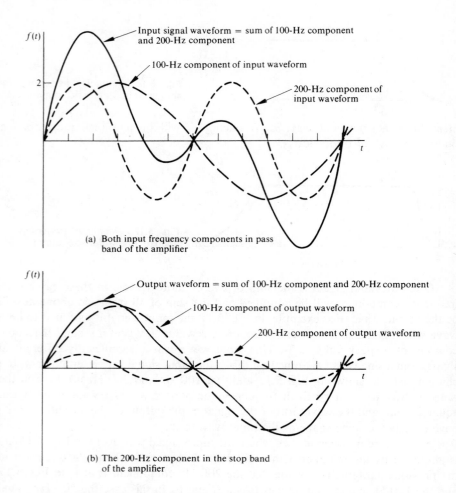

Fig. 5.18. Adding two different sinusoidal waves.

drift when its amplification varies in this way. Drift refers to a gradual shift or change in the output over a period of time due to changing conditions or the aging of circuit components (all other variables being constant). Drift can be reduced by using high-quality components and negative feedback in the amplifier.

Feedback is an operation in which a part of the output signal is fed back into the input and added to the signal being amplified (Fig. 5.19). The feedback signal V_{fb} cancels out part of the source signal V_s. Therefore, V_{in} may be much smaller than V_s. This is negative feedback. The overall amplification is then

$$A = \frac{V_{out}}{V_s} = \frac{1}{B + 1/A_v},$$
(5.4)

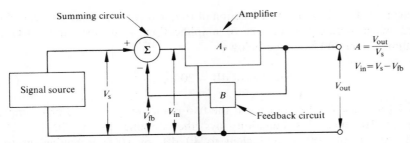

Fig. 5.19. Block diagram of a feedback amplifier.

where $B = V_{fb}/V_{out}$. If A_v is very large, the overall amplification becomes approximately equal to $1/B$. This means that any small variation in the amplification A_v will have essentially no effect on the overall amplification A; the amplification will not vary or drift appreciably. The B factor is usually obtained from a voltage-divider circuit that contains resistors or resistors, capacitors, and inductors. These components are much more stable than transistors or vacuum tubes.

Consider the following example. Assume that an amplifier has a voltage amplification A_v of 10^6 without negative feedback and a voltage amplification A of 1000 is needed in a particular measurement system. By the equation given above, B is 0.001. A feedback circuit is connected to the amplifier to produce a B of 0.001. An overall amplification A of 1000 will result. Assume that with age the voltage amplification A_v decreases by a factor of 10 to 0.1×10^6. According to the above equation, the overall amplification will now drop to 990, which is only a 1% change. In other words, when A_v changes by a factor of 10, the overall amplification only changes by a factor of 0.01. Thus a significant reduction in the variation of overall amplification has been achieved. Negative feedback also decreases distortion significantly.

Selection Criteria for Amplifiers

Certain specific characteristics are sought in amplifiers to be used in measurement systems. These desired characteristics depend on the signal source and the signal to be amplified. Three different types of output signals may be needed from the system: a large signal voltage, a large signal current, or a large signal power. An amplifier that can deliver a large output voltage may not be able to deliver a large output current, or vice versa. An amplifier that can deliver a large output power signal to a low impedance load may not be able to deliver a large output power signal to a high impedance load. The proper amplifier must be chosen depending on the type of function to be amplified. Do you want a current amplifier, a voltage amplifier, or a power amplifier? Specific characteristics to be considered when selecting an amplifier are given below.

Amplification and gain. The amount of amplification required may be a factor of 2, 5, 10, or any number up to 10^6 or more in a particular application. Voltage amplification $A_v = V_{out}/V_{in}$ is a function of frequency. Sometimes the decibel unit is used when stating the amount of amplification. A decibel unit (dB) is a logarithmic function as defined below:

$$\text{Number of dB} = 20 \log_{10}\frac{V_2}{V_1}, \qquad (5.5)*$$

where V_1 and V_2 are the voltages at the two points in question. For example, if $V_{out}/V_{in} = 10$, then this equation says the amplification is 20 log 10 or 20 dB. An A_v of 100 is equivalent to 40 dB, of 1000 is equivalent to 60 dB, of 10^6 is equivalent to 120 dB. Current amplification can also be given in decibels with the aid of this equation by substituting I's for V's.

The power gain of the amplifier is defined to be the ratio of the output power over the input power. It is given in dB by the following equation:

$$\text{Number of dB} = 10 \log_{10}\frac{P_2}{P_1}, \qquad (5.6)*$$

where P_1 and P_2 are the powers at the two points in question.

When the value of A_v or A_i drops to 0.707 times its maximum value, the amplification is said to be 3 dB down. When P_2 drops to one-half of P_1, the power gain is said to be 3 dB down. In any application the amplification at a particular frequency of interest must be large enough to produce a usable output.

Frequency-response characteristics.   An amplifier is not capable of amplifying all frequencies equally, as indicated in Fig. 5.17. Some frequency components in the signal will be amplified more than others. When this happens within the band of frequencies contained in the signal, distortion of the waveshape occurs (Fig. 5.18). It is important to know which frequencies are contained in the signal and to use an amplifier that will equally amplify all of these frequencies so that there will be no waveshape distortion. It is common practice for the manufacturer to state the range of frequencies over which the voltage amplification A_v or the current amplification A_i does not vary by more than 0.293 of its maximum value (3 dB).

Bandwidth.   The *bandwidth* of an amplifier is the range of frequencies within which performance with respect to some characteristic falls between specified limits. For example, the bandwidth of an amplifier may be specified to be 10 kHz between the 3-dB down frequencies. The amplifier with the characteristics shown in Fig. 5.20 has a bandwidth of 10 kHz between the 3-dB down frequency limits of f_1 and f_2.

Input signal level.   The signal level to be amplified must be known in general terms. A particular amplifier is designed to accommodate a specified range of input voltages or currents without producing excessive distortion of the output signal. If the input signal is too small, the amplifier may not have enough amplifi-

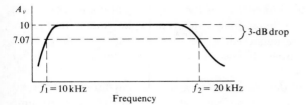

Fig. 5.20. Frequency response characteristic of an amplifier.

cation to provide the level of output signal required of the system. If the input signal exceeds the amplifier rating, either the waveshape of the output signal will be distorted or the amplifier will be damaged or both will occur.

Input impedance.   The input impedance of the amplifier has an effect on the amplitude of the signal that will appear at the input terminals of an amplifier. Reference to Fig. 5.21 will help bring out this important point. The source is shown to be an ideal sinusoidal signal generator, with internal resistance R_{int}, connected to the input of an amplifier. The input circuit of the amplifier is shown to be just a resistor. This is a voltage-divider circuit. As the input impedance (a resistance R_{input} in this case) decreases relative to the internal resistance of the source, the voltage at the input to the amplifier decreases. The largest value of V_{in} will occur when the input resistance of the amplifier is much larger than the internal resistance of the source.

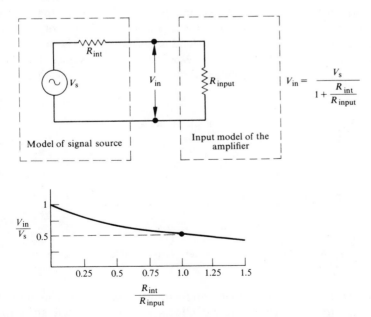

Fig. 5.21.   Simplified model of ac source connected to an amplifier.

Output impedance. The output impedance of the amplifier, in conjunction with the load impedance connected to the amplifier, determines the voltage level, current level, or power that can be delivered to the load without distortion of the signal waveform. The manufacturer will specify the load impedance the amplifier is capable of driving.

The amplifier may be considered as having an input and an output circuit consisting of a source and an output impedance, as shown in Fig. 5.22. Assume that we have the problem of determining the proper value of R_L to use so that the maximum power possible for a given V_{in} will be delivered to the load resistor. Let us assume that the internal impedance is a resistance of 1000 Ω. Then

$$I = \frac{kV_{in}}{Z_{out} + R_L} = \frac{kV_{in}}{1000 + R_L}.$$

The power dissipated in a resistor is given by

$$P = I^2 R$$

so

$$P = \left(\frac{kV_{in}}{1000 + R_L}\right)^2 R_L.$$

This equation can be solved for R_L, and a curve can be plotted for P vs. R_L, as shown in Fig. 5.23. The maximum power delivered to the load resistor occurs when the load resistance equals the output resistance of the amplifier. When these two resistors are equal, the load is said to match the source and maximum power is transferred to the load. When the load resistance and the output resistance are not equal, the amplifier and load are said to be mismatched.

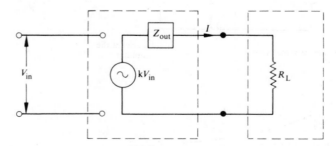

Fig. 5.22. Output circuit model of an amplifier connected to a load resistance.

Distortion. Distortion of the signal being amplified may be very undesirable in a scientific measurement. Two different effects may occur when an amplifier is operating nonlinearly and producing distortion. If a single frequency is being

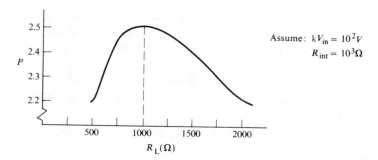

Fig. 5.23. Output power vs. R_L.

amplified and the waveshape is distorted, harmonics of the signal frequency will be produced.

Harmonic distortion is defined in the following way:

$$\text{Distortion factor} = \left(\frac{\text{Sum of the squares of amplitudes of all harmonics}}{\text{Square of amplitude of the fundamental frequency}}\right)^{1/2}. \quad (5.7)*$$

Consider this example. A sine wave input signal is large enough to produce a distorted wave at the output. Measurements indicate that the input signal frequency, the fundamental, is 200 Hz. The amplified signal at the output is measured and found to be made up of the following components.

$10 \sin 2\pi (200)t$ (the fundamental component),
$2 \sin 2\pi (600)t$ (the third harmonic),
$1 \sin 2\pi (800)t$ (the fourth harmonic).

Therefore, the distortion factor is

$$\left(\frac{2^2 + 1^2}{10^2}\right)^{1/2} = 0.223.$$

Intermodulation distortion is another effect that can occur when an amplifier is operating nonlinearly and there are two or more different frequency components in the signal being amplified. When it occurs the output signal will contain frequencies not present in the input signal: harmonics of each input frequency, frequencies equal to the sum of the input frequencies, frequencies equal to the differences between input frequencies, and the input frequencies. Needless to say, these harmonics along with the sum and difference frequencies in the output are not desirable if waveshape is important. They are indications that the amplifier is operating nonlinearly.

Output signal level. The amplifier will be able to produce output signals up to some rated maximum value without producing distortion greater than a specified amount. Beyond that maximum value, the signal will become significantly distorted. As an example, assume that an input signal is 1 mV and is fed into an amplifier with an A_v of 1000 and a rated maximum output of 2 V with less than 0.05% distortion (distortion factor = 0.0005). Under these conditions the output voltage will be 1 V and distortion should be less than 0.05%. If the input signal is increased to 10 mV, the output of A_r times 10 mV will exceed 2 V. This cannot happen without severe distortion.

Noise. All amplifiers generate *noise*. If the signal level is much greater than the noise, the latter will not have very damaging effects. Thus the ratio of the signal to the noise is the important thing. If the signal to be amplified is 1 mV or more, amplifier noise will probably not be too much of a problem. If the signal level is 10 μV, then there is a good chance that the amplifier noise will overshadow the signal unless special filtering or other procedures are used. If the signal to be amplified is less than 1 mV, it will be important to make sure that the amplifier being used generates very little noise. Sometimes an amplifier will come with a specification of equivalent input noise voltage. This value can be compared to the expected input signal voltage. If the equivalent input noise voltage is not much smaller than the input signal voltage, special filtering or processing must be introduced to detect the signal at the output of the amplifier.

Consider an amplifier with an observed output noise voltage of 10 mV rms. The voltage amplification is 40 dB or $A_v = 100$. The signal to be measured is 0.1 mV rms at the input. Will it be possible to detect the signal at the output of the amplifier? The equivalent noise level at the input can be determined by dividing the output noise by the voltage amplification: 10 mV/100 = 0.1 mV. The signal to be amplified will be 0.1 mV at the input to the amplifier. The signal and the noise will be superimposed on each other in the amplifier. Since they have the same rms voltage, the output signal plus noise will have a waveshape significantly different from the signal waveshape (see Fig. 5.24). Therefore, the measurement

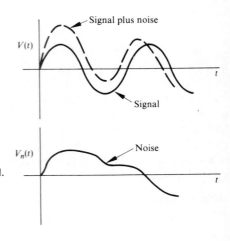

Fig. 5.24. Effects of adding noise to a signal.

will probably be of questionable value. (See Chapter 10 for a more detailed discussion of noise problems.)

Drift. In applications where fixed amplifications are required, the drift·characteristics of amplifiers becomes very important. Drift refers to the change in voltage amplification, current amplification, or power gain during a specified period of time in a particular environment. For example, the drift specification may state that the voltage amplification in the band of frequencies from 100 Hz to 10,000 Hz will vary less than 0.05% in a 24-hour period when operating in a temperature range between 70° and 90°F with a power line voltage varying no more than 10% from 115 V.

Summary of Amplifier Characteristics That Must Be Considered

1. Amplification or gain: adequate to provide useful output?
2. Frequency-response characteristic: flat or varying?
3. Bandwidth: includes the band of frequencies to be amplified?
4. Input signal level: large enough to accept input signal without producing distortion?
5. Input impedance: properly matched to source impedance?
6. Output impedance: properly matched to load impedance?
7. Distortion: does it distort the signal even when the input signal level is not exceeded?
8. Output signal level: large enough to be useful?
9. Noise: noise level due to the amplifier much less than the signal level?
10. Drift: amplification stays constant over the period of time of the experiment?

5.4 FILTERS

An *electric filter* is a filter designed to separate electric waves of different frequencies. A filter introduces relatively small loss to waves in one or more frequency bands in the pass band and relatively large loss to waves of other frequencies in the stop band. This is a very handy building block to have available to a scientist. For example, suppose that in a particular experiment the signal frequency is 2 kHz and the power line current produces a significant amount of 60-Hz noise. This noise causes distortion in the waveshape of the signal. A filter can be used to attenuate (introduce a large loss to) the 60-Hz noise while leaving the 2-kHz signal intact. The output of the filter will contain both the 2-kHz signal and the 60-Hz noise, but the noise will be very small compared to the signal. Thus error in the measurement will be diminished.

There are three major types of filters: low pass, high pass, and band pass. A *transfer function* is used to help describe the characteristics of these filters;

it is the ratio of the output response of a circuit to the input signal to the circuit:

$$\text{Transfer function} = \frac{\text{Output signal voltage as a function of frequency}}{\text{Input signal voltage as a function of frequency}}. \qquad (5.8)*$$

This ratio can be plotted as a function of frequency, as in Fig. 5.25.

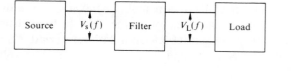

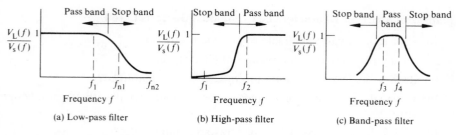

(a) Low-pass filter   (b) High-pass filter   (c) Band-pass filter

Fig. 5.25. Transfer functions for basic filters.

Low-pass Filter

A low-pass filter will pass frequencies from dc up to f_1 (pass band) from the source to the load with very little attenuation. At frequencies above f_1 (stop band) the output signal voltage $V_L(f)$ delivered to the load will drop off as frequency increases. This type of filter is appropriate when the signal falls in the band from dc to f_1 and there are noise frequencies above f_1. If the noise frequency is f_{n1}, the output voltage will contain a significant amount of noise in addition to the signal. If the noise frequency is f_{n2}, the ouput voltage will contain essentially no noise and the signal will be readily observable.

High-pass Filter

The high-pass filter is designed to attenuate all frequency components below f_2 while passing to the load all frequencies above f_2 with little or no attenuation. This is the type of filter to use if the signal being observed is much higher than 60 Hz and the noise is a 60-Hz sine wave induced from the power line into the specimens being tested, i.e., if $f_1 = 60$ Hz and the signal frequency is higher than f_2.

Band-pass Filter

The band-pass filter will pass signals in a band of frequencies from f_3 to f_4 to the load with little or no attenuation. All other frequency components are attenuated.

This type of filter is useful when the noise spread is from dc to much above f_4 and the signal to be measured is in the band from f_3 to f_4. The noise in this band will appear at the load along with the signal, but noise of other frequencies will not be as prominent. The standard AM radio uses a band-pass filter to help select the particular station you want to listen to and reject all of the other stations that are broadcasting at the same time but transmitting at different frequencies.

Tunable Filter

Any one of the three types of filters described above may have provisions for varying the critical frequencies f_1, f_2, f_3, and f_4. This tuning capability can be very handy. As an example, suppose you are searching for a small signal in a relatively narrow band of frequencies that is being generated by a test specimen in the presence of a large amount of noise. The noise is much larger than the signal so that the signal cannot be detected. A tunable band-pass filter can be used to search for the signal. The bandwidth of the filter $f_4 - f_3$ must be as wide as the signal frequency band. The filter will then reject most of the noise. If it is tuned to a frequency outside the signal band, only noise will be detected. If it is tuned to the signal band frequencies, most of the noise will be filtered out and there is a chance that the signal will be larger than the noise in the signal band frequencies.

Selection Criteria for Filters

The performance of a filter in a particular application is dependent on its transfer function characteristics. The criteria for selecting one filter over another filter can be embodied in three questions.

1. Is the pass band of the filter's transfer function flat enough so that all frequency components that are to be passed by the filter are passed without any change in their relative amplitudes?
2. Is the attenuation of frequency components in the stop band sufficient so that these components will not cause problems at the output of the filter?
3. Will the filter characteristics change in an undesirable way when the filter is connected to the source and the load? Will these characteristics change with the load impedance?

The pass-band region of the filter's transfer function curve must be flat if there is to be no waveform distortion of the signal passing through the filter. Reference to Figs. 5.17 and 5.18 will reveal what happens when this curve is not flat. Assume the A_v curve to be a transfer function curve. The degree to which this curve may deviate from a flat curve depends on the amount of signal waveform distortion that can be tolerated and still provide useful results.

The major purpose of the filter is to reduce the amplitude of all the frequency components in the input wave that are not part of the desired signal. The transfer function curve of filters gradually changes between the pass band and the stop band. This means that frequencies near the knee of the curve in the stop band will be passed with almost the same amplitude as frequencies in the pass band. If there is a particularly critical component that must be filtered out (attenuated) in the stop band, it is essential that the filter have a large amount of attenuation at that frequency. Once again Figs. 5.17 and 5.18 will show this effect. Assume that these are transfer function curves. In Fig. 5.17 the frequency f_3 may be considered to be in the stop band of a band-pass filter. This frequency component is attenuated significantly compared to the frequencies between f_1 and f_2. In Fig. 5.18 we see that the 100-Hz component may be considered the desired frequency while the 200-Hz component may be considered the undesired frequency or the noise. The waveform in Fig. 5.18(b) shows that the output wave will look almost like the 100-Hz wave. A relatively small amount of distortion is present in the output wave. The amplitude of the components passing through the stop band that can be tolerated by the experimenter depends on the problem being studied.

Most filters are designed to be driven by a source of a specified output impedance and have a load impedance of a specified value. If either of these impedances change from the specified values, the transfer function between the input of the filter and the output may change. A filter used in one application successfully may not be effective in another application if these impedance factors are not considered.

5.5 SIGNAL SOURCES

Another major building block that is used in many measurement systems is the signal source. This is a piece of equipment that generates a particular waveshape needed to operate or test the item or specimen being investigated. This source may generate a sine wave voltage, a square wave, a ramp, a triangular wave, or a pulse wave. There are other possibilities, but they will not be discussed in this book.

There are five characteristics that must be considered when using any of the sources discussed below.

1. Purity of wave shape
2. Amplitude variation
3. Frequency drift
4. Output impedance
5. Maximum output signal level

All of the signal sources to be discussed generate periodic waves (those which repeat a particular waveshape once every period). The signal is fed into a circuit or specimen which will have some effect on the signal. A modified signal is present at the output of the circuit or specimen which contains some information about the circuit or specimen. It is important that the original source signal does not change its character over the interval of time during which the experiment is being run. Changes that are sensed in the modified wave should be due to the circuit or specimen and not due to the signal source. Thus it is important that the waveshape not be subject to distortion by the source and that it maintain purity of waveshape even though the input impedance of the circuit or specimen may change. Also the amplitude of the wave should not change from one period to the next, and the period of the wave should be constant for a particular setting of the signal source.

The output impedance must be known because that will help determine the signal level that can be produced at the input to the circuit or specimen.

Oscillators

The most common signal source is the sine wave *oscillator*, which generates sinusoidal voltage waves. The oscillator is usually equipped with controls for varying the frequency and amplitude of the oscillations. Frequencies from a fraction of a hertz to 40 gigahertz can be generated. Each oscillator has a specified band of frequencies over which it can be tuned; for example, from 1 Hz to 100 kHz in 5 overlapping bands.

There are many different types of circuits used to generate sine wave voltages. However, they all have the common feature of using positive feedback from the output to the input of an amplifier, as shown in Fig. 5.26. When the oscillator power is turned on, the signal at the output may begin to increase. A portion of this increasing voltage is fed back to the input of the amplifier so that the output will increase still further. The increased output causes a larger input, which in turn causes the output to increase. If this process were to continue without abatement, the output voltage would become infinitely large. This is impossible because of the limitations imposed by the power supply voltage level. The amplifier will cease to operate linearly and eventually a point will be reached when further increases in the voltage at the input can cause no more increases in the output volt-

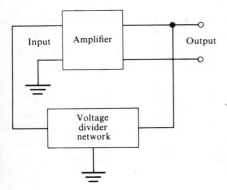

Fig. 5.26. Oscillator consisting of an amplifier with positive feedback.

age. The output will drop off causing the voltage fed back to the input to decrease which in turn will cause the output to decrease even more. This decline of output will continue until the output reaches about zero, and then the process will repeat itself.

If the feedback is positive (reinforcing as described above) and there is sufficient amplification, oscillations will occur at some frequency whether or not the amplifier is designed for this purpose. The particular frequency of oscillations is dependent on the component values in the circuit. Oscillations are not uncommon in amplifiers in which adequate care is not taken to prevent their occurrence.

The oscillator usually has a frequency dial that can be hand set to the desired frequency. This dial may be calibrated linearly or nonlinearly depending on the way the oscillator was designed. The frequency generated at a particular setting will vary somewhat but will usually fall within 1% to 3% of the frequency setting. If greater accuracy than this is required, an electronic frequency counter can be used to measure the actual frequency or a frequency synthesizer source can be used.

There are oscillators designed to be electrically swept through a specified range of frequencies as a function of time (Fig. 5.27). This type of oscillator is called a sweep oscillator. It is a useful source when the frequency response of a circuit or speciman is to be measured. The oscillator will generate a constant amplitude sine wave for all of the frequencies through which it sweeps. The output of the circuit or specimen is observed by noting the variation in amplitudes of the response as the input signal sweeps through the frequencies.

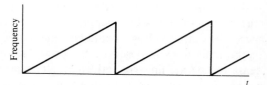

Fig. 5.27. Output frequency vs. time for a sweep oscillator.

The harmonic distortion (see the distortion factor equation in Section 5.3) for the output waveform for typical oscillators used in scientific work ranges from 0.1% to 5%. The amount of distortion is sometimes determined by the impedance of the load that is connected to the oscillator. Occasionally severe distortion occurs for certain combinations of load impedance and settings of the amplitude control on the oscillator. If the waveform is critical, it should be observed with the aid of an oscilloscope.

The output from an oscillator may be connected to the load in one of several ways. There is a power line ground connection to the oscillator through the grounding wire in the power cord. This grounding wire is connected to the metal frame of the oscillator and is brought out to a terminal on the front panel of the oscillator. Through this grounding wire, this terminal can be connected to the ground terminals of any other instrument or component in the measurement system. Problems may arise on account of these ground wires if the system is not set up properly. In Fig. 5.28 the measurement wanted is the voltage across the load resistor. An ac voltmeter, powered by the 60-Hz power line, is connected across the load resistor. This voltmeter reading will be incorrect because the two power cord ground wires will short out the resistor R_1 through the power line ground conductor. Such "hidden" short circuits through the power line ground circuit must be avoided.

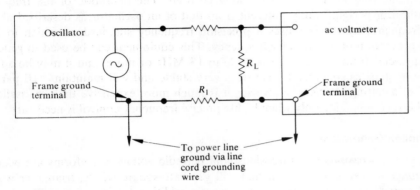

Fig. 5.28. Measurement circuit with a grounding problem.

Some oscillators have what is called a floating output which is not connected directly to the frame ground. If an oscillator with this feature is used in the circuit of Fig. 5.28, the resistor R_1 will not be short-circuited. In other oscillators the impedances between both output terminals and the ground terminal are equal (Fig. 5.29). This type of oscillator is said to have a balanced output. Some oscil-

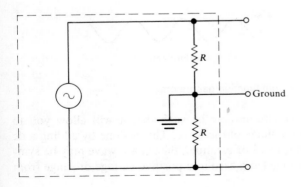

Fig. 5.29. Oscillator with output terminals connected to equal resistors connected to ground.

lators are battery operated. They have the advantage of not being affected by the power line ground and thus are not subject to grounding problems such as illustrated in Fig. 5.28.

Frequency Synthesizer

An oscillator provides moderately good frequency accuracy and relatively small drift from the frequency at which it is set. There are situations where very precise sine wave frequencies are needed and almost no drift can be tolerated. In these situations *frequency synthesizers* may be used. The operation of the frequency synthesizer is significantly different from that of an oscillator as described above. A frequency synthesizer uses a precision frequency standard on which to base the generation of a particular frequency. This equipment can be used to generate frequencies from a fraction of a cycle to 13 MHz or more, and it may be adjustable in steps as small as 0.1 Hz. It is very stable and will maintain ±10 parts in 10^6 of a setting per year. However, it is much more expensive than an oscillator and is recommended only when highly precise frequency control is necessary.

Function Generators

There are occasions when nonsinusoidal periodic voltage waveforms are wanted. A *function generator* is a unit that will generate square waves, triangular waves, and sometimes ramp or sawtooth waves in addition to sine waves. These types of waves are shown in Fig. 5.30. The frequency of these waves may be varied as may their amplitude. There is equipment which can generate these waves from a fraction of a cycle per second up to the megahertz range.

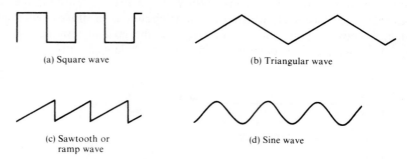

(a) Square wave

(b) Triangular wave

(c) Sawtooth or ramp wave

(d) Sine wave

Fig. 5.30.   Output waveforms from function generators.

The output of a function generator may be such that it will allow you to establish the zero-reference-level voltage of the wave. This is done by adding a dc voltage to a symmetrical square wave. For example, the square wave may be symmetrical about zero voltage or range from zero to a positive voltage or range from zero to a negative voltage, as in Fig. 5.31. Note that the waveforms in (b) and (c) are the same as that in (a) except for a dc voltage component.

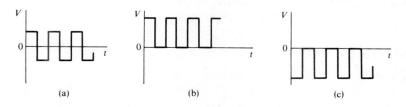

| (a) | (b) | (c) |

Fig. 5.31.   Square waves with different zero-voltage levels.

Pulse Generator

A *pulse generator* is designed to produce rectangularly shaped pulses of relatively narrow width compared to the period of the pulses, as in Fig. 5.32. Both the pulse-repetition rate and the width of the pulse may be varied in addition to the amplitude of the pulse. Generators with a pulse width as small as a fraction of a microsecond are available. Other generators are designed to produce specific sequences of pulses which are then followed by zero output for periods of time before the sequences are repeated. A pulse generator may be used to periodically trigger a set of operations in an experiment. The rate at which the operations are to be triggered can be set by the pulse repetition control on the pulse generator.

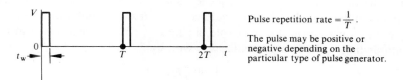

Pulse repetition rate $= \dfrac{1}{T}$.

The pulse may be positive or negative depending on the particular type of pulse generator.

Fig. 5.32.   Output waveform from a pulse generator.

Summary of Signal Source Characteristics That Must Be Considered

1. Waveshape: Is the waveshape of the output signal pure or is it distorted under some load conditions?

2. Amplitude: Is the amplitude of the output signal the same for all periods of the wave?

3. Frequency: Does the frequency of the output signal drift from the desired frequency over a period of time?

4. Output impedance: Is the output impedance large or small and will it appropriately match the load impedance?

5. Output signal level: Can the output signal level be adjusted to as large or as small a value as needed for the experiment?

5.6 MODULATORS

Modulation is the process by which some characteristic of a wave is varied in accordance with a modulating wave. The modulating wave contains the information of interest, such as temperature, position, pressure, voice conversations, etc. *Demodulation* is the process by which that which was done in modulation is undone and the original modulating wave is once again formed. Devices which produce modulation and demodulation are called *modulators* and *demodulators,* respectively. (Demodulators are also called detectors in some cases.)

Modulators are used when it is not possible to transmit an information signal in its original form to the point of its use, as when signals are to be telemetered or combined with other signals and transmitted along a single pair of wires, a *coaxial cable,* or through the air. For example, if the general location of a fish in a river is to be determined, a small transmitter could be fastened to the fish. This transmitter would send a radio signal to the surface of the water and then through the air to be detected by a standard radio receiver. So long as the distances are relatively short, this procedure would work.

In order to more fully understand the effects of modulation on a signal, it will be helpful to note that electrical signals can be described in either of two domains: the time domain or the frequency domain. The time domain is one in which the amplitude of the variable, voltage or current, is some function of time that describes a waveform. For example, a sine wave may be expressed in terms of amplitude that varies in a particular way with time:

$$f(t) = A \sin 2\pi f_1 t,$$

where f_1 is the frequency and t is time. The waveform of this function is called a sinusoidal wave. The same function can also be described by saying that $f(t)$ is a sinusoidally varying function of time with a frequency f_1 and amplitude A. Thus $f(t)$ may be described graphically in each of the two domains, time and frequency, as in Fig. 5.33.

Often the signal contains a continuous band of frequencies, as in Fig. 5.34. A voice wave is a good example. A small child's voice signals have frequencies in a higher-frequency band than an adult male's voice signals.

Two general types of modulation are commonly used: *amplitude modulation* and *frequency modulation*. Amplitude modulation is the process by which the amplitude of a carrier wave is varied as a function of a modulation wave. This is the type of modulation used in standard AM broadcasting stations. Frequency

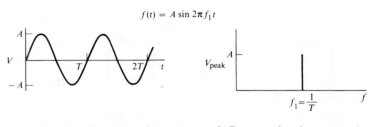

$$f(t) = A \sin 2\pi f_1 t$$

(a) Time domain representation   (b) Frequency domain representation

Fig. 5.33. Time- and frequency-domain representations of a sinusoidal wave.

modulation is the cyclic or random dynamic variation, or both, of instantaneous frequency about a mean or carrier frequency.

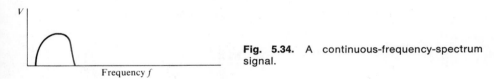

Fig. 5.34. A continuous-frequency-spectrum signal.

Each of these types of modulation may be used to translate the band of frequencies of a signal to another band of frequencies. This is a particularly useful capability when similar sources are generating signals that must be transmitted to a remote location over a common pair of wires or by radio waves.

As an example, consider four different signal sources simultaneously producing frequencies ranging from 100 Hz to 1000 Hz. These signals provide information about the environment in a small remote region of forest. The environmental parameters are temperature, humidity, light intensity, and soil moisture. In each case the particular value of the parameter is automatically measured at the test site and converted to a frequency; for example, a frequency of 100 Hz represents 0°F, 200 Hz represents 20°F, and so forth.

At a particular instant, assume that the four frequencies generated are as shown in Fig. 5.35. These four frequencies are translated into radio frequencies as shown and transmitted to the data-collection point several miles from the test site. Amplitude modulation is used to obtain this frequency translation to shift the signals up to the radio frequency band. It is a characteristic of this type of modulation to produce the sum and difference frequencies shown on either side of each carrier frequency. A specific carrier frequency is used for each signal source and they are labeled f_{c1}, f_{c2}, f_{c3}, and f_{c4}. The four groups of frequencies are transmitted simultaneously to the receiver. This process is called frequency-division multiplexing when sources are combined in this way. The receiver contains a demodulator that translates each of the groups back to their original frequencies so that the

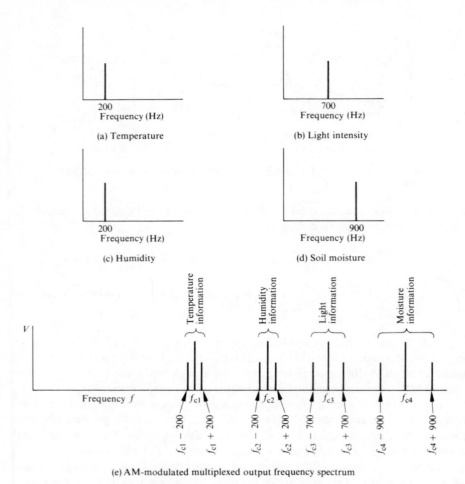

(e) AM-modulated multiplexed output frequency spectrum

Fig. 5.35. Frequency-domain information for the telemetering problem using amplitude modulation.

specific values of temperature, humidity, etc. can be obtained. Frequency modulation could also have been used in this example.

Other types of modulation are also available; the most generally useful ones are listed in Table 5.1.

TABLE 5.1
Useful types of modulation

Type	Major function	Comments
AM (amplitude modulation)	Produces frequency translation	Used in standard AM radio broadcasting and in frequency-division multiplexing; not particularly good in noisy environment unless high power is used; relatively inexpensive to implement
FM (frequency modulation)	Produces frequency translation	Used in standard FM radio broadcasting; reasonably good performance in noisy environment; relatively inexpensive to implement
FSK (frequency shift keying)	Produces discrete values of frequency that are related to discrete signals	Commonly used in binary systems
PSK (phase shift keying)	Produces discrete values of phase angle of a wave; the phase angle is related to discrete signals	Commonly used in binary systems
PCM (pulse code modulation)	Produces coded sequences of pulses that are related to the amplitude of a continuously varying signal.	Used in time-division multiplexing, as in telephone systems; very good performance in noisy environments; relatively expensive to implement

5.7   REVIEW QUESTIONS AND PROBLEMS

5.1   What does the term "voltage regulation" mean? What is the equation that is used to calculate the numerical value of voltage regulation?

5.2   What is meant by the term "short circuit" as compared to the term "open circuit"?

5.3   What is meant by the term "ripple" as related to a power supply output of voltage or current?

5.4   Is it desirable to have a power supply with a high or a low internal resistance?

5.5   What are the differences between dc power sources and ac power sources?

5.6   A precision measuring instrument has been imported from a foreign country.

It is designed to operate on 220 V at 50 to 60 Hz. It requires 18 W of power to operate. How can this instrument be modified so as to operate on 120-V 60-Hz power lines in the laboratory?

5.7   What is the difference between an ordinary transformer and an autotransformer?

5.8   What are the major differences between the outputs of a half-wave rectifier and a full-wave rectifier?

5.9   What are the characteristics of a diode?

5.10   What is the purpose of the filter in a full-wave rectifier?

5.11   What are the desirable characteristics of a regulated dc power supply? Why are they considered desirable?

5.12   What is meant by the term "current limiting" when related to dc power supplies?

5.13   Describe the major differences between a linear amplifier and a nonlinear amplifier?

5.14   What characteristics must a control device have if it is to be used as an amplifier?

5.15   In an amplifier, is it essential that the control device be connected in series with a resistor (or inductor, or capacitor, or transformer) and a power source? Why or why not?

5.16   What can cause waveshape distortion in an amplifier?

5.17   If the frequency response characteristic curve for an amplifier is not flat, what kinds of problems may occur when using the amplifier?

5.18   What are the advantages of having an amplifier that has negative feedback built into it?

5.19   A particular amplifier is said to have a power gain of 30 dB. What does that mean? How does this differ from an amplifier that has a voltage amplification of 30 dB?

5.20   What is meant by the term "bandwidth" of an amplifier?

5.21   If the frequency response of an amplifier is said to be 3 dB down, what does that mean?

5.22   In what way does the input impedance of an amplifier affect the performance of an amplifier when it is connected to a signal source?

5.23   In what way does the output impedance of an amplifier affect the performance of an amplifier when it is connected to a high-impedance load, as compared to a low-impedance load?

5.24   What information does the "distortion factor" of an amplifier provide?

5.25   Under what conditions will noise in an amplifier cause problems? What difficulties arise because of these problems?

5.26   The output noise voltage of an amplifier is measured to be 30 mV rms. The amplifier has a voltage amplification of 60 dB. A sine-wave signal voltage in the range from 0.1 mV rms to 1 mV rms is to be amplified using this amplifier. Will the output noise voltage be large enough to overshadow the output signal voltage?

5.27   What is meant by the term "transfer function"?

5.28   What are the major characteristics of a filter that must be considered when selecting a filter for a particular application?

5.29   What general types of filters are available to be used in scientific work?

5.30   A sine-wave signal source is needed to produce an audio signal for testing the hearing capabilities of a particular animal. This source is to be connected to an amplifier which will drive a loudspeaker. What characteristics of the signal source must be considered along with the characteristics of the amplifier if an effective system is to be set up?

5.31   Two different signal sources are available to do a particular job. Each source will produce an output signal voltage of the desired amplitude and frequency. However, one of the sources has one of its output terminals connected to the power line ground wire and the other source has its two output terminals isolated from the power line ground wire. Under what conditions would one of these sources be better than the other source?

5.32   What differences, if any, exist between the output waveshapes of a sine-wave generator, a function generator, and a pulse generator?

5.33   What is the physical difference between a coaxial cable and an ordinary wire?

5.34   What is the difference between the time and the frequency domain representations of a signal?

5.35   Assume that two different information sources have very similar output signals and that these signals are produced simultaneously. A system to transmit the information to a remote location has been proposed as shown in Fig. R5.1. What functions must be performed in signal processor 1 and in signal processor 2?

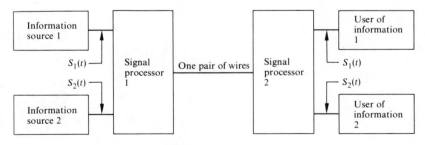

Fig. R5.1

6

transducers
and their application

6.1 OBJECTIVES

There are many experiments in which we want to measure a parameter such as temperature, light intensity, position, humidity, etc. In each of these cases a device called a transducer or sensor is used to produce an electrical signal which is related to the desired parameter. This chapter provides an introduction to some of the transducers that are commonly used in many fields of endeavor. Both passive and active transducers are discussed along with methods of designing simple circuits which can be used to produce the monitored or recorded signal. Characteristics which should be ascertained when searching for an appropriate transducer are stated briefly.

The basic operation of simple series and parallel circuits has been explained. The reader may now want to know how to design relatively elementary measurement circuits. Circuit design examples will be given to show how the transducers can be used to produce electrical signals.

In this chapter we will begin with the definitions of the general terms used in connection with transducers. Then we will take note of the quantities to be measured, discuss the general methods of using transducers, briefly describe specific transducers along with design examples, and finally examine the characteristics to look for when seeking a transducer. Precision measurements require close attention to many little factors. What follows will provide only a background for further study of this important aspect of measurement. The reader is urged to study the references cited to gain a more complete understanding of this subject.

6.2 THE TRANSDUCER

A *transducer* or sensor, as it is sometimes called, is a device which provides a usable output in response to a specified physical quantity, property, or condition which is measured. It is used in a general way, as shown in Fig. 6.1. The *mea-*

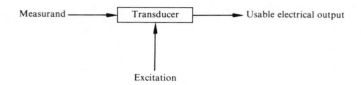

Fig. 6.1.   Input and output terminology.

surand is the physical quantity, property, or condition which is measured. The *excitation* is the external electrical voltage and/or current applied to a transducer for its proper operation. The *output* is the electrical quantity, produced by a transducer, which is a function of the applied measurand.

The transducer has a *transfer function,* which is a mathematical, graphical, or tabular statement of the influence which a system or element has on a signal or action; it is stated in terms of measurements at the input and output terminals. A graphical representation of a transfer function is shown in Fig. 6.2. A transfer function may be either linear or nonlinear, as shown in this figure. Ideally a particular measured value should always produce exactly the same output. Unfortunately, real devices may not work so well. Error will occur even in the absence of vibration, shock, or acceleration. The output may show a band of values when a given measurand value is applied repeatedly, as shown in the figure. If the device is linear, the characteristics of the device will determine the slope of the transfer function curve. If the device is nonlinear, the particular shape of the transfer function curve may be considerably different from the one shown in the figure. The shape of the curve is determined by the properties of the device.

The sensitivity of the transducer is most important. It tells how large an output will be produced for a given change of the measurand. *Sensitivity* is defined to be the ratio of the change in transducer output to the change in measurand. The *threshold value* of the measurand is defined to be the smallest change in the measurand that will result in a measurable change in transducer output. If the measurand becomes smaller than the threshold value for the transducer, no measurable output signal change will be noted.

Consider the following example, which points out the characteristics described above. Information is to be obtained on the reaction of an animal to a flickering light. The particular reaction to be observed is the animal's response to the light by placing his paw on the ground as in walking or running. The number of times the paw touches the ground and the rate at which it is done are to be determined in relation to the flickering. Two different sensing problems must be solved. A measurement must be made to determine the change in light intensity where the animal is located. The measurand in this case is light intensity. As yet what the output should be has not been determined: current, voltage, or something else. Similarly, whether or not excitation is required will not be known until a particular transducer has been chosen. The second problem is to determine

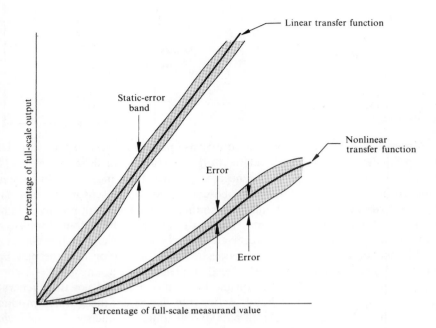

Fig. 6.2.   Output-measurand relation of the transfer function.

when the paw has touched the ground. A pressure transducer may be installed on the paw so that a usable output occurs whenever the animal puts his weight on the paw. The measurand is then the pressure. The output and excitation are also unknown quantities until a specific pressure transducer is chosen.

In this example it may be convenient to have a light-sensing transducer that is a linear function of the light intensity. This device will make it easy to determine the specific light intensity, but it need not be linear if there is a way of calibrating a transfer function scale. To do so, a standard light-intensity measuring instrument is placed alongside the light-sensing transducer and the output of the transducer is calibrated against this standard instrument for light-intensity levels that will occur during the experiment.

One type of light-sensing device that may be used is a photoconductor. This is a device whose resistance changes with the intensity of the light that strikes it. The measurand is the light intensity and the output of the transducer is resistance. If an ohmmeter is available, it is possible to measure the resistance of the photoconductor and calibrate a scale to relate ohms to light intensity. If the photoconductor is used in this way, no excitation has to be applied to the photoconductor besides what is in the ohmmeter. There is a method of producing an output even when an ohmmeter is not available. The photoconductor can be placed in series with a fixed resistor and a voltage source, as shown in Fig. 6.3. The voltage across R_p will change as the light intensity changes R_p.

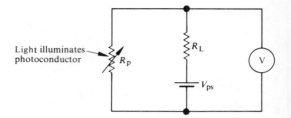

Fig. 6.3. Photoconductor transducer with excitation and an output-sensing voltmeter.

A piezoelectric device may be used to sense pressure in this experiment. The device produces a voltage that is related to the pressure applied to the device. No excitation is required and all that is necessary is a voltage-measuring instrument of appropriate sensitivity. Wires must be connected to the sensor and a means provided to run these wires to a voltmeter so that the animal is not restricted in his movements. A radio transmitter may be used to transmit the output response of the piezoelectric transducer to a receiver. In this case linearity of the output is probably not too important. All that is needed is an indication that the paw has been lifted from the ground and then placed on the ground once again.

Transducers may be classified on the basis of whether or not they generate a voltage in response to a measurand. *Active transducers* are those which produce a voltage without an excitation from an external source of energy. *Passive transducers* are those which are electrically sensitive to the application of a measurand, but they do not produce any voltage; the quantity affected may be resistance, inductance, or capacitance. These quantities can be measured with appropriate circuitry.

6.3   QUANTITIES TO BE MEASURED

There are many different types of experiments in which the information to be obtained is related to one of the following items:

1. Light

2. Temperature

3. Force or pressure

4. Deformation or strain

5. Position or dimension

6. Humidity

The needed measurement may not have to be very exact. For example, maybe all that is needed is to determine whether or not a light intensity is less than or greater than a particular threshold value. How much below or above this threshold may be of no interest. This type of measurement is a go/no-go determination. If the quantity is above the threshold value, a buzzer will be turned on; and if the quantity is below the threshold value, the buzzer will be turned off. A transducer will be needed to produce an output that can be compared to the threshold value.

In many cases it is important to know the specific value of the quantity being measured. The specific temperature in a controlled environment may be needed along with the specific humidity. The specific strain that may exist in a material may be needed along with the position of the item being tested. In each of these situations the relationship between the two quantities involved may be needed for the experiment to provide significant results. The level of error that can be tolerated must be established and appropriate transducers chosen that will safeguard this level of tolerance.

Many different types of transducers can be used to measure variables of interest to the experimenter. The table below gives a partial listing of some of the commonly used transducers and indicates the basic type of measurement for which they can be used.

TABLE 6.1
Measurement and transducer types

Type of measurement	Transducer
	(Passive type: resistance)
Force and deformation of a material	Strain gage
Position and dimension	Linear potentiometer
Light intensity	Photoconductor
Temperature	Thermistor
Force or pressure above a threshold	Microswitch (go/no-go output)
Moisture in air	Humidity sensor
	(Active type)
Light intensity	Photovoltaic cell
Temperature	Thermocouple
Sound	Microphone
Pressure change	Piezoelectric crystal

6.4 USE OF PASSIVE TRANSDUCERS: CONTROL-DEVICE DESIGN METHOD

There are many transducers which do not produce a voltage or current without external excitation. These transducers are called passive devices. Examples of such devices are strain gages, photoconductors, thermistors, and linear potentiometers, the details of which will be given in Section 6.7. If these devices are to be used, some external source of energy must be provided to excite them. Each of the above-named devices utilizes a resistance which varies with the measurand. There are two common ways of detecting change in the transducer resistance. In this section a *control-device* method of designing the detection circuit will be given. In Section 6.5 we will discuss the bridge-circuit method.

A transducer with a variable resistance may be excited as shown in Fig. 6.4. The output voltage can be calculated if the resistance of the device is known for each value of the measurand.

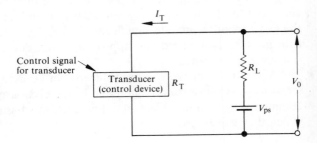

Fig. 6.4. A resistance-type transducer excited by a dc voltage source in series with a resistor. The measurand is the control variable.

The passive type of transducer can be thought of as a control device when it is used in a circuit such as that shown in Fig. 6.4. As the measurand changes and thus changes the resistance of the transducer, the flow of current in the circuit changes. We say that the flow of current through this circuit is controlled by the measurand; i.e., as the resistance of the transducer increases, the output voltage increases. The measurand could be light, strain, temperature, position, or any of a number of other parameters, depending on the particular measurement to be made. We have

$$V_o = \frac{1}{1 + R_L/R_T} V_{ps}, \tag{6.1}$$

where R_L is the load resistance, R_T is the transducer resistance, and V_{ps} is the power supply voltage

The specific characteristics of a transducer are often given in graphical form as a function of the measurand. It is possible to determine the transducer resistance for any value of the measurand on the basis of these characteristic curves. However, this is usually not the easiest method of determining the output voltage for a particular load resistance. There is a graphical method which will provide a good estimate of the performance of a particular transducer with a minimum of effort.

Study the characteristic curves for a photoelectric cell, as shown in Fig. 6.5. A family of curves is given for different light intensity levels. The photoelectric cell operates on the principle of photoemission: as the intensity of the light striking the cell increases, the current that can flow in the cell increases. This device requires the use of an excitation voltage to produce an output voltage. Three questions immediately come to mind when this cell is placed in a circuit, as shown in Fig. 6.4.

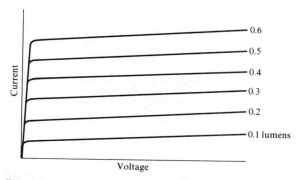

Fig. 6.5. Characteristic curves for a photoelectric cell.

1. What value of power supply voltage V_{ps} should be used?
2. What value of load resistance R_L should be used?
3. What values of output voltage V_o can be expected?

There is a relatively simple procedure for determining the answers to these questions. The procedure is very general and can be used with any device that is described by a set of characteristic curves relating the output voltage, the output current, and the measurand. The choice of a power supply voltage is first. The device, the photoelectric cell in this example, has a maximum voltage rating which must not be exceeded. The power supply voltage should be less than this maximum rating. The largest possible output signal voltage usually occurs when the power supply voltage is near the maximum value. However, a large output signal voltage is not always needed. Therefore, the choice of the power supply voltage may be somewhat arbitrary and depends on the supplies that are available in the laboratory.

The second step in the design procedure is to determine a load resistor value. A load line is drawn on the characteristic curves based on the equation for current flow in this circuit:

$$I = \frac{V_{ps}}{R_T + R_L}. \qquad (6.2)$$

If the transducer resistance happens to be infinite, the current flow through the transducer will be zero (point 1 in Fig. 6.6). If the resistance of the transducer is zero, the current flow will be determined by the supply voltage V_{ps} and the load resistance R_L, so that $I = V_{ps}/R_L$ by Eq. (6.2). This is point 2 in Fig. 6.6. When the transducer resistance equals the load resistance, the current flow through the transducer is exactly half the value at point 2. This can be verified by using Eq. (6.2). The voltage from the vertical axis to V_{ps}, point 1, is the sum of the voltage across the transducer and the voltage across the load resistor. The load line will always be a straight line when linear scales are used. The value of the load

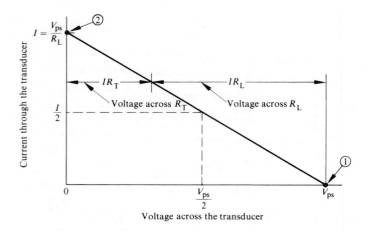

Fig. 6.6.   Construction of a load line.

resistance determines the slope of this straight line. In Fig. 6.7 three different values of load resistance are shown. Note that as the load resistance increases, the load line rotates about point 1 and approaches a horizontal line.

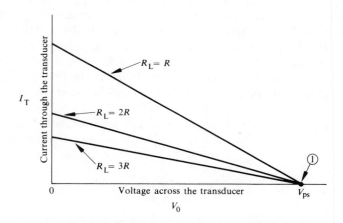

Fig. 6.7.   Change in slope of the load line as the load resistance increases.

The output voltage is the voltage across the transducer and can be found from the characteristic curve with the load line. For example, Fig. 6.8 shows a set of curves for a photoelectric cell that is connected in series with a 2-MΩ load resistor and a 100-V power supply. When the light intensity is 0.1 lumens, the voltage across the transducer is given by the intersection of the load line and the 0.1-lumen curve, which is 80 V.

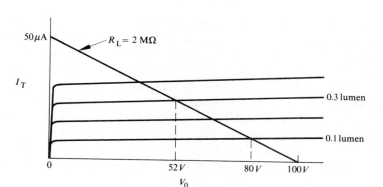

Fig. 6.8. Characteristic curves for a photoelectric cell and an associated load line.

If the light intensity increases to 0.3 lumens, the voltage across the transducer is given by the intersection of the load line and the 0.3-lumen curve, which is 52 V. The output voltage is always given by the intersection of the measurand curve and the load line.

The procedure described above can be used to determine the output voltage of any type of passive transducer for which a set of characteristic curves can be obtained. The specific output voltage obtained for a particular value of the measurand is dependent on the power supply voltage and the load resistance picked by the circuit designer. Usually there is a reasonable range of power supply voltages and load resistances that can be used. Let us look at the curves for a photoconductor and see what happens when different values are used for these variables. Figure 6.9 shows the load resistance being held constant and the power supply voltage being varied. When the power supply has a value of V_{ps1} and the

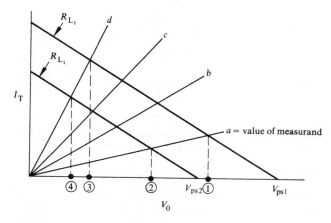

Fig. 6.9. Characteristic curves for a photoconductor and associated power supply and load resistor.

measurand varies from a to d, the output voltage varies from ① to ③. When the power supply voltage is V_{ps2} and the measurement varies from a to d, the output voltage varies from ② to ④. Note that the change from ① to ③ is greater than the change from ② to ④. Thus the choice of power supply voltage will affect the magnitude of the output voltage change.

Another factor must be considered when designing this circuit. Every transducer of the passive type has a maximum-current and a maximum-power dissipation rating. These must not be exceeded if the transducer is to perform well; they establish the boundary conditions within which the transducer must operate. Figure 6.10 shows these boundaries along with two different load lines. The maximum-power-rating curve is plotted by calculating the current that can flow through the device for a particular voltage across the device. Recall that power equals current times voltage: $P = VI$. For the curve, $I = P_{max}/V$. Note that the load resistance R_{L_1} is too small and its load line crosses the maximum-power-dissipation curve. This is not an acceptable load, because if light intensity should be b or c, the transducer would become overheated and damaged. The load line for R_{L_2} falls within the acceptable limits of operation and indicates that R_{L_2} could be used safely.

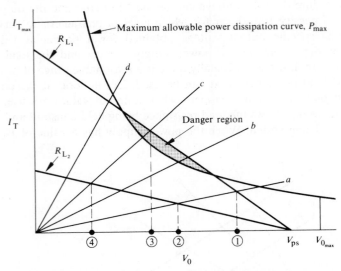

Fig. 6.10. Photoconductor characteristics including maximum allowable limits of current, voltage, and power dissipation.

A point to remember

A wide range of power supply voltages and load resistances can be used unless a specific output voltage is required for a particular value of the measurand.

More examples will be given in Section 6.7 to show how the control method of designing excitation circuits can be done for passive transducers. A second method is introduced in the next section.

6.5   USE OF PASSIVE TRANSDUCERS: BRIDGE-CIRCUIT METHOD

There are many instances in which the variation of the transducer resistance is quite small so that the control-device method discussed in Section 6.4 will be inadequate for detecting changes in the transducer output. More sophisticated circuitry is required, and the most common one is the *Wheatstone bridge* (Fig. 6.11). (The basic bridge circuit will be discussed again in Section 7.6 and in problem 9.6.)

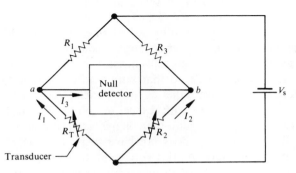

Fig. 6.11.   The Wheatstone bridge circuit used to determine the resistance of a transducer.

In the bridge circuit one of the resistors is the transducer and the other three resistors can be varied so as to produce zero voltage across points a and b, called a null condition, which brings the bridge into balance. Current I_3 will be zero when the bridge is in perfect balance. Then current I_1 is determined by R_T and R_1:

$$I_1 = \frac{V_s}{R_T + R_1}. \tag{6.3}$$

Similarly,

$$I_2 = \frac{V_s}{R_2 + R_3}. \tag{6.4}$$

Also,

$$I_1 R_T = I_2 R_2. \tag{6.5}$$

Combining these equations, we obtain the equation for the transducer resistance:

$$R_T = \frac{R_1}{R_3} R_2. \tag{6.6}$$

Assume that R_2 is the balancing resistor that is adjusted to produce a null response from the *null detector* (a device or circuit that can detect very low voltage or currents). If the three resistors R_1, R_2, and R_3 are known, then R_T can be determined. Precision variable resistors are used in bridge circuits so that minute changes in the transducer resistance can be measured.

If the transducer resistance is to be very accurately determined and if the bridge is to be responsive to very small changes in resistance, extreme care must be taken in the design and construction of the bridge circuit. Errors can result from temperature changes, moisture, thermoelectric-contact potentials caused by dissimilar metal junctions, too high a current flowing through the transducer, and other factors. The details of these kinds of problems are widely publicized and the reader is directed to the references on Wheatstone bridges if more information is required.

The null detector may be a sensitive galvanometer or a sensitive digital voltmeter if the ground of the signal source can be isolated from the ground of the voltmeter. The galvanometer is a current-measuring instrument that has its zero setting at the center of the scale so that both positive and negative values of current flow can be detected. Note that as the balancing resistor is varied, point a may be either positive or negative with respect to point b. When the bridge is out of balance and Eq. (6.6) is not valid, the voltage between points a and b may be quite large and the null detector does not have to be very sensitive during this part of the balancing procedure. As this voltage becomes closer to zero when the balancing resistor is being adjusted properly, the sensitivity of the null detector must be increased. For example, if the voltage V_s is 20 V, the null detector should be set on the ±20-V scale at the beginning of the balancing operation. When the voltage between a and b is about 0.4 V, it will be difficult to determine whether or not there has been a change when the balancing resistor is varied by a small amount. At that time the voltage scale of the null detector should be lowered to approximately ±1 V. As further balancing is done, it may be necessary to change the voltage scale of the null detector to ±0.01 V for a particularly sensitive balance. The scale needed will depend on the accuracy needed in the measurement and the tolerance of the resistor.

6.6   USE OF ACTIVE TRANSDUCERS

Some transducers will produce an electrical signal in response to the measurand and in the absence of any excitation source. They are called active transducers. Microphones and record player pickups are examples. A display or recording device is used with the transducer to present information about the measurand to the experimenter. If the amplitude of the signal generated by the transducer is large enough, a direct connection can be made between the transducer and the display or recording device, as shown in Fig. 6.12.

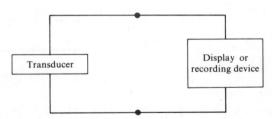

Fig. 6.12. The signal level from the transducer is large so that a direct connection can be made between the active transducer and the display or recording device.

Not all of the active transducers can be connected directly to a display or recording device and produce a large enough signal to make a measurement. Sometimes it is necessary to place some type of coupling circuit or an appropriate amplifier between the transducer and the display or recording device, as shown in Fig. 6.13.

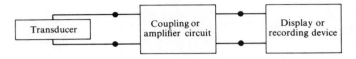

Fig. 6.13. Transducer with coupling circuit to display or record.

In Chapter 2 we discussed the problems of coupling a source to a load. The important thing to remember is that the internal impedance of the source must be known along with the input impedance of the load that is connected to the source. If the source impedance differs significantly from the load impedance, the maximum power that the source is capable of delivering to a load cannot be achieved. This maximum power transfer can be achieved only when the source impedance is equal to the conjugate of the load impedance. (Complex impedances are discussed in Chapter 9.) When the impedances consist only of resistance components, the maximum-power-transfer relationship says that the source resistance must equal the load resistance. The source matches the load. (Refer to Fig. 5.23 for an example of maximum power transfer.)

Consider the example of a microphone that is being used to measure sound in a particular experiment. Assume that the internal impedance of the microphone is 100 kΩ and that a display device has an input impedance of 10 kΩ. Also assume that for a particular sound level the microphone generates an internal voltage of 10 mV and that the microphone is connected directly to the input of the display device, as shown in Fig. 6.14(a). The voltage V_{in} at the input to the display device can be determined by reference to Fig. 6-14(b) and use of Eq. (4.16); it is 0.91 mV. Figure 6.14(c) shows a transformer being used to match the microphone impedance to the display-device input impedance. The impedance looking into the transformer must be 100 kΩ in order to obtain maximum power transfer from the microphone to the display device. If we assume that the transformer is lossless, which may be reasonable for a good transformer, all of

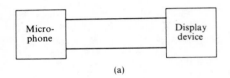

(a)

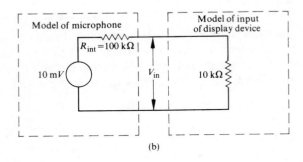

(b)

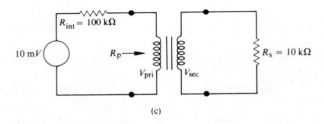

(c)

Fig. 6.14. Microphone connected to a display device.

the power delivered to the input of the transformer is transferred to the input of the display device. The impedance ratio must be 10 for maximum power transfer:

$$\frac{Z_{pri}}{Z_{sec}} = \frac{100 \text{ k}\Omega}{10 \text{ k}\Omega} = 10.$$

Note that all impedances in this example are pure resistances. Refer to Section 4.7 for more information about transformers.

The voltage that will appear at the input to the display device can be calculated as follows:

P_{pri} is the power into the primary of the transformer,

P_{sec} is the power out of the secondary of the transformer,

$P_{pri} = P_{sec}$ under the assumption that the transformer is lossless,

$$P_{pri} = \frac{V_{pri}^2}{R_p},$$

$$P_{sec} = \frac{V_{sec}^2}{R_s},$$

$R_p = R_{int}$ for maximum power transfer.

Then

$$\frac{V_{pri}^2}{R_p} = \frac{V_{sec}^2}{R_s},$$

$$V_{pri} = \frac{10 \text{ mV}}{2} = 5 \text{ mV} \quad \text{when } R_p = R_{int},$$

$$V_{sec} = \sqrt{\frac{(25 \times 10^{-6})\,(10^4)}{10^5}} = 1.58 \text{ mV} = V_{in}.$$

We note that this value of V_{in} obtained with a transformer is larger than the value 0.91 mV which was calculated without the use of the transformer. Thus a transformer can be used to increase the signal level obtained from a transducer.

There are transducers that generate signals too low to be usable even with a transformer. An amplifier must then be used to increase the signal amplitude. Usually the amplifier is most effective when the transducer internal impedance is matched to the amplifier input impedance. If the amplifier has more amplification than is necessary, however, a mismatch between the transducer internal impedance and the amplifier input impedance can be tolerated.

6.7 PASSIVE TRANSDUCERS: RESISTANCE TYPE

Several different types of transducers were introduced in the previous section to show how a circuit could be designed to respond to a transducer output. The main emphasis was to show how a transducer could be used in a circuit. In this section we will look at some specific transducers, listed in Table 6.1, to see what they are capable of measuring. However, as a sidelight, examples will be given to provide the reader with a review of the methods described in the previous two sections. All of the transducers discussed in this section will be of the passive type and the variable controlled by the measurand will be the resistance. For a comprehensive treatment of transducer characteristics the reader is referred to the *ISA Transducer Compendium* [14, 15], which gives detailed information on hundreds of transducers of all types.

Strain Gage: A Resistance-type Transducer

A *strain gage* is a transducer which is used to measure the deformation of a material that has been acted on by a force. The gage is made up of a resistance or semiconductor material. In its normal state, with no force acting on it, it has a nominal value of resistance. In a measurement, the gage is fastened to a material that is being subjected to a force. This force causes a deformation of the material and hence a dimensional change of the gage. As the gage is stretched or compressed, its resistance changes. Thus it acts like a variable resistor. The change in resistance due to this deformation is then recorded or displayed for use by the experimenter. The *gage factor* is a measure of the ratio of the relative change of resistance to the relative change in length of a resistive strain gage.

One type of strain gage is made of a fine wire laid out in a pattern, as shown in Fig. 6.15. The wire is mounted on a flexible backing substance, which is then cemented to the material that is to be deformed by a force. When the material being tested is subjected to a stretching force and becomes deformed, the fine wire in the gage stretches and becomes smaller in cross-sectional area. Resistance is inversely proportional to the cross-sectional area of a wire, so that when the wires are stretched, the resistance of the gage increases. There is a limit to how much the gage can be stretched and still return to its original shape when the strain is removed. This limits the maximum change in gage resistance that can be obtained to approximately 0.1–1% of the nominal gage resistance. Because of this relatively small resistance change, a sensitive measuring circuit is required. The Wheatstone bridge is often used to make this measurement.

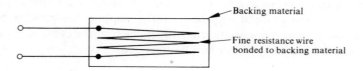

Fig. 6.15.   A wire strain gage.

Example 6.1   Strain gage application.   Consider an experiment in which a diaphragm is used to help measure the air pressure inside an environmental chamber. With any pressure change in the chamber, the diaphragm changes shape. One method of detecting this latter change is to cement a wire strain gage to the surface of the diaphragm. As the diaphragm is deformed, the gage will become stretched or compressed and its resistance will change. This change in resistance can be detected with very sensitive circuits and the information can be recorded for later use.

Assume that a strain gage is available with a nominal resistance of 120 Ω and that this resistance changes at most by ±0.25 Ω with diaphragm deformation. How sensitive must a detecting circuit be if this small change in resistance is to be measured and related to pressure change?

There are at least two different ways of measuring the strain gage resistance. A precision resistance-measuring bridge may be used. Usually this type of bridge must be manually operated and the resistance value read off the dials by the operator. Any temperature change will cause the resistance of the gage to change even when there is no deformation of the diaphragm. This will lead to incorrect readings unless temperature is taken into consideration.

A second method of measuring the resistance is to use a Wheatstone bridge. The temperature problem noted above can be solved by using two strain gages in the bridge, one on the diaphragm and the other located in the same temperature zone but not connected to anything that will become deformed. Both gages will change by the same amount due to temperature differences and their changes will be balanced out by the bridge. This arrangement is shown in Fig 6.16. The nominal resistance of the two strain gages should be the same, 120 Ω in this example. Set R_3 and R_4 also to 120 Ω. When the diaphragm is at its nominal position, the voltages at points a and b will be equal. If the temperature should increase, the resistance of both gages would increase by a like amount and the voltages at points a and b would still be equal; no error would result from temperature changes.

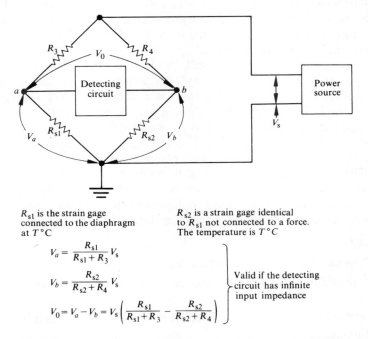

R_{s1} is the strain gage connected to the diaphragm at $T°C$

R_{s2} is a strain gage identical to R_{s1} not connected to a force. The temperature is $T°C$

$$V_a = \frac{R_{s1}}{R_{s1}+R_3} V_s$$

$$V_b = \frac{R_{s2}}{R_{s2}+R_4} V_s$$

$$V_0 = V_a - V_b = V_s\left(\frac{R_{s1}}{R_{s1}+R_3} - \frac{R_{s2}}{R_{s2}+R_4}\right)$$

Valid if the detecting circuit has infinite input impedance

Fig. 6.16. Identical strain gages used to balance out temperature effects.

To determine the sensitivity requirement for the detecting circuit, we must determine the voltage between points a and b. The largest voltage change will correspond to the largest diaphragm deformation. Assume that the gage resistance has changed to 120.25 Ω due to the deformation of the diaphragm. V_a is equal to $+0.50052V_s$ according to the equation in Fig. 6.16. V_b is equal to $0.5V_s$. The voltage at the detector is $0.00052V_s$. If $V_s = 100$ V, the voltage at the detector is 0.52 mV. The detector must be sensitive to voltages in this range. We must be careful, however. If the power supply voltage were to change at the same time as the gage resistance, there would be no way of knowing which effect was responsible for the change in the detector input because V_o is directly proportional to V_s. If V_s does not change and R_3 is varied to bring the detector voltage to zero, $R_{s1} = R_3$ from $R_{s1} = R_{s2} R_3/R_4$. This balancing of the bridge by varying R_3 can be done manually or automatically with a feedback control system.

If a chart recorder is used as the detecting circuit and no balancing of the bridge is done, the full-scale reading of the recorder must be 0.52 mV when the gage resistance is 120.25 Ω and $V_s = 100$ V. When the gage resistance is at the other extreme, 119.75 Ω, V_o will be -0.52 mV. These values were obtained by using the equation in Fig. 6.16. Thus the recorder must have a zero center scale reading. The variation of the power source voltage must be much less than 0.50 mV if accurate readings are to be given by the recorder. It should also be apparent that any action which causes one of the branches of the bridge to change in the range from ± 0.25 Ω will cause errors.

There is another effect that will produce erroneous results. A small electrical potential can be generated by two dissimilar metals being connected together in some circumstances. This effect is called the *thermocouple effect*. In the case of the bridge circuit, the following may happen. If the wires used to connect R_{s1} to the detecting circuit and R_3 are of different materials from those used to connect R_{s2} to the detecting circuit and R_4, an electrical potential may be generated between points *a* and *b*. This potential will throw the bridge out of balance. The bridge must be rebalanced to produce a null condition on the detecting circuit, but this balance will now occur at the wrong value of resistance so that an incorrect value will be given to the unknown resistance. (See the discussion of thermocouples in Section 6.8 for more details.)

Points to remember

1. Changes in strain-gage resistance are very small.

2. Temperature effects can be canceled out if two strain gages are used in a Wheatstone bridge circuit.

3. Very sensitive detecting circuits must be used when measuring changes in strain-gage resistance.

Linear Potentiometer: A Resistance-type Transducer

A *linear potentiometer* is a transducer that is used to measure position. It is a resistor made of a material that has uniform resistance along the full length of the resistor. Connected to the resistor is a movable tap which can be positioned by a mechanical linkage to the physical device whose position is desired. As the physical device moves, the tap moves along the resistor within the limits of the length of the resistor (Fig. 6.17). The resistance between the tap, labeled 1, and one of the terminals, say 2, is linearly related to the distance between the end and the tap. Thus the position of the physical device being measured is linearly

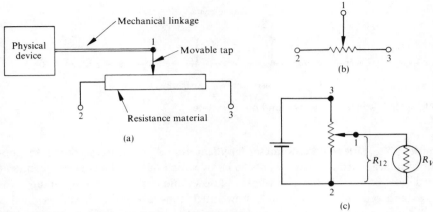

Fig. 6.17. Configuration of a linear potentiometer.

related to the resistance between the tap and one of the terminals. Position can be determined by a resistance measurement between points 1 and 2. If a voltage is applied across the potentiometer, the voltage at the tap (1) may also be linearly related to the position of the tap. When using the voltage method of determining position, the linear relation between voltage at the tap (1) and position depends on the equivalent input resistance R_v of the voltage-measuring device. Note that R_v is in parallel with the resistance between points 1 and 2. Recall that the parallel equivalent resistance for this combination is

$$\frac{R_{12}\,R_v}{R_{12} + R_v},$$

where R_{12} is the resistance between terminals 1 and 2. This is not a linear function of R_{12}. R_v should be much larger (10 to 100 times) than the total resistance of the potentiometer if good linear response is required.

A voltage-measuring device, such as a voltmeter, a chart recorder, or a cathode-ray oscilloscope, can be used to measure this voltage and give an indication of the position of the physical device connected to the tap. The ability to accurately resolve the position of the physical device depends on the type of material used for the resistance medium. If a straight piece of wire of uniform composition is used, the tap will always be in contact with the wire and there will be infinite resolution. If wire is wound around a core such that the tap makes contact with the wire only once every turn, then it will not be possible to detect position on a continuous basis. The electrical analogy of this arrangement is shown in Fig. 6.18. The change in resistance from point to point comes in steps of resistance equal to one turn of wire. Highest resolution will occur when the step resistance is very small.

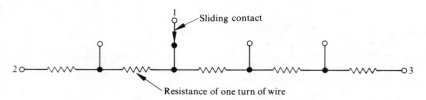

Fig. 6.18.   Model of a wire-wound potentiometer.

Example 6.2   Linear-potentiometer application. A scientist studying the behavior of a large bird in a cage wants to know which part of the cage environment the bird most prefers. In part, he wants to know which part of a perch the bird prefers to stand on and approximately how much time every day it stands on this part. A linear potentiometer can be used to help obtain this information.

A hinged perch that is supported by a spring can be used. The linear potentiometer is connected to the end of the perch, as shown in Fig. 6.19. When the bird stands near the hinge, very little pressure is applied to the spring and the tap on the linear potentiometer is near the top of the resistor. As the bird moves toward the left end of the perch, more pressure is exerted on the spring and the perch moves down causing the tap to move and pick off a lower voltage to be recorded. Position relative to voltage can be calibrated for a bird of a given weight. Some physical damping may be required to keep the perch from moving too much as the bird makes minor movements while standing on a particular part of the perch.

The choice of a particular value of potentiometer resistance is not critical. It should not be so low as to cause excessive current drain from the power source. If loading effects of the chart recorder are to be avoided, the potentiometer resistance should be much lower than the input resistance of the recorder. A compromise between these two factors must be made. The resolution obtainable by this system is dependent on the stability of the power source voltage, the incremental resistance change along the surface of the resistor tapped by the moving contact, and the smoothness of the operation of the perch.

Photoconductor: A Resistance-type Transducer

A *photoconductor* is a transducer that is used to measure light intensity. It is a resistor made of a semiconductor material that is sensitive to light intensity. In the absence of light the photoconductor has nominal value of resistance. As light intensity increases, the conduction properties of the semiconductor increase and the resistance of the photoconductor decreases. The resistance change may not be a linear function of the incident illumination in footcandles. The semiconductor materials used can be made to be sensitive to different wavelengths of light. It is important to know the particular wavelength of light to be measured so that an

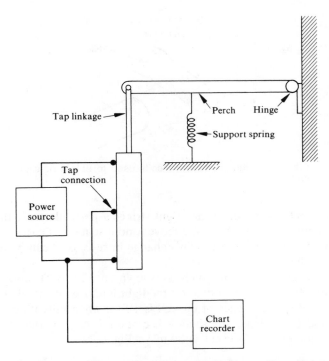

Fig. 6.19. System indicating perch position with a linear
potentiometer.

appropriate photoconductor can be used. The rate at which the light intensity
fluctuates must also be taken into consideration when picking an appropriate
photoconductor. Photoconductors do not respond instantaneously to changes in
light intensity.

The photoconductor resistance can be measured directly to provide an indication of the incident light intensity. A photoconductor can be excited with an
external source of power, as described in Section 6.4, and a voltage measurement
can be taken to provide an indication of incident light intensity. When external
excitation is used, care must be taken to ensure that the maximum-power-dissipation rating of the photoconductor transducer is not exceeded. The resistance of
this type of transducer is dependent on temperature as well as on light, so that
changes in ambient temperature, as well as temperature changes due to power
dissipated by the device, will affect the performance of the transducer.

Example 6.3   Photoconductor application.   A study is to be made of the physiological tremor of a person's finger. The rate at which the finger moves as well as
the total excursions of the finger are to be determined.

One method of obtaining the data is to use a light source in conjunction with
a photoconductor, as shown in Fig. 6.20. A set of very narrow photoconductive

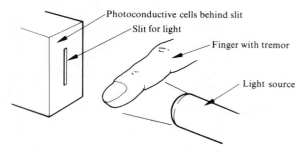

Fig. 6.20. Photoconductive cells used to obtain data on finger tremor.

cells is located behind the slit. When light strikes a particular cell, the resistance of the cell becomes low. As the finger moves and a shadow is cast on the cell, the resistance of the cell will increase. This change in resistance can be detected and the location of the shadow identified.

A signal-detection scheme such as shown in Fig. 6.21 may be used to produce an output that is dependent on the light intensity at the photoconductive cell. Assume that the resistance of the cell is 100 Ω when fully illuminated by the light source and 1 kΩ when a full shadow is cast on it. Assume that the maximum-power-dissipation rating of the cell is 50 mW (Fig. 6.22).

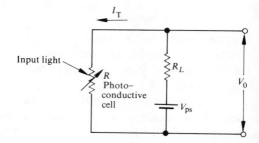

Fig. 6.21. Detecting circuit for one of the photoconductive cells.

The choice of the load resistance may be somewhat arbitrary, so that two different values are given to serve as examples. If the load resistance R_L is 1 kΩ, the voltage V_o will vary from V_a to V_c when the cell lighting changes from full illumination to full shadow. If the load resistance is 0.25 kΩ, the voltage V_o will vary from V_b to V_d, exceeding the maximum-power-dissipation rating. The voltage variation obtained with the 1-kΩ load may be adequate, depending on the particular type of detector circuit used. The *time constant* for the photoconductors must be small enough to allow the output to follow the movements of the finger.

One method of obtaining the rate information required is to feed the voltage V_o into an analog computer and let the computer calculate the rate at which this voltage varies. This can be done simultaneously for each of the cells, and the

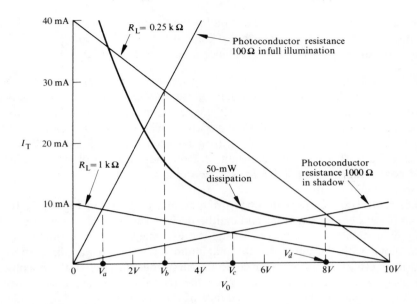

Fig. 6.22. Characteristic curves for photoconductive cell: two load resistor lines and the maximum-power-dissipation line.

rate can be plotted on a chart recorder to be studied at a later date. Maximum excursions can be determined by noting the outputs of the various cells.

A second method of obtaining the required information is to feed the voltage V_o into an *analog-to-digital converter* and then take the digital data obtained from the converter and process them with a digital computer. It is possible to store the digital information for later recall as well as to calculate the rates and excursions required.

Thermistor: A Resistance-type Transducer

A *thermistor* is a transducer used to measure temperature. It is constructed of materials whose conduction properties are temperature sensitive. As the temperature varies, the resistance of the thermistor changes. This resistance change can be sensed directly with a resistance-measuring device or by exciting it with an external source of power and measuring a voltage across the device as described in Section 6.4. If external excitation is used, power will be dissipated by the thermistor due to this source and a temperature rise will result. This will produce measurement errors unless corrections are made or the excitation current is kept low enough so that no appreciable heating takes place in the thermistor due to the excitation.

There is a maximum rate at which a thermistor will follow temperature changes. A thermistor of small mass is required for measurements of high rates of change of temperature. The time constant for the thermistor must be known before we can determine whether or not a particular thermistor will do an accurate job of producing an output change in resistance following temperature change.

Example 6.4   Thermistor application.   A growth chamber has been set up with a temperature-cycling system to simulate normal daily temperature fluctuations. The project leader would like to install several temperature monitors in various parts of the chamber to record the temperatures. The temperature range is 20°C to 50°C. A thermistor is available with a resistance of 14.5 kΩ at 50°C and 100 kΩ at 20°C. It has a time constant of 2 seconds and can dissipate 0.7 mW. A 9-V power supply is available as is a recording voltmeter. What value of load resistance should be used?

The thermistor temperature-measuring system is shown in Fig. 6.23. It is a very simple system to construct and can be designed in accordance with the discussion in Section 6.4. The curves for the two extreme values of resistance can be drawn, along with the curve for the maximum allowable power dissipation, as shown in Fig. 6.24. The load resistance R_L curve must fall below the maximum-allowable-power-dissipation curve. When the recording voltmeter is connected across the thermistor, the input impedance of the voltmeter must be considered. If this impedance is very large compared to R_L and the thermistor resistance, the effects of the voltmeter can be neglected, as is done in Fig. 6.24. From the curves in Fig. 6.24 it can be seen that V_o varies from 6.9 V to 3 V when the temperature varies from 20°C to 50°C.

Although the voltmeter input impedance has been neglected, it may nevertheless produce a drastic change in the readings if it is comparable to the thermistor resistance. Consider the situation where the voltmeter has an input resistance of 10 kΩ. Note that the voltmeter is directly in parallel with the thermistor. At 20°C the parallel combination of these two resistances is 9.1 kΩ, while at 50°C the parallel combination is 5.93 kΩ. Thus the voltmeter input resistance overshadows most of the change in thermistor resistance over this temperature change (Fig. 6.25).

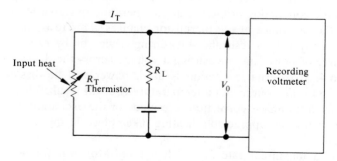

Fig. 6.23.   Thermistor temperature-measuring system.

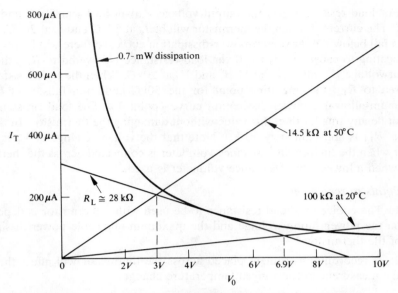

Fig. 6.24. Curves for the thermistor temperature-measuring system.

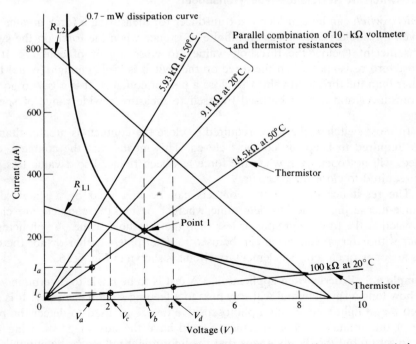

Fig. 6.25. Loading effects caused by voltmeter input resistance connected in parallel with the thermistor.

For load resistance R_{L1} the output voltage V_o will be V_a at 50°C and V_c at 20°C. The current through the thermistor will be I_a at 50°C and I_c at 20°C. These points fall below the maximum-power-dissipation curve, so there will be no excessive heating to cause problems. If the load resistance is lowered to R_{L2}, then the output voltage V_o will be V_b at 50°C and V_d at 20°C. When the load resistance is lowered to R_{L2}, the operating point for the 50°C condition falls right on the maximum-allowable-power-dissipation curve (point 1). The load resistance R_L cannot be any smaller than this value without damaging the thermistor. In this example, R_{L1} is approximately 30 kΩ. Note that the voltage change of V_o is much larger when the high-input-resistance voltmeter is connected across the thermistor than when a lower-input-resistance voltmeter is used.

Points to remember

1. The choice of a load resistance to be used with a thermistor is dependent on the power supply voltage and the maximum allowable power dissipation of the thermistor.

2. A recording instrument placed across the thermistor will affect the voltage measurement for a given temperature change.

Microswitch: A Resistance-type Transducer

A *microswitch* can be considered a transducer for measuring a force greater than a given threshold value. It has an infinite resistance when the force on the switch is insufficient (below the threshold value) to close a pair of contacts. It has almost zero resistance when the force on the switch is large enough (equal to or greater than the threshold value) to close a pair of contacts. It is a go/no-go type of transducer and cannot be used by itself to measure a wide range of specific forces.

In most switches, the force required to close the contacts is greater than the force required to keep the contacts closed. This means that the contacts, once closed, will not open even when the force has been reduced to a value less than that required to close the contacts.

The resistance between the contacts can be measured by a standard resistance-measuring device to determine whether or not the contacts are closed and whether the force is greater or less than the threshold value. A voltmeter together with external excitation can be used to determine whether or not the contacts are open or closed. An elementary circuit is shown in Fig. 6.26.

Example 6.5   Microswitch application.   A test is to be made to determine when and how long a small animal will stay next to a feeding station each day. It is suggested that a light source and a photosensitive device be used to detect the presence of the animal. This arrangement would have the advantage of being very easy to set up but the disadvantage that the light might influence the animal's behavior. A second method involves building a platform adjacent to the feeding

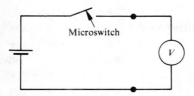

Fig. 6.26. Detecting the open or closed condition of a microswitch.

area and supporting it on a microswitch, as shown in Fig. 6.27. A microswitch is available that has the following specifications. A 6-oz. force is required to close the contacts. Once closed, the contacts will remain closed until the force on the switch actuating button becomes less than 2 oz. The actuating button for the switch moves $\frac{1}{32}''$ between the on and off positions. Will this switch be acceptable?

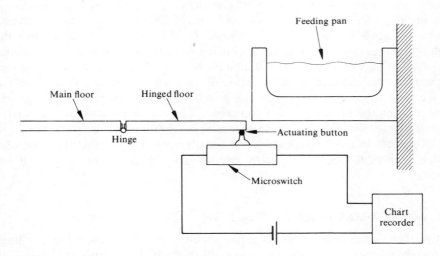

Fig. 6.27. Microswitch application to determine the presence of an animal at a feeding station.

To answer this question, it will be necessary to consider the mechanical aspects of this problem. When there is no animal on the pivoted section of the floor, the weight of this section will be supported equally by the hinge and the microswitch. After the switch has been closed, it will remain closed until the force is less than 2 oz. Therefore, the force that the floor exerts on the microswitch must be less than 2 oz. without the animal. Assume that this section of floor weighs $3\frac{1}{2}$ oz., thus exerting a force of $1\frac{3}{4}$ oz. on the microswitch. The spring in the microswitch will lift the floor, open the contacts, and shut off the voltage to the chart recorder.

When the animal is on the pivoted section of the floor, the combined weight of the floor and the animal must produce a force on the switch-actuating button in excess of 6 oz. As the animal first steps on the floor next to the hinge, little force change will be experienced at the microswitch. As the animal moves to the feeding pan, more force will be exerted on the microswitch-actuating button. The minimum weight of the animal required to operate the microswitch will depend on how the weight is distributed over the length of the animal. If all the weight of the animal could be concentrated directly over the actuating button, the minimum animal weight would be 4¼ oz. plus. A concentrated weight at this point is not possible, so that the minimum weight of the animal must be greater than this amount.

Humidity Sensor: A Resistance-type Transducer

A *humidity sensor* is used to detect the moisture in the air. One type of humidity sensor uses a material that changes its conduction properties with the absorption of moisture. This material is placed between conductors of very low resistance. As the moisture is absorbed in the material, the conducting path through the material between the low-resistance conductors will increase and the resistance between the two terminals of the humidity sensor will decrease. This resistance change can be detected with a standard resistance-measuring device, or the device may be excited externally and a voltage measurement taken to get an indication of the humidity. Care must be taken not to pass too much current through the sensor, because that would cause self-heating and dry the sensor.

Response to change in humidity is usually very slow, so that this type of a device is prone to error. It is useful only when a high degree of accuracy is not required.

6.8   ACTIVE TRANSDUCERS

Active transducers require no excitation, being capable of generating a voltage or current whenever a measurand is applied to them. The transducers discussed in this section are only a few of the many different types that are available.

Photovoltaic Cell: An Active-type Transducer

A *photovoltaic cell* is a transducer used to measure the intensity of light. It is constructed of a material capable of generating a voltage when light strikes its surface. This voltage may not be a linear function of light intensity, but with appropriate calibration the relation between light intensity and voltage across the cell can be determined.

If a resistor is connected across the terminals of the photovoltaic cell, current will flow in the circuit. The amount of current flow is dependent on the light intensity, the surface area of the cell, the material used in the cell, and the temperature of the cell. A current-sensing device or a voltage-sensing device may be used to detect the output of the photovoltaic cell.

Example 6.6   Photovoltaic-cell application.   Light intensity is to be tested. When it is greater than a specified threshold value, an elapsed-time recorder is to be turned on. When it is less than this threshold value, the recorder is to be turned off.

A photovoltaic cell is to be used to sense the light intensity and a threshold detector will turn on the elapsed-time recorder, as shown in Fig. 6.28. The photovoltaic cell available has a set of characteristic curves as shown in Fig. 6.29. The first step in designing the circuit is to work with the characteristic curves of the cell and the load resistor, as shown in Fig. 6.29. Note that the voltage across the cell will drop as the current flow through the cell increases, as shown by the circular curves. The cell will respond as if it has a nonlinear internal resistance. The cell and the load resistor R_L are in parallel, so that the voltage developed by the light energy is applied to R_L, as shown in Fig. 6.30. Assume that the threshold light intensity to be detected is L_b and that R_{in} of the threshold detector is infinite. Further assume that the threshold voltage needed by the detector is V_{T1}. A vertical line can be drawn at that voltage to determine the current that will flow when L_b is present. The intersection of this line and the curve for L_b is at I_1. I_1 will flow through R_L, so the load resistance can be determined by the equation

$$R_L = \frac{V_{T1}}{I_1}.$$

The input resistance of the threshold detector was assumed to be infinite in the above example. This input resistance R_{in} is in parallel with R_L and must be considered if its value is not much greater than R_L.

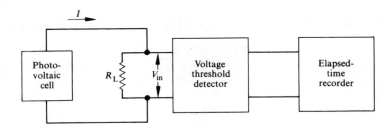

Fig. 6.28.   Threshold-detector measuring system, for light intensity.

Consider a second case where the threshold voltage needed is V_{T2} and R_{in} is not infinite. Drawing the vertical line at this voltage, we find that the current flow through the parallel combination of resistances R_{Lp} is I_2. Then

$$R_{Lp} = \frac{V_{T2}}{I_2}.$$

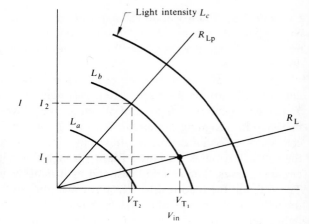

Fig. 6.29. Characteristic curves of photovoltaic cell and load resistor.

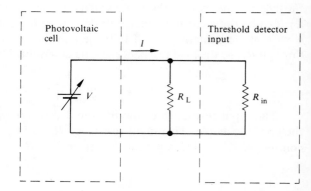

Fig. 6.30. Model of a photovoltaic-cell measurement circuit.

If R_{in} is known, then the value of R_L required can be obtained by the equation

$$\frac{V_{T2}}{I_2} = \frac{R_L R_{in}}{R_L + R_{in}}.$$

We have

$$R_L = \frac{V_{T2} R_{in}}{I_2 R_{in} - V_{T2}}.$$

Thermocouple: An Active-type Transducer

A *thermocouple* is a transducer used to measure temperature. It is constructed of two wires of dissimilar materials joined at one point. This joining of two dissimilar metals produces an electric potential, a few mV or less, which can be measured with a very sensitive voltmeter. No external excitation is required to produce a voltage that is related to the temperature of the junction.

Larger output voltages can be obtained by connecting a group of thermo-couples in series. Such a connection is called a *thermopile*. A thermopile has the advantage that the voltmeter used for detecting its temperature-related output need not be as sensitive as that needed for just one thermocouple.

The thermocouple effect may appear where it is not wanted whenever two dissimilar wires are connected together. Thus the wires connecting the thermo-couple to the voltage-measuring device may also produce a thermoelectric voltage which can affect the voltage reading. These voltages may be as high as 40 to 60 $\mu V/°C$ in the temperature zone between 0° and 100°C. Therefore, care must be taken to ensure that the temperature of the wire junctions at the measuring device do not change from the ambient temperature used when the thermocouple mea-suring system was calibrated. If these temperatures do change, errors will result. One method used to overcome this type of error is shown in Fig. 6.31. With this system the voltage between points 1 and 2 will be zero when the measuring thermocouple is at 0°C. At this temperature the thermally generated voltages at the two junctions will cancel each other out: when the temperature of the measuring junction changes from 0°C, a different voltage will appear across ter-minals 1 and 2.

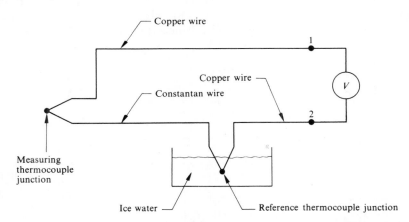

Fig. 6.31. Use of a reference thermistor when making temperature mea-surements with a thermistor.

The current that flows through the junction will affect the measurement by changing the temperature of the junction. It is desirable to use a voltage-measuring device that will draw as small a current as possible. Potentiometric measurements are used when very high-input-impedance voltmeters are not available.

The time it takes the thermocouple to respond to changes in temperature is dependent on the physical size of the wires used. When a rapid response is desired, the wires must be very small. The smaller the wires, the shorter is the time required for the junction to reach thermal equilibrium with its immediate environment.

Example 6.7 Thermocouple application. The temperature of a rabbit is to be monitored while it is under the influence of a drug. A sealed thermocouple will be implanted in the part of the rabbit where the temperature is to be measured. The animal will be asleep and not moving during the experiment. How can the measurement be made?

Two thermocouples can be used and placed in series, as in Fig. 6.32. For the temperature range expected and the thermocouple materials used, an output voltage of approximately 1 mV is expected. One of the thermocouples is kept at a reference temperature in an ice bath. The other is to be implanted in the rabbit. The voltage will be measured by the potentiometer. The tap on the variable resistor is moved until the null detector indicates no measurable voltage difference between points a and b. No appreciable current will be flowing through the wires to the thermocouples to cause heating or voltage drop problems. The position of the tap can be calibrated in °C prior to implanting the thermocouple by placing the measuring thermocouple in a controlled environment of known temperature.

The power supply that is available has a regulated output voltage of 10 ± 0.05 V. The voltage at point c with respect to ground is to be 2 mV so that the expected voltage at null condition will fall near the center of the range of R_1.

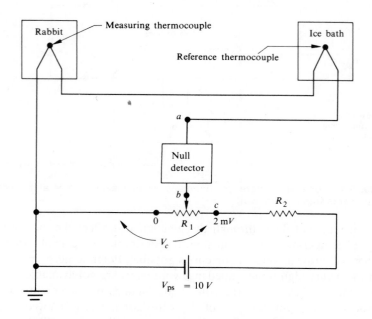

Fig. 6.32. Measuring temperature with thermocouples and using a null condition for detecting the thermocouple voltage.

A 1,000-Ω four-turn potentiometer is used for R_1. What should R_2 be and what effect will the variation in power supply voltage and resistor tolerance have on the temperature calibration?

By the voltage-divider equation we can obtain the value of R_2:

$$V_c = \frac{R_1}{R_1 + R_2} V_{ps},$$

$$R_2 = \frac{R_1(V_{ps} - V_c)}{V_c} = \frac{10^3(10 - 2 \times 10^{-3})}{2 \times 10^{-3}} \cong 5 \times 10^6 \ \Omega.$$

Assume that a resistor of $\pm 1\%$ tolerance is used for R_2. What effect will it have on the voltage at point c as it varies from $5 \times 10^6 \ \Omega$? We have

$$V_c = \frac{10^3}{10^3 + 5.05 \times 10^6} (10) = 1.98 \ \text{mV} \quad \text{when } R_2 \text{ is } 1\% \text{ high},$$

$$V_c = \frac{10^3}{10^3 + 4.95 \times 10^6} (10) = 2.02 \ \text{mV} \quad \text{when } R_2 \text{ is } 1\% \text{ low}.$$

The error at point c caused by this variation in R_2 is about 1%.

What error will result when the power supply voltage varies by $\pm 0.5\%$? We have

$$V_c \cong 0.2 \times 10^{-3} (10.05) = 2.01 \ \text{mV} \quad \text{when } V_{ps} \text{ is } 0.5\% \text{ high}.$$
$$V_c \cong 0.2 \times 10^{-3} (9.95) \ \ = 1.99 \ \text{mV} \quad \text{when } V_{ps} \text{ is } 0.5\% \text{ low}.$$

The error caused by this variation in R_2 is 0.5%.

The calibration of temperature in respect to the position of the four-turn potentiometer tap should be done at normal operating temperatures and with the actual resistors and power supply that will be used in the measuring system.

Piezoelectric Crystal: An Active-type Transducer

A *piezoelectric crystal* transducer is used to measure force. It is constructed of a crystal with the property that an output voltage is produced when a force is applied to the crystal. This type of transducer has a high internal electrical impedance and must be connected to a high-impedance detecting circuit with low shunt capacitance if maximum power is to be delivered to the detecting circuit. It will not generate a steady-state output response, although it may respond to frequencies as low as 2 Hz. The high-frequency response of the piezoelectric crystal transducer is limited by the mechanical properties of the transducer. Frequency response specifications for specific transducers should be obtained from the manufacturer.

Microphone: An Active-type Transducer

A *microphone* is a transducer capable of measuring pressure; it is most commonly used to measure sound pressure waves. Certain microphone characteristics should be obtained before selecting a microphone for a particular application: output impedance, frequency response characteristics, mechanical ruggedness. The input impedance of the amplifier to be used with the microphone must be known so that a proper impedance match can be obtained to yield maximum power transfer from the microphone to the amplifier.

There are many different types of microphones: carbon granual microphones, electrodynamic microphones, capacitance microphones, crystal microphones, ribbon microphones, hot-wire microphones. Microphones may be much more sensitive to sound coming from one direction than from another direction. For example, the electrical output of the microphone may be one unit of magnitude when a sound source of a particular intensity is placed directly in front of the microphone at a distance of 3 ft. If the same sound source is placed 3 ft. from the microphone but off to one side, the electrical output may be only half that noted in the other position. This effect can be shown graphically as in Fig. 6.33. If this sensitivity pattern is cardioid or heart-shaped, the microphone has the greatest sensitivity to sound striking the microphone from sources directly in front of the microphone and tends to reject sound that comes from the side or rear of the microphone. A microphone with this type of sensitivity pattern is sometimes called a unidirectional microphone. There are other microphones which have omnidirectional sensitivity patterns which respond almost equally well to sounds from all sides of the microphone.

Example 6.8 Microphone application. A high-quality microphone of low impedance (150 Ω), is to be used with a tape recorder to record the chirps of

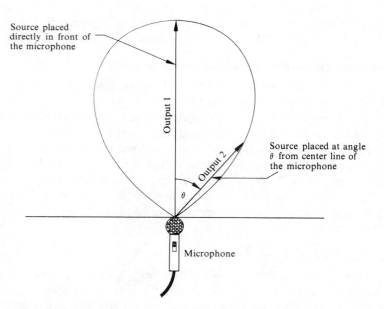

Fig. 6.33. A directional-sensitivity pattern for a particular microphone.

crickets. The tape recorder was tested with a constant voltage at the input and found to give a frequency response characteristic curve that is flat from 50 Hz to 30 kHz. The input impedance of the recorder is 50 kΩ. Should the microphone be connected directly to the tape recorder input?

The microphone will deliver the maximum power to the amplifier when its internal impedance is matched to the load to which it is connected. The maximum power can be delivered to a load from a source when the real part of the source impedance, the resistance, equals the real part of the load impedance, and when the imaginary part of the source impedance, the reactance, equals the negative of the imaginary part of the load impedance. (Refer to Chapter 9 for more information on reactance.) A transformer can be used as an impedance-matching device, as discussed in Section 4.7. A transformer with a flat frequency response characteristic curve should be used to couple the microphone to the tape recorder. The transformer should have a primary-side impedance specification of 150 Ω and a secondary-side impedance specification of 50 kΩ to match the 150-Ω microphone to the 50-kΩ amplifier.

6.9 OTHER TYPES OF TRANSDUCERS

In the previous section a brief introduction was given to some of the very commonly used transducers as examples of the types of things that can be done. The reader may wish to refer to other references in search of more detail on the various types of transducers. Table 6.2 on the following page lists some types of transducers not previously described to help the reader's search for additional information.

6.10 CHARACTERISTICS TO LOOK FOR IN A TRANSDUCER

The success of any electrical measurement depends in part on using a transducer that has the best possible characteristics needed for the particular measurement. Table 6.3 beginning on the following page lists some important characteristics and the considerations which must go into the selection of a transducer for purposes of measurement.

TABLE 6.2
Other transducers

Name	Measurand
1. Photodiode	Light
2. Phototransistor	Light
3. Photomultiplier	Light
4. Photoelectric cell	Light
5. Magnetostriction device	Pressure
6. Ionization gage	Pressure
7. Semiconductor strain gage	Pressure
8. Capacitance diaphragm	Pressure
9. Variable-reluctance gage	Pressure
10. Differential-transformer gage	Pressure
11. Electrodynamic generator	Sound pressure
12. Hydrophone	Water pressure variations
13. Force-balance transducer	Pressure, acceleration
14. Differential transformer	Position
15. Rotary potentiometer	Position
16. Variable inductance	Position
17. Variable capacitance	Position
18. Induction flow meter	Flow
19. Hot-wire anemometer	Rate of flow, fluid velocity
20. Bolometer	Radiant heat

TABLE 6.3
Characteristics to be considered when selecting a transducer

Characteristic	Considerations
1. Measurand	Which physical quantity, property, or condition is the transducer to sense?
2. Sensitivity	How much change in transducer output can be obtained for a given change of the measurand?
3. Threshold	What is the smallest change in the measurand that will result in a measurable change in the transducer output?
4. Excitation	What type of external power source, if any, must be used with the transducer to produce a transducer output which is related to a measurand input?
5. Output	What is the amplitude of signal that can be obtained from the transducer? Is this signal a current or a voltage? What effect will the input impedance of the detecting circuit have on the signal at the output terminals of the transducer?

TABLE 6.3 (Continued)
Characteristics to be considered when selecting a transducer

Characteristic	Considerations
6. Static-error band	How much variation in output signal can be expected under conditions of normal room temperature and in the absence of mechanical stresses?
7. Repeatability	How much variation in output signal will occur when the same measurand value is applied repeatedly, under the same conditions and in the same direction?
8. Transfer function	What is the relation between the measurand input value and the transducer output signal over the allowable range of input values?
9. Overload	What is the maximum amplitude of the measurand that can be measured without causing damage to the transducer and without causing the transducer output to exceed the specified tolerance?
10. Frequency response	What is the shape of the curve of transducer output signal amplitude vs. the frequency of the measurand signal when the amplitude of the measurand signal is held constant?
11. Time constant	What is the length of time required for the transducer output to rise to 63% of its final value as a result of a step change in the measurand?
12. Stability	How well will the transducer retain its performance characteristics throughout its specified operating life and storage life?
13. Operating life	What is the minimum length of time over which the specified continuous and intermittent rating of a transducer will apply without change in transducer performance beyond specified tolerances?
14. Storage life	What is the minimum length of time over which a transducer can be exposed to specified environmental conditions without changing its performance beyond specified tolerances?
15. Adjustability	What provisions are there for making calibration adjustments?
16. Physical Characteristics	What are the spatial dimensions and weight of the transducer? What provisions have been made for mounting the transducer?

6.11   REVIEW QUESTIONS AND PROBLEMS

6.1   What is meant by the term "transducer"?

6.2   What is the major difference between an active and a passive transducer?

6.3   A light-sensing device has the characteristic curves shown in Fig. R6.1. This device is connected in series with a dc power supply of 200 V and a 20-MΩ resistor. Determine the range of output voltages that can be obtained across the light-sensing device if the light varies from 0.1 lumens to 0.4 lumens.

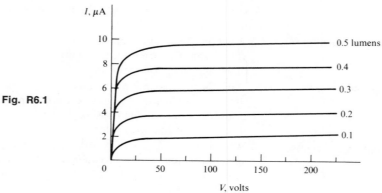

Fig. R6.1

6.4   A light-sensitive resistor acts as a linear resistor if the light illuminating the resistor does not change its intensity. Its resistance is decreased by a factor of two whenever the light intensity doubles. When the light intensity is L_1, the resistance is 10 kΩ. The maximum voltage that can be applied across the device is 20 V and the maximum current that can flow through the device is 10 mA. The maximum power dissipation for the device is 50 mW. Design a circuit that uses this device to produce an output voltage signal of maximum possible amplitude when the light intensity varies from L_1 to $4L_1$. What is the maximum voltage variation that can be produced by your circuit?

6.5   A Wheatstone bridge circuit is to be used to determine the resistance of a temperature-sensitive resistor. For the range of temperatures to be measured, this resistor varies from 1000 Ω to 100 Ω. A regulated dc power source is available to produce 30 V. A microammeter which reads ±50 μA maximum and has an internal resistance of 300 Ω is available to use as a null detector.

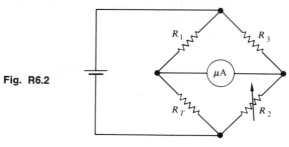

Fig. R6.2

What size variable resistor should be used for R_2 in Fig. R6.2 if R_1 and R_3 are each 500 Ω? What will the needle of the ammeter do if the circuit is not balanced? How should the circuit be operated to determine the resistance of the temperature-sensitive resistor?

6.6   A physician would like to monitor the movements of a tiny baby lying on a mattress. He has proposed to place the mattress on a board that is suspended on springs. Whenever the baby moves, the board will start to rock slightly. Attached to the board will be a linear potentiometer. As the board moves, the tap on the potentiometer moves. The resistance from end to end of the potentiometer is 1000 Ω. Its power rating is 1 W. The tap on the potentiometer moves a maximum of 1 cm. The board moves a maximum of 0.5 cm. Design a circuit that can be used to produce an output voltage that is proportional to the position of the board. What is the maximum voltage variation that your system will produce?

6.7   A light-sensing resistor has been designed into a bridge circuit as shown in Fig. R6.3. It occupies the R_{s1} position. If its resistance varies from 100 to 300 Ω while the other resistors are held constant at 200 Ω, what variation of voltage V_0 will occur? Assume the input impedance of the detecting circuit is essentially infinite. If R_{s1} varies from 100 to 300 Ω while R_{s2} is 200 Ω and R_3 and R_4 are each 300 Ω, what variation of voltage V_0 will occur? Is there any combination of resistance values for R_{s2}, R_3, and R_4 that will produce a maximum variation of voltage V_0?

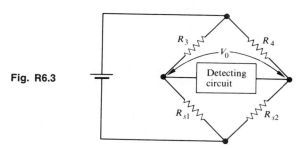

Fig. R6.3

6.8   A measuring system such as that shown in Fig. R6.4 is set up to measure the temperature inside a test specimen. The difference in voltage between that gen-

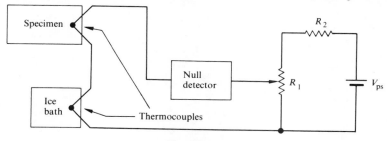

Fig. R6.4

erated by the thermocouple in the specimen and that generated by the thermo-couple in the ice bath is 0.2 mV. Assume that a sufficiently sensitive null de-tector is available to enable the operator to balance the circuit. If the value of V_{ps} is 6 V, what values of the resistors R_1 and R_2 should be used? What type of a resistor would you recommend for R_1?

6.9 A photovoltaic cell is available that has a characteristic curve as shown in Fig. R6.5. A voltmeter with an input resistance of 10k Ω is connected across the cell. What voltage will be read on the voltmeter when the cell is illuminated with light intensity L_1?

Fig. R6.5

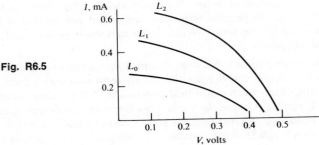

6.10 What major characteristics must be considered when picking a transducer?

7
basic display and storage building blocks

7.1 OBJECTIVES

As was pointed out in Chapter 1, the final result of almost any research investigation is an accumulation of measurement data. All the data must be displayed on some device before the biologist can make use of them. In this chapter we will describe some of the devices used to display the desired data.

Before choosing a display device, the biologist must understand and recognize its properties so that he can use it efficiently. The following questions should be asked: Is the device accurate? Does it have a range and sensitivity suitable to the desired measurement? Does it fulfill the needs for correctly displaying the data? How rapidly does the signal change and does the device display the actual signal or does it distort the signal? Does the scientist want a steady-state visual display such as found in meters? Does he want a temporary or time-related visual display such as on the cathode-ray oscilloscope? Does he want a permanent record, and if so, will he choose a strip-chart recorder, magnetic-tape recorder, or an electronic or mechanical counter?

If data are to be collected over an extended period of time, the scientist may wish to record these data as a permanent record either by using a strip-chart recorder or a magnetic-tape recorder. If the data are to be used in a computer, he may wish to record the information on magnetic tape. It is important, therefore, for the scientist to carefully select his display device. In nearly all cases involving biological measurements, accuracy and sensitivity of the display device are of paramount importance. For example, if one wishes to measure the length of time required to cleave the bonds of a protein by an enzyme, the display device must be accurate; it must be sensitive and have a rapid response.

Many of the basic display devices that may be chosen in biological measurement systems will be discussed in this chapter. We shall not indulge in any extended discussion of the physical principles involved in the operation of display devices. If the reader desires to more clearly understand the mechanics and the complex electronics of these devices, he may want to consult the books that are cited in Appendix 4 or refer to manufacturer's information sheets for specific instruments.

7.2 METERS: dc ANALOG TYPE

Measurement of dc Current

The basic meter used widely in electronics today is the *moving-coil* or *D'Arsonval meter*. This meter converts electrical energy to the physical displacement of a pointer by means of a mechanism shown in Fig. 7.1. A coil of fine wire is wound on a frame which is placed between the poles of a permanent horseshoe magnet. Pivots are attached to the frame which rotate in jeweled bearings with minimum friction. A pointer is attached to the coil frame and a spring allows the pointer to return to a fixed reference point. These are the movable parts of the meter. When current flows through the coil, a magnetic field is developed which interacts with the magnetic field of the permanent magnet and causes the coil to move or rotate.

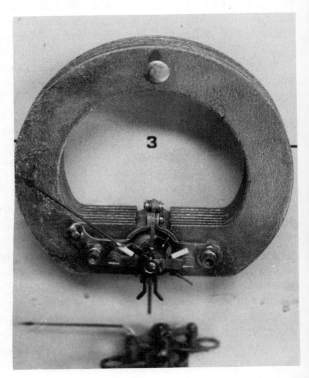

Fig. 7.1. Moving-coil or D'Arsonval meter movement.

The direction of rotation depends on the direction of current flow. The magnitude of current determines the final deflection of the pointer.

This moving-coil meter is the heart of the dc milliammeter. A very common dc milliammeter requires 1 mA to produce full-scale deflection. However, each individual meter is constructed to measure a basic range of current. Typical values for full-scale current are 50 μA, 1 mA, 10 mA, 100 mA, 1 A, 5 A, and 10 A. A good selection of other values is also available. Although meters with almost any range of current can be purchased, it is often less expensive and simpler to use a meter already on hand. The current range may be extended by adding a resistor in parallel with the meter. This resistor is called a shunt. If the meter range is less than required, a shunt of the correct value can be connected across the meter terminals to obtain the desired range (Fig. 7.2).

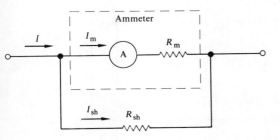

Fig. 7.2. Required circuit modification for changing the range of currents measured by an ammeter.

The principle of the shunt is to provide a path through which part of the current I can flow, while the remainder flows through the meter. The fraction flowing through the meter may be very small compared to I. The shunt resistance R_{sh} can be calculated by means of Ohm's law. The voltage across the ammeter is the same as the voltage across the shunt:

$$I_m R_m = I_{sh} R_{sh}, \quad \text{where} \quad I_m + I_{sh} = I.$$

Using these two equations, we can obtain the following:

$$R_{sh} = \frac{I_m R_m}{I - I_m}, \tag{7.1}*$$

where I_m = full-scale meter current, I = maximum current to be measured, and R_m = resistance of meter movement. This calculation is based on the desired full-scale reading for the modified ammeter.

Example 7.1   Modifying a dc milliammeter to measure higher currents.   A particular experiment requires the use of an ammeter that will measure a maximum current of 20 mA dc. On hand is a meter that will measure 1 mA dc full scale. The meter-movement resistance is 100 Ω. An appropriate circuit modification can be made to provide a full-scale reading of 20 mA dc.

In this example, $I = 20$ mA, $I_m = 1$ mA, $R_m = 100$ Ω. We have

$$R_{sh} = \frac{10^{-3}\,(100)}{20 \times 10^{-3} - 1 \times 10^{-3}} = 5.263 \ \Omega. \tag{7.1}$$

This amount of resistance is not available in a standard fixed resistor so that a precision variable resistor must be used for the shunt. One possibility is to use a resistance bridge (Wheatstone bridge) to measure the variable resistor. Set the resistance bridge to the desired value and then connect the variable resistor to the bridge. Move the contact on the resistor until the bridge is balanced. Make sure the contact is not again moved once the setting has been made. A second method is to use a dc power supply and a precision resistor (Fig. 7.3).

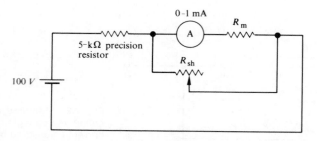

Fig. 7.3. Method of setting the value of shunt resistance needed to modify a dc milliammeter.

The parallel combination of R_{sh} and R_m is much less than 5 kΩ. Thus the current that flows from the battery will be determined by the battery voltage and the 5 kΩ resistor. In this case, this current is the desired 20 mA. The shunt resistance is set to 0 Ω before the dc voltage is turned on. After the dc voltage is turned on, the resistance of the shunt is increased until a full-scale reading is obtained on the meter. For this value of shunt resistance the full-scale reading corresponds to a current of 20 mA. The original scale on the 1 mA meter movement must be multiplied by 20 when this shunt resistor is connected.

A series of shunts may be calculated and the resistors placed across the meter individually by switching so that the moving-coil meter may be used for measurement of a wide range of currents. Such a series of shunts is collectively called an Ayrton shunt and is shown in Fig. 7.4. Specific values of resistances to be used can be determined by means of Ohm's law, as was done in the previous example.

A point to remember

A basic moving-coil meter can be modified by the use of one or more shunts in parallel with the meter, to extend the range of this meter.

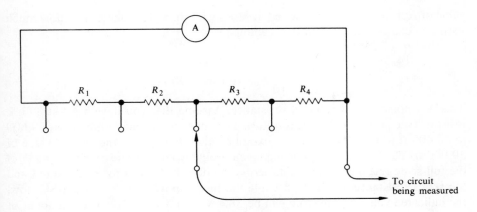

Fig. 7.4.   An Ayrton shunt connected across an ammeter.

Measurement of dc Voltage

The ammeter, with modifications, can be used to measure dc voltages. If a large resistor is placed in series with the meter, a dc voltmeter is produced, as in Fig. 7.5. To make a voltage measurement, we place this dc voltmeter across the terminals of the unknown voltage source. We can calculate the series resistance needed to convert a basic ammeter to a voltmeter.

The formula is as follows:

$$V = I_m \, (R_m + R_{ser})$$

$$R_{ser} = \frac{V}{I_m} - R_m. \qquad\qquad (7.2)*$$

Example 7.2   Modifying a dc milliammeter to measure dc voltages.   A milliammeter with a full-scale reading of 1 mA and a resistance of 100 Ω is available in the laboratory. A dc voltmeter is needed with a full-scale reading of 40 V. What

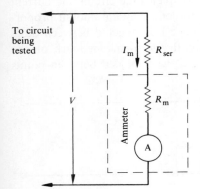

Fig. 7.5. Ammeter modified into a voltmeter.

value of resistance should be added in series with the milliammeter and how much variation can be expected in the readings?

By Eq. (7.2) we have

$$R_{ser} = \frac{40}{10^{-3}} - 100 = 39{,}900 \ \Omega.$$

This is a nonstandard value of resistance. Assume that you have a 40-kΩ $\pm 1\%$ resistor. One percent of 40 kΩ is 400 Ω. Thus this resistor may range from 39,600 to 40,400 Ω when new. These two extreme values fall outside the desired value of 39,000 Ω. The basic meter movement will probably be accurate to within $\pm 3\%$ of the full-scale reading at any point across the dial. If 40 V is to be measured and the series resistance is 1% high while the meter movement is reading 3% low, the indicated value on the scale will be 38.4 V or 4% low. This is the amount of error that can be expected; it may be even higher if the reading is on the lower end of the scale.

A voltmeter of this type is described as having X number of Ω/v. This is a figure-of-merit rating. The higher the value of X, the higher is the resistance of the voltmeter. In most cases this figure of merit should be as high as possible. In Example 7.2 the total resistance is 40 kΩ and the voltage rating is 40 V. This means that $X = 40$ kΩ/40 V or 1 kΩ/V.

A point to remember

A voltmeter can be constructed by connecting a resistor of appropriate value in series with an ammeter.

Measurement of Resistance

The basic moving-coil meter can be used to construct a circuit that can measure the resistance of an unknown component. Such a circuit is called an *ohmmeter*. A simple series-ohmmeter circuit is shown in Fig. 7.6. The unknown resistor is connected between points 1 and 2. This resistor completes the circuit and current will flow through the meter, causing the pointer to deflect by an amount proportional to the value of resistance. When no resistance is connected between these two points, the pointer does not deflect and thus the zero-current mark on the scale represents infinite resistance. If a short circuit were placed between points

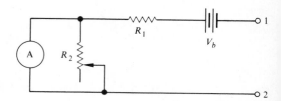

Fig. 7.6. A series-ohmmeter circuit.

1 and 2, the resistance R_2 must be adjusted to give a full-scale deflection of the pointer. Thus this point on the scale represents zero resistance. Any value of resistance connected between points 1 and 2 will result in a deflection of the pointer to a position between the two endpoints. This ohmmeter scale will be nonlinear.

Example 7.3   Modifying a dc ammeter to measure resistance.   A chemical solution is to be monitored to make sure that its electrical resistance falls in the range of 100 to 200 Ω. The lab assistant would like to use his digital ohmmeter for this measurement, but unfortunately this instrument cannot be tied up for long periods of time for the experiment. The alternative is to build a simple ohmmeter and calibrate the scale for the region between 100 and 200 Ω.

Two moving-coil meters are available for use in this experiment as well as a regulated dc power supply:

Microammeter	0–50 μA	300-Ω resistance
Milliammeter	0–10 mA	2-Ω resistance
Power supply	0–10 V	100 mA maximum

Assume that any current less than 10 mA flowing through the solution will not have any detrimental effects on the solution. Which of the two meters should be used?

Let us first try the 50-μA meter in the simple circuit shown in Fig. 7.7. (The zero-resistance adjustment R_2 has been deleted.)

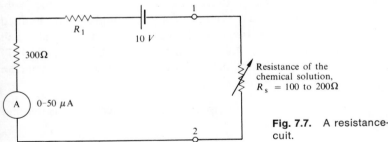

Resistance of the chemical solution, R_s = 100 to 200Ω

Fig. 7.7.   A resistance-measuring circuit.

Assume that we want the microammeter pointer to be at midscale when the solution resistance is 150 Ω. The pointer will move up or down the scale as the solution varies from this amount. What should be the value of R_1? How far will the pointer move as the resistance is varied from 100 to 200 Ω?

By Ohm's law we find that R_1 has a value of 400 kΩ to cause a current flow of 25 μA (midscale reading) when the power supply is set at 10 V. Note that the 150 Ω of the chemical solution is so small compared to R_1 that it has essentially no effect on the position of the pointer. In fact, any variation of the solution resistance from zero to 5 kΩ will have little effect on the position of the pointer. Therefore, this meter and circuit are not satisfactory for this application.

Consider the 10-mA meter together with a 1-V power supply, as in Fig. 7.8.

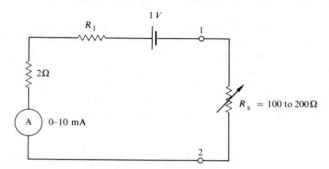

Fig. 7.8. A circuit for measuring solution resistance.

For a midscale reading of 5 mA, R_1 must be 48 Ω when the solution is 150 Ω. If the solution resistance increases to 200 Ω, the current will decrease to 4 mA. If the solution resistance decreases to 100 Ω, the current will increase to 6.67 mA. Thus there is a good displacement of the pointer in the range of interest. A word of caution: Note what would happen if the solution were to become a short circuit, with zero resistance. The total series resistance would be 50 Ω. For the 1-V source Ohm's law would indicate a flow of 20.0 mA. This value exceeds the 10-mA full-scale reading of the meter and could be disastrous. A better answer to the problem would be to make $R_1 = 98$ Ω. Then terminals 1 and 2 could be short-circuited without damaging the meter. The consequence of increasing R_1 to this value will be to have the range for 100 to 200 Ω fall between 5 mA and 3.33 mA. This will yield a smaller deviation than that in the previous design, but it is still acceptable.

A point to remember

An ohmmeter can be constructed by appropriately connecting resistors and a voltage source to an ammeter.

7.3 METERS: ac ANALOG TYPES

Measurement of Voltage or Current

Not all signals that are to be measured are direct current, so that another class of instruments must be available when making a measurement of voltage or current at a particular frequency. There are several different types of meter movements used for ac measurements. Many of them have a nonlinear scale as compared to the linear scale of moving-coil meter. It is important that the scale not be too compressed in the range of the signal being measured. For example, a reading for a

35-V input could not be read accurately on the voltmeter scale shown in Fig. 7.9.

An ac signal may contain a single frequency, such as 60 Hz, with the information of the signal being related to the amplitude of the voltage or current at that frequency. Another ac signal may have a frequency of 1 kHz that is held constant while the amplitude of the voltage or current is varied. A meter that is capable of measuring a 60-Hz signal may not be able to measure a 1-kHz signal, even though the voltage or current range is the same for both signals. It is important to look at the specifications for the particular meter being used to determine whether or not accurate readings can be made at the given signal frequency. Some ac voltmeters are capable of making accurate measurements over a frequency range from 10 Hz to 10 MHz, while others may have only a range of 30 Hz to 300 Hz.

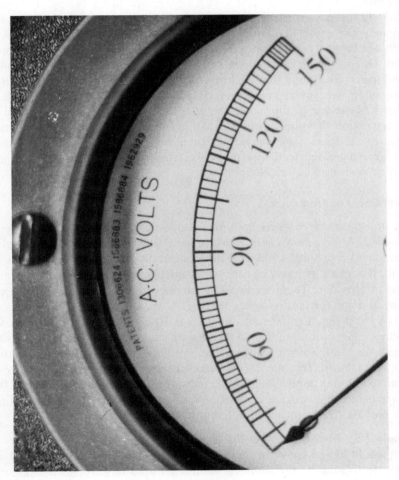

Fig. 7.9. Nonlinear scale on an ac voltmeter.

Example 7.4   Measurement of the 60-Hz power line voltage.   In a laboratory the technicians noted that the vacuum tubes in their oscilloscopes and voltmeters were burning out at a much higher rate than seemed reasonable. Also their incandescent light bulbs were burning out often. These two phenomena indicated the possibility that the power line voltage was having large fluctuations. Obviously higher than normal voltages would heat up the filaments excessively and thus hasten their failure. (Recall that power is a function of the square of the voltage: $P = V^2/R$ for a resistive circuit.) A measurement of the line voltage was therefore called for. (The power line frequency is usually within a small fraction of a percent of the specified value.)

An ac voltmeter capable of measuring at 60 Hz was connected across the power line. The voltage was 120 V at 8 A.M. on the first morning. The voltmeter was left in the power circuit and the technicians noted the line voltage reading throughout the day. The reading stayed fairly constant. Since 120 V was within the ratings for the oscilloscopes, excessive filament heating should not have occurred. One of the technicians worked through the evening and kept monitoring the voltmeter. She found that the line voltage rose to 137 V by 10 P.M. The same phenomenon was found every evening and the mystery was solved. This high voltage was capable of shortening the life of the filaments and was caused by the poor regulation of voltage supplied to the building. A means of regulating the voltage in the laboratory was implemented and the lives of the tubes and light bulbs were increased to the normally expected span. A simple ac voltage measurement proved to be very helpful.

Measurement of Frequency

There are special cases where both the voltage amplitude and the signal frequency are needed. A *wave analyzer* is an instrument designed specifically to provide this measurement capability. Unlike the devices just discussed, it is not a simple meter. Instead, it consists of many circuits which enable it to obtain both frequency and voltage information. There are two dials on the wave analyzer: one for the voltage reading and one for the frequency reading.

The input signal voltage may vary from 10 μV to 100 V or more. A variety of voltage ranges are available on the instrument, so that accurate readings can be taken across the full range of allowable input voltages. The frequency setting involves two factors. The band of frequencies that are measured simultaneously is determined by one control, and this bandwidth may range from 2 Hz to 100 Hz for a typical instrument. The center frequency may be tuned to anywhere between 20 Hz and 50 kHz by means of different band settings.

Example 7.5   Measurement of the temperature environment of a rabbit.   A biologist would like to know the temperature range in which a certain breed of rabbits like to live during the summer. He has set up a large, penned-in area in the natural habitat of this rabbit. The area contains sunny spots and shady spots of both grass and sand. There are shrubs and trees throughout the area. The rabbit has a burrow in which it spends part of its time. As the rabbit moves from place to place, it may be in a warm or cool region. The study requires plotting out temperature in relation to time of day at the point where the rabbit is located. How is this to be done?

A miniature FM radio transmitter can be attached to the rabbit. The information signal generated by the transmitter can be made proportional to the temperature of the rabbit. The information is translated into the frequency that is related to the temperature. The transmitter can send a radio signal containing this information to an FM receiver at the perimeter of the pen. As the rabbit moves from sun to shade, the temperature will change and cause the frequency of the information signal to change. The FM receiver can then be used to detect this information signal. The output of the FM receiver can be fed into a stable magnetic-tape recorder to be analyzed at a later date.

The recorded information signal can be analyzed by means of a wave analyzer. In this example, the voltage amplitude of the signal is of no importance. The information about temperature is contained in the frequency of the signal. If the rabbit stays in one temperature zone for four or five minutes, there will be a satisfactory recording of one frequency to enable the biologist to measure that frequency with a wave analyzer. He will play the tape recording into the wave analyzer, set the voltage amplitude on a scale that will give a good reading on the output meter. He will then tune the wave analyzer to the frequency of the information signal. Probably he knows the approximate frequency, so that he can tune the wave analyzer to the right range before starting the recording. At first he should use a large bandwidth setting, for example 50 Hz, so that it will be relatively easy for him to "tune in" the information signal. When he begins to get a reading, he can then change to a narrow bandwidth, for example 5 Hz, and make the specific frequency reading from the dial. Much finer tuning can be made while using the narrow bandwidth setting compared to the large bandwidth setting.

This system should be calibrated before the transmitter is attached to the rabbit. The transmitter should be placed in a particular temperature zone; a temperature should be taken with an auxiliary thermometer, and a recording made at the output of the FM receiver. This procedure must be repeated for every zone in the full range of temperatures to be measured. The resulting recording must then be analyzed and the temperature-vs.-frequency data correlated.

This method of gathering data will result in ten or twelve hours of recording per day if continuous recordings are made. If playback is done at the same speed as the recording was made, much time will be required for analysis of the data. One method of reducing playback time would be to record at a very slow speed and play it back at a much higher speed. This is a satisfactory procedure so long as the speed control mechanism of the recorder is very stable.

If a wave analyzer is available, the procedure described in the example above will yield the proper results. Another solution to this problem would be to use a frequency counter to measure the frequency at the output of the tape recorder. (See Section 7.10.) This type of instrument usually has a digital, direct numerical readout and is very easy to use when only a single frequency is present at one time. The wave analyzer is capable of measuring each particular frequency component of a periodic wave that contains many different frequencies.

7.4   METERS: VOM, VTVM

Commercially constructed meters can be purchased for measuring more than one variable with a single meter. A *multimeter* or VOM is one such meter. The acronym VOM stands for volt-ohm-milliammeter. As the name implies, you may measure voltage (ac or dc), dc current, and resistance with a VOM. The VOM usually has an input impedance figure-of-merit rating of about 10,000 Ω/V on the ac settings and 20,000 Ω/V on dc settings.

Another meter that is commonly used to measure voltage and resistance is called a *vacuum tube voltmeter* or VTVM or *vacuum tube multimeter*. This meter was designed and developed so that it would bring a very high input impedance to the applied voltage. The VTVM usually has an impedance of at least 1 $M\Omega$. It is able to measure voltage very accurately. Keeping the discussion of impedance in Chapter 2 in mind, one can see that the VTVM draws an extremely small amount of current when connected across a circuit. This feature enables the VTVM to be used as an accurate measuring instrument. The VTVM will measure both ac and dc voltages.

7.5   METERS: DIGITAL TYPE

In recent years, with the advent of solid-state circuitry, digital readout meters have become available at reasonable cost. The major differences between these meters and those discussed so far lie in the method of displaying the output and the obtainable accuracies. In place of a pointer that moves along a scale, numbers will light up in a digital readout meter to show the registered voltage, current, or resistance value. This is a particularly desirable feature because it removes the need to estimate what number should be written down when the pointer falls between two calibration points on the scale. The digital readout numbers may have from three to eight digits on the digital meter. This means that much greater accuracy is possible with this type of meter than with the analog type.

Digital meters can be purchased that will measure only one variable—voltage, current, resistance, or time—or they may be of the multimeter type which can be used to measure two or three different variables depending on the setting of a function switch on the meter. They come in a full range of values for any of the variables to be measured. Many of these meters are battery powered in addition to being powered by the ac power line.

A digital voltmeter or ammeter may be used as a visual display device in a measurement system. The data may be directly read from the digits displayed on the instrument. Many of the *analog-to-digital conversion systems* on the market at the present time use meters of this type to visually display the voltage or current fluctuations. However, the data can also be permanently recorded on punched tape, magnetic tape, or printed on paper. The basic analog-to-digital converter systems are usually equipped with at least five channels for recording data. Although the costs of these devices have been reduced in recent years, they remain quite high. However, they have the unique advantage of recording data quickly and accurately in a form that is compatible with a computer input. Therefore, the tedious process of transposing analog data to digital information or to some other usable form is eliminated. Most of the commercial systems have extremely high input impedances and are easy to use.

7.6 STRIP-CHART RECORDERS

There are many *strip-chart recorders* on the market. Most of them use some form of paper chart dispensed from a roll. The data may be recorded by means of a pen on paper, by pressure, or by heat from a special stylus on some type of sensitized paper. The ink-pen chart recorder is the most common and usually the least expensive to buy and operate.

The most common strip-chart recorders usually fall under one of the following basic types: movable-coil meter and potentiometric. These two types of recorders record the data in an analog form. The moving-coil recorder is structured in a similar way to the D'Arsonval meter discussed earlier in this chapter. This type of recorder may display the information in either a curvilinear or a rectilinear form. Because the rectilinear display is easier to read and to measure, this type of recorder is the most commonly available on the market today. The movement of the pen is in a direction perpendicular to the movement of the paper. Figure 7.10 shows recordings made on a rectilinear type of recorder. The moving-coil recorder usually has a very rapid response to the input signal and should be chosen when this feature is wanted.

The potentiometric strip-chart recorder utilizes a servomechanism that moves a sliding contact of a linear potentiometer so as to always produce a zero control voltage (Fig. 7.11). The motor moves the tap on the potentiometer whenever a voltage appears between points 1 and 2. If this voltage is of one polarity, the motor will rotate in one direction. If the polarity changes, the motor will rotate in the other direction. This voltage is the resultant of the input signal V_{13} and the potentiometer voltage V_{23}. When the voltage between 1 and 2 is zero, the system is said to be in balance or at a null point. If the input voltage then increases, the

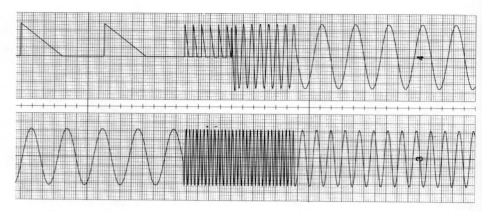

Fig. 7.10.   Recordings made by a rectilinear-type of chart recorder.

voltage V_{12} will increase in a positive direction and the motor will drive the contact to a higher voltage. When a balance is again obtained, the motor will stop. There may remain very small input voltage changes which are insufficient to operate the motor. Thus there is a "dead" region. When the motor is operating, the pen is moved a distance proportional to the movement of the tap on the potentiometer. Many of these instruments have a slow response.

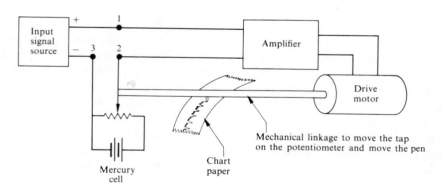

Fig. 7.11.   Simplified diagram for a potentiometric strip-chart recorder.

Selection Criteria

As with the selection of a proper meter, it is important to select the correct strip-chart recorder for the type of signal to be recorded. The following must be considered before purchasing a strip-chart recorder for a measurement system.

1. Accuracy of the instrument: Since data are extremely important to the scientist, she or he must know if the displayed information closely approximates

that which is actually being generated. Typical linearity across the scale ranges from 0.1% to 3% of full scale, depending on the quality of the recorder. Resettability also ranges from 0.1% to 3% depending on the quality of the recorder.

2. Sensitivity of the instrument: The sensitivity of the instrument is usually given in terms of the voltage required to produce a given displacement of the pen. It may range from 0.1 mv to 500 v for every full span of the chart. It may have a current-measuring sensitivity as low as 0.2 mA per inch of displacement.

3. Range of the instrument: It is necessary to know the ranges of the output signal voltage or current so that a recorder may be purchased that is calibrated for these ranges. Most companies offer a voltage divider at the input of the recorder so that several ranges are available with the turn of a knob. Since many signals will vary in amplitude with time, a method by which range adjustment can be quickly changed is very useful. Some recorders may have only one range for the full displacement of the pen. Others may have up to 20 different ranges, so you may select the particular one that will best display the signal levels being measured. A convenient feature of some recorders is a dc displacement control that allows you to add or subtract a dc voltage to the signal being measured. For example, assume that the signal varies from 20 to 22 V and you need to see in detail the waveshape of this variation. If a full-span range of 25 V were used, the variation of 2 V would be less than 10% of the full-scale value. If the recorder would subtract 20 V from the input signal and display the difference, a full-span range of 5 V could be used. The variation of 2 volts would fill 40% of the span and much more detail of the signal could be seen than on the 25 V range. In effect, signal magnification is obtained.

4. Rapidity of pen movement: What is the time rate of change of the signal to be measured? Will the recorder react quickly enough to accurately display the signal? If the response time of the pen is slower than the changes in the input signal, then some of the desired data will not be recorded. For example, in the aphid experiment described in Chapter 1, very short-duration impulses were shown. If a chart recorder had been chosen that would not respond to these rapidly varying signals, the impulses sought would not have been displayed and the experiment would not have proved satisfactory. Choice of the proper recorder is essential. Many biologically related signals do not change rapidly, so that many recorders are adequate for recording this type of data.

    The response time may be from ¼ sec or more for a full-scale displacement. Oscillographic strip-chart recorders may have a response rise time of 7 msec to a step-change input. Rise time means the time required for the response to move from 10% to 90% of maximum deflection on the chart.

5. Frequency of the input signal: Most strip-chart recorders are designed to measure slowly varying or dc signals. The rapidity of pen movement deter-

mines the signals that can be accurately displayed. Consequently, the signal must be close to 0.0 Hz. If the input signal does have a frequency component, the biologist must purchase a recorder that will respond accurately to this frequency. Oscillographic strip-chart recorders will accurately measure signals from dc to 150 Hz and possibly even higher frequencies. Other strip-chart recorders are designed to measure the rms value of ac signals ranging from 1 Hz to 500 kHz. When an ac strip-chart recorder is not available, sometimes it is possible to rectify the ac signal and record the dc component of the output of the rectified signal.

6. Maximum allowable resistance of the source being measured: Some manufacturers will give a specification of the maximum allowable source resistance. If this resistance is exceeded, the recorded value of the signal will be in error. This value is related to the input resistance of the strip-chart recorder. It may be important to choose a recorder with a high input resistance in order to avoid loading down the circuit being tested and getting a voltage that is lower than it would be without the chart recorder. Table 7.1 shows the effects of loading on the measured voltage. The input resistances of the two main types of chart recorders usually range from 1 MΩ to 10 MΩ.

Table 7.1
Loading effects of a chart recorder*

R_{cr}/R_{out}	V_{cr}/V_{actual}
10	0.909
100	0.990
1000	0.999

*R_{cr} = input resistance of chart recorder, R_{out} = output resistance of circuit being measured, V_{cr} = voltage at input to chart recorder, and V_{actual} = actual voltage at test point without chart recorder.

7. Chart speed: Strip-chart recorders are usually constructed to provide variable rates at which the chart paper can pass under the recording pen. Typically, the rates range from 2 in/sec or more down to 2 in/hr or less. A wide variety of intermediate speeds is available. The particular chart speed needed is determined by the rate at which the signal being measured varies, the need for fine detail of the changes of signal level and the length of time the experiment is conducted.

Example 7.6   Monitoring a dog's muscular response to a moving platform.
A physiologist wanted to study the postural control of a dog in response to
standing on a moving table. This involved measuring the pressure exerted by each
paw, the electrical response to muscle action at various points in the dog's body
synchronized with other recordings, and taking moving pictures of the dog
standing on the moving table.

Many channels were required to record all of these data simultaneously. A
multichannel strip recorder was used that had a flat frequency response characteristic in the range of frequencies produced by the various transducers. The recorder
had to be synchronized with the movie camera so that correlation studies could
be done to determine the dog's posture in relation to her muscular response to the
moving table. The recorder was able to record the information accurately, but the
time required to manually take the information off the strip chart was extensive.
Therefore the physiologist added a multichannel magnetic-tape recorder to
record the data so that they could be automatically transferred to a computer for
processing.

7.7   X-Y RECORDERS

There are many experiments in which the scientist wants to know how a signal
variable changes with the control variable. In such situations it is helpful to have
a plot of the signal variable vs. the control variable. The *X-Y recorder* is a
machine that will drive a pen in both the horizontal and vertical directions in
response to two signals applied at its inputs. The pen writes on ordinary blank
paper or graph paper. An example will bring out some of the features of the
X-Y recorder that must be considered when designing an experiment.

Example 7.7   Valve opening vs temperature.   Fresh air is to be blown into an
enclosure in which small animals are living. A temperature-sensitive valve opens
and closes a port to allow more or less air to flow through the enclosure depending
on the temperature. The position of the valve will help determine the air flow.

Suppose that we would like to record the position of the temperature-
sensitive valve as a function of temperature. A transducer that measures position
could be connected to the valve to generate an electrical signal that is proportional
to the valve position. This signal could be connected to the *Y*-axis input of the
recorder. A temperature-sensitive transducer could be connected appropriately to
generate an electrical signal proportional to temperature. This signal would then
serve as the input to the *X*-axis of the recorder. As the temperature is moved up
and down, the recorder pen would plot out the response of the valve and show
whether or not the valve responds linearly with temperature and whether or not it
always gives the same position for a specific value of temperature.

Several questions come to mind.

1. What is the range of voltages that will be generated by the valve-position-sensing transducer?

2. What is the range of voltages that will be generated by the temperature-sensing transducer.

3. What is the maximum rate at which the valve-position voltage will change?

4. What is the maximum rate at which the temperature signal voltage will change?

Answers to these questions will provide the information needed to help determine the specifications required of the X-Y recorder.

Y-Axis Options

The amplifiers that drive the pen along the Y-axis usually have controls which allow you to select a range of input settings, for example 10 mV/in, 20 V/in, etc. Some recorders have plug-in amplifiers, so that you have a choice of several ranges. They may also provide a differential amplifier input, so that you may record the difference between two signals.

X-Axis Options

The X-axis input of the recorder may contain an amplifier and controls identical to those of the Y-amplifier. If so, you can obtain graphs with identical scales on both the horizontal and vertical axes. In some applications this is a very desirable feature. There are other applications in which the X- and Y-input signals have radically different levels, so that totally different ranges are required of the X-axis amplifier and the Y-axis amplifier.

There are occasions on which an input signal varies with time rather than with some physical parameter. In these cases it is desirable to have an X-Y recorder that has a time-base generator to drive the pen in the X direction. Recorders with this feature are available which provide a range of pen displacements per unit of time. You may want to have the pen move linearly at a rate of 1 in/min for 10 min and then stop. In another experiment you may need a rate of 1 in/sec for 10 sec and then have the pen stop. X-axis time-base units are available for many different rates of pen movement. Note that when the recorder is used in this way, it will provide the same type of recording that a strip-chart recorder would give, except that it has a limited time span. Usually the X-Y recorder will take a standard 8½ × 11 in. sheet of paper or an 11 × 17 in. sheet.

Computer X-Y Recorders

Your experiment may involve feeding the data directly into a computer so that you can process the data before making a chart of the desired information. Proper equipment is needed for this process. If an analog computer is used, the signals may be fed directly into the computer amplifiers if they are not too large and if the source and amplifier resistances match properly. The output of the analog computer then drives an *X-Y* recorder.

If a digital computer is used, an analog-to-digital converter will be needed to interface with the computer. This converter changes the analog signal from the source to the appropriate digital format needed by the computer. *X-Y* recorders are available that take the digital output directly from the computer and move the pen in accordance with the digital signals. This equipment makes it quick and easy to produce charts and graphs, and therefore is convenient to have when many of them are needed. They are quite expensive, however, and must be used with a computer that has the proper digital output.

7.8   TAPE RECORDERS

Information that is to be stored can be in analog form or digital form depending on the type of system generating the information. Information in analog form can be recorded by magnetic-tape recorders, while that in digital form can be recorded by means of either magnetic- or paper-tape recorders. In general digital recorders are more expensive than analog recorders, although the price also depends on the frequency characteristics of the signal to be recorded.

Magnetic-tape Recorders

There are many types of magnetic-tape recorders on the market. The quality of the recording is dependent on the frequency response of the recorder, and the recorders are priced accordingly. In most cases the scientist wants a faithful reproduction of the signal applied at the input of the recorder. The ideal recorder is one which will amplify all the frequency components present in the signal by an equal amount. The frequency response is said to be flat in the range in which this condition is obtained. This type of curve is shown in Fig. 7.12. In addition, the phase relationships between the various frequency components in the signal should not be changed in the recording. If the phase differences are changed, that is, if there is a phase shift, the waveshape of the signal at the output will not be the same

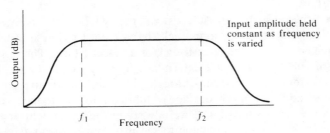

Fig. 7.12.   Flat frequency response curve from f_1 to f_2.

as the signal waveshape at the input. (Refer to Section 11.3 and Fig. 11.12 for comments on phase shift.) Then the scientist may misinterpret the recorded information.

Quite often the frequency response of a recorder has the vertical scale calibrated in decibels, as in Fig. 7.12:

$$\text{Number of decibels (dB)} = 10 \log_{10} \frac{P_{out}}{P_{in}}$$

$$= 20 \log_{10} \frac{V_{out}}{V_{in}}$$

where P_{out} = output power, P_{in} = input power, V_{out} = output voltage, and V_{in} = input voltage. The vertical scale is a logarithmic scale and is nonlinear when given in decibels.

Tape recorders designed for home use rarely have a flat frequency response over a wide range of frequencies. They are usually built to "sound good" rather than to accurately reproduce the input signal. Also, they have treble and bass controls so that you may change the sound. How these controls are set can have a very radical effect on the shape of the frequency response curve. In general this type of machine will not produce accurate reproductions and should be used with caution in scientific work if the information sought is contained in the waveshape of the signal. The frequency range of such recorders falls in the audio frequencies between 20 Hz and 20 kHz.

The input to the tape recorder may be generated by a microphone or some other type of transducer. If the signal is acoustic, a microphone will be needed. Unfortunately, the microphone adds one more element to the system that can produce poor frequency response characteristics. For example, it may not respond to the low and high frequencies that are to be measured. If so, poor or completely inadequate information may be recorded. The choice of microphone to be used with a particular recorder must be done carefully to ensure that it is compatible with the recorder in terms of matching impedance and frequency response. Instrument-quality microphones are expensive, costing as much as $700 or more. However, without the proper microphone, the highest-quality recorder will not give satisfactory results.

There are occasions when the scientist can get by with a relatively low-quality recorder, such as a two-track or four-track stereo recorder. These usually require ¼-in. wide magnetic tape, a tape cartridge, or a cassette tape. The tapes come in a wide range of qualities which are determined by their frequency response characteristics, background noise, print-through characteristics (tape on one layer magnetizing the adjacent layer of tape), lubrication (to reduce record-head wear), and storage characteristics. Carefully study the manufacturers' specifications and then try several types of tape to see if they will adequately serve your needs before purchasing large quantities of a particular brand and type. Recorders for scientific use may give specifications for the particular types of recording tape that should be used for your application.

Noise is always present in a tape recording. It cannot be eliminated completely because some of it is generated by the tape itself and is in the band of frequencies that is to be recorded. If the signal level is relatively small, noise may be very significant compared to the signal. In this case be sure to get a low-noise tape. Sometimes you may have some control over the noise, because it is generated in the playback recorder. If the signal is recorded at a low level, it may be necessary to use the maximum amplification of the playback amplifier. When this is done, the amplifier noise may become large enough compared to the signal to be objectionable. This problem may be eliminated by increasing the recording level when the recording is originally made. If the recording amplifiers are not noisy, the signal-to-noise ratio on the tape will be high, and lower amplification will be needed during playback. The noise of the playback amplifiers will be less objectionable than before. Noise can also be produced by dust on the tape. Figure 7.13 shows an oscillogram of the output of a recorder with a constant input. Note the nonuniformity of the signal in relation to time. The decreases in signal level are

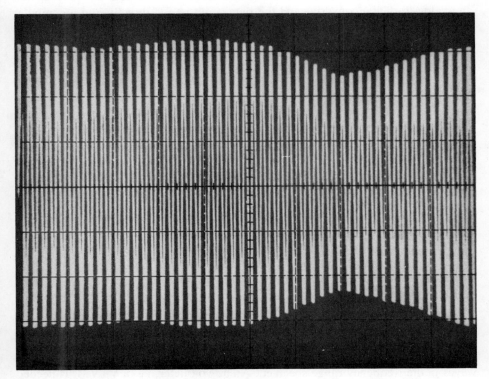

Fig. 7.13.   Effects of noise on the output of a constant-input tape recording.

heard as snaps and pops on the loudspeaker. They are probably caused by dirt on the tape. This dirt changes the spacing between the magnetic material and the recording or playback head. Another cause may be nonuniformity of the magnetic material on the tape as produced by the manufacturer. Obviously this type of noise is undesirable.

Distortion of signal amplitude, such as described above, can be very detrimental to an experiment. To overcome this problem, frequency-modulation (FM) tape recorders may be used. In these recorders the information contained in the amplitude of the signal is translated into various frequencies. These frequencies are recorded on the tape instead of the varying-amplitude signal. When amplitude noise appears on the tape, it has little effect on the output signal because the FM recorder is not sensitive to amplitude variations. The electronic device required to change amplitude into frequency is contained in the recorder. On the other hand, the recorder will change frequency back to amplitude so that the output signal from the recorder is the same as the original amplitude-varying input signal. In Example 7.6, where a strip-chart recorder was originally used to record the data, the experimenter found that an FM tape recorder was much more satisfactory because the output of the FM recorder could be played into an analog-to-digital converter and the data could be fed directly into a computer for analysis. The FM recorder had multichannels and provided accurate results.

Important points to remember

1. Make sure that the tape recorder has an adequate frequency response characteristic for the signal to be recorded.

2. Make sure that the input source, a microphone or some other transducer, is compatible with the recorder in terms of impedance and frequency.

3. Use a tape that has low noise and has adequate frequency response characteristics.

4. Keep the tape clean.

5. Make sure that the tape recorder has adequate tape-speed control.

Example 7.8   Measuring the response characteristics of a recorder.   A biologist has two tape recorders available and she would like to measure the frequency response characteristics of both at different settings of their tone controls. She would like to use the recorder with the flatter response in the frequency range of 500 Hz to 9 kHz. The response she needs is from the input of the recorder to the output terminals that are connected to the loudspeaker. How could she make the measurements?

Several pieces of equipment are required to make this test. A sinewave signal generator is needed which is capable of producing constant-amplitude sine waves in the frequency range specified. An ac voltmeter, i.e. a VTVM, is needed to measure the signal level. The system should be connected as shown in Fig. 7.14

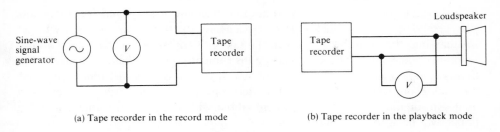

(a) Tape recorder in the record mode   (b) Tape recorder in the playback mode

Fig. 7.14. Monitoring the signal during recording and playback.

when the signal is being recorded. Set the signal generator at the desired frequency and then set the amplitude level of this signal such that a good recording (with no discernible distortion) is obtained with the tone controls set as desired. Measure the level of the input signal with the ac voltmeter. Change the frequency setting of the generator to the next frequency to be tested and leave the amplitude, as monitored with the ac voltmeter, unchanged. Make the recording of this frequency without changing any settings on the recorder. Repeat this process for as many frequencies as needed. This will ensure that the input signal level is the same for all frequencies. In each instance make a long enough recording so that you can get a good measurement of the recorded signal.

Next, set the recorder on playback and set the tone controls at the desired positions. At this point you probably will not know where these positions are. A little trial and error will be required. Once you have established a setting, do not change it until you have measured all the frequencies recorded when playing back the recording. This measurement is made by connecting the ac voltmeter across the terminals of the loudspeaker connected to the recorder. At each frequency make an output measurement. Plot these output voltages against frequency on a graph paper. If these points indicate a horizontal line with respect to the frequency axis, then the response is said to be flat. Chances are that this will not happen.

Paper-tape Recorders

Some digital readout instruments have an output that can be used to operate a paper-tape punch. The data are punched onto the paper tape, so that they may be used at a later date. The information on the tape can be reproduced by a typewriter with a paper-tape reader, such as those commonly used with digital computers. The rate at which data can be recorded is determined by the punching speed of the particular recorder. It is essential that the rate at which you are generating the data does not exceed the maximum input rate allowable for the particular recorder.

This method of recording has the special advantage that the data are in the proper form to be used by a computer; it has no need for manually keying in the data that have been read visually from an instrument or strip-chart recorder output. The computer can quickly perform whatever operations are necessary to get the data into the form the user needs. To take full advantage of these capabilities, you must make sure that the measuring instruments you purchase have an output that is compatible with a paper-tape punch. If the measuring instrument provides an analog output and does not have an appropriate digital output signal, an analog-to-digital converter that is compatible with both the instrument and the punch will have to be obtained.

7.9   OSCILLOSCOPES

The *oscilloscope* is a key instrument in many laboratories where electrical measurements are made. It is an instrument primarily for making visible the instantaneous values of one or more rapidly varying electrical quantities as a function of time or of another electrical or mechanical quantity. There are two major types of oscilloscopes: general-purpose oscilloscopes and storage oscilloscopes. The general-purpose oscilloscope will display a voltage waveform whenever an electrical signal is present at the input terminals. The display is on the screen of a cathode-ray tube (CRT). The storage oscilloscope is capable of storing or retaining the display on the screen of a storage CRT after the signal has vanished from the input to the oscilloscope. This storage feature is a definite advantage. On the other hand, storage oscilloscopes are more expensive than general-purpose ones. A storage oscilloscope is shown in Fig. 7.15.

The CRT screen is the display element of the oscilloscope and is in the upper left-hand corner of the instrument in Fig. 7.15. The screen is marked with horizontal and vertical lines so that waveforms can be easily measured on the screen. The CRT is similar to a TV picture tube in that an *electron* beam is used to strike the screen of the tube to produce light. The position of the beam is controlled by signals that are fed into the horizontal- and vertical-axis amplifiers. The position of the beam is varied in proportion to these two signals. The vertical signal causes the beam to move up and down, while the horizontal signal causes the beam to move along the horizontal axis. As these voltages vary, the beam moves across the face of the screen and traces out a path of light. Figure 7.13 shows a waveform produced in this way. It is a photograph of a voltage waveform that was displayed on the screen of a CRT in an oscilloscope.

The picture produced by an oscilloscope is similar to that produced by an *X-Y* recorder. The major difference lies in the fact that the pen can move only relatively slowly, whereas the electron beam can move very rapidly. In special-purpose oscilloscopes, the beam may move as fast as 1 cm in 500 picosec.

There are controls to set the intensity of the light the beam produces on the screen and the focus of the spot size of the beam. When the horizontal amplifier is connected to a time-base generator, the beam can be made to sweep across the

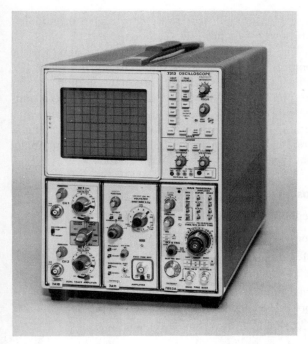

Fig. 7.15. Storage oscilloscope with plug-in units.

screen from left to right to trace out a line of light. A single trace across the screen can be made as a result of a single triggering of the time-base generator. Periodic sweeps can be made to display waveforms by periodically triggering the time-base generator. When the period of this sweep is the same as the period of the incoming signal to the vertical amplifier, a stationary waveform is displayed on the screen. This is the usual way of using the oscilloscope to display a periodic waveform. Fig. 7.16 shows the blocks of the oscilloscope that provide these features.

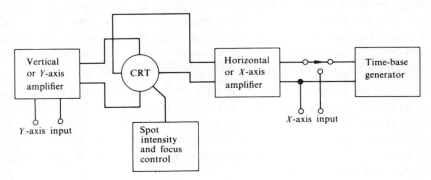

Fig. 7.16.   Simplified block diagram of an oscilloscope.

Most high-quality general-purpose oscilloscopes are constructed in modules. The main frame consists of power supplies, the cathode-ray tube, the spot intensity, and focus controls. The frame has provisions for plug-in units for the horizontal- and vertical-axes inputs. The oscilloscope shown in Fig. 7.15 is of this type. The bottom half of the instrument has space for three plug-in units. In this model the individual units are numbered 7A18, 7A11, and 7B53A. These units can be pulled out individually and replaced with other units. The main frame may also include a time-base generator if there is no provision for this to be a plug-in unit. This plug-in feature allows you to select an input unit that has the capability needed to display the particular type of signal that you wish to study.

The General-purpose Oscilloscope

The general-purpose oscilloscope has the following capabilities:

1. It will display periodic time-varying voltage waveforms.
2. It will accept input signal voltages from about 10 mV to 500 V. Special units are available for voltages as small as 10 μV or as large as 12 kV.
3. It will provide a time scale ranging from 1-μsec/division to 12-sec/division or longer. Special units provide a time scale as small as 500 picosec/division.
4. It can be used to display X-Y plots of two time-varying voltages.
5. It may be able to display two to four time-varying voltage waveforms simultaneously if multitrace input amplifiers are available for the oscilloscope. A few of the oscilloscopes have a dual-beam CRT, so that two simultaneous, independently driven traces can be displayed.

The operation of this type of oscilloscope is described below. General-purpose oscilloscopes are sufficient for displaying most of the electrical signals that are measured.

General operation of an oscilloscope.   The use of an oscilloscope to its fullest capacity requires that you carefully study the manufacturer's operating manual to learn how to use the special features of the particular model you will be operating. The following steps provide a very brief introduction to some of the major controls that must be adjusted to obtain a useful display on the screen.

1. Turn on the power and adjust the intensity and focus control so as to get a small bright spot on the screen. If the spot is too bright, the screen may be damaged by the burning of the phosphor coating. It may be necessary to turn the horizontal and vertical position controls to bring the spot onto the screen.
2. Turn the horizontal and vertical position controls to move the spot or line to the desired position on the screen.
3. Connect the signal to be observed to the vertical input terminals.

4. Set the vertical amplifier *deflection factor* control to the appropriate v/div position so the signal to be displayed will fill one quarter to three quarters or more of the screen. (The deflection factor is the ratio of the input signal amplitude to the resultant displacement of the indicating spot on the screen of the CRT.)

5. Set the sweep trigger control to the appropriate position.

   (a) Free running: The beam makes a sweep across the screen and then automatically repeats the sweep without reference to the input signal. This usually produces traces that look like a jumble of lines and may not be useful.

   (b) Internal trigger: The beam is started at a particular time that is related to the voltage level of the signal being observed. This voltage may be selected to be a positive or a negative voltage of various magnitudes, depending on the setting of the controls. This setting will produce traces that overlap one another so that a stationary waveform appears.

   (c) External trigger: The beam is started at a particular time that is related to the time that a trigger signal is applied to the external trigger input of the oscilloscope. If repetitive trigger signals occur, repetitive sweeps will be produced.

   (d) Single sweep: In response to a single-trigger signal a single sweep of the beam is produced. No further sweeps will occur until the trigger circuit is activated again.

6. Adjust the time-base-rate control to give the appropriate sec/div sweep rate of the beam so the detail of the waveform can be observed.

7. Readjust the vertical-amplifier setting and the time-base setting so as to make the waveform observed larger or smaller in amplitude and expanded or compressed in time as desired.

Figure 7.17 shows an example of the CRT display when the triggering controls are not synchronized with the sine wave being viewed, giving rise to multiple traces.

The Storage Oscilloscope

There are many occasions when a signal appears only briefly; it is not periodic so that the image that is presented on the screen of a general-purpose oscilloscope cannot last any longer than the persistence of the phosphor used on the screen. This results in an image of very short duration. It is difficult to study such a short-lived visual image. The *storage oscilloscope* is designed to overcome this limitation and to make available the capability of retaining displayed waveforms for a long time.

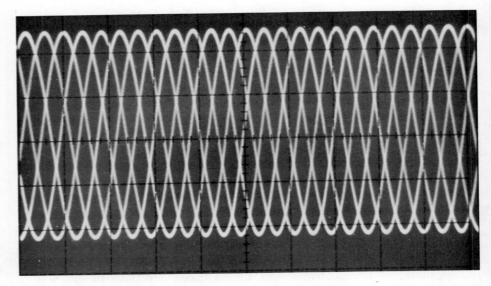

Fig. 7.17. Oscilloscope waveform of a sine wave when the sweep is not synchronized with the sine wave.

All of the features of the general-purpose oscilloscope are present in the storage oscilloscope. The only difference is the latter's ability to retain the image on the screen. This feature enables you to view a transient signal for a long period of time; it enables you to trace out two or more signals simultaneously or separately so that they may be retained for study and comparison.

The operation of the storage oscilloscope is the same as that described above, except for the storage controls. There are three different ways of using this type of oscilloscope. The oscilloscope may be put in the nonstored mode, in which the screen displays signals exactly as viewed on a general-purpose oscilloscope. The stored mode is the second way of using the storage oscilloscope. The screen of the storage CRT is split so that the upper and lower halves may be used independently in the stored mode. In this mode you can display single-shot signals (those that occur only once) by means of the storage feature. The trace can be placed in the upper or lower half of the screen or in both halves. When the trace is no longer needed, you push the erase button and the screen is cleared and made ready for the next trace which can be initiated as desired by an appropriate triggering operation. When using the oscilloscope in this way, it is possible to store one trace on the top half of the screen and then store a second trace on the bottom half of the screen so that they may be compared. One or the other or both may be erased when no longer needed.

The third way of using the storage oscilloscope is to operate it in the auto-erase mode. In this mode the signal is stored for display for a preset period of time and then is automatically erased and a second trace is produced by the triggering signal. The viewing time may be set for the length of time desired depending on the waves being studied. There are other special features available on storage oscilloscopes and these should be sought out from the manufacturers.

Horizontal-axis Plug-in Options

Time-base plug-in. The most common unit used to drive the beam in the horizontal direction is the time-base generator. (See the lower right-hand plug-in unit in Fig. 7.15 and also Fig. 7.18.) This generator causes the beam to repetitively move linearly across the screen. The rate at which the beam sweeps across the screen can be controlled by a knob with 25 positions ranging from 0.05-μsec/div to 5-sec/div. The screen may be 10 divisions wide. Oscilloscopes that have time-base plug-in units may utilize several different plug-ins that can be picked for specific applications. For example, one plug-in may have a range of 0.1-μsec/div to 1-sec/div in 22 knob positions. Another plug-in may have a range of 50-nanosec/div to 1-sec/div in 23 knob positions with a "times 100" expander which magnifies the waveform on the screen.

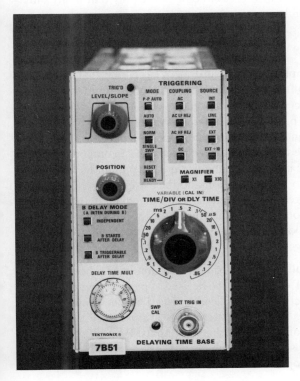

Fig. 7.18. Horizontal-axis time-base plug-in unit.

Another type of plug-in may have a delayed-sweep generator with 23 different sweep rates. This delayed-sweep generator is convenient to have when you want to start the sweep at some specified time after a trigger signal is received. For example, a periodic trigger may indicate the initiating of a specific event which will not occur for 10 msec. When the specific event does occur, its duration is only 10 μsec long. The variations of the signal are not to be observed during the 10-msec interval because they might be misinterpreted to be the specific signal. In this case the delay time could be set to 10 msec and the sweep rate for the delayed sweep set at 2-μsec/div. Good resolution would be obtained for the 10-μsec interval of the specific signal.

Horizontal-axis amplifier.   If the oscilloscope is to be used as an X-Y-display unit, an amplifier input must be available for the horizontal deflection system. Some oscilloscopes have such an input terminal associated with the time-base generator, but the amplifier may have different characteristics than the vertical-axis amplifier and thus may produce phase errors between the two signals being studied.

Other oscilloscopes have provisions for plugging in an appropriate amplifier in place of the time-base unit. In this case an amplifier with similar characteristics to the vertical amplifier can be used. There is a variety of amplifiers available. The details of these will be given in the next section. Suffice it to say that many different deflection factors are available.

Vertical-axis Plug-in Options

Basic amplifier.   The basic amplifier, shown in Fig. 7.19, is one that provides a beam-positioning control, a control to provide a variable-deflection factor, and a single input for either ac or dc. The ac input setting will not pass the dc component to be displayed but will pass the ac portion of the signal. The dc input setting will pass both ac and dc signals to be displayed. This is a convenient feature if the input signal contains a large dc component and a small ac component. If the major point of interest is the ac component, the dc component can be blocked or rejected by setting the control to the ac position and then using a small deflection factor setting to produce a large display of the small ac signal. If these adjustments were not made, the dc component would produce the larger displacement on the screen and the ac component would produce a very small displacement which would be hard to view accurately.

Dual-trace and four-trace amplifiers.   The dual-trace amplifier, shown in Fig. 7.20, enables a single-beam CRT oscilloscope to be used to produce two apparently simultaneous traces across the screen. This is accomplished by electronic switching circuits in the plug-in unit. Two signal-input terminals are provided on the unit. There are separate positioning controls for each of the inputs. Four different modes of operation are possible. The signal from channel 1 or channel 2 can be displayed by itself. This mode of operation allows you to use the oscilloscope as a

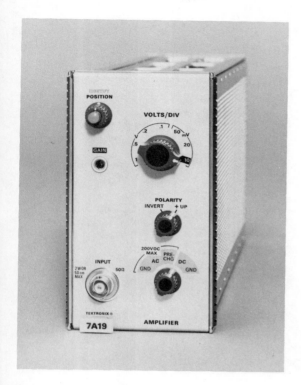

Fig. 7.19. Basic vertical-axis plug-in unit.

single-trace oscilloscope. All of the features of the basic amplifier are present.

In the second mode of operation, the *alternate* mode, the two input signals are displayed for a complete sweep across the screen on an alternating basis. First, a complete sweep is made with the channel 1 signal causing deflection of the beam. Then the beam is automatically displaced by a set amount as controlled by a positioning knob and the channel 2 signal is displayed on the next sweep of the beam. This mode of operation is repeated automatically so that there appear to be two simultaneous traces. Since the two traces are not occurring at exactly the same time, the time relation between the two signals may be lost. This error can be corrected by following the manufacturer's operating instructions for triggering.

The third mode of operation is called the *chopped* mode. In this mode the two input signals are displayed alternately within one sweep of the beam; i.e., channel 1 is displayed for 5 μsec and then channel 2 is displayed for 5 μsec and then channel 1 is displayed for 5 μsec, and so forth until the end of the sweep time. So long as the period of the sweep is very much longer than the 5 μsec, both signals will appear to be presented simultaneously and the time relationship between them is retained. In reality a series of dots of light make up each trace; but when these dots are close enough together, they appear to be a continuous line.

The fourth mode of operation is called the *added* mode. In this mode the two

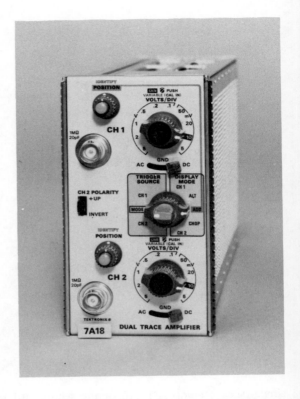

Fig. 7.20. Dual-trace plug-in unit.

input signals can be added or subtracted from each other and the sum or difference is displayed on the screen.

The four-trace amplifier operates on the same general principle as the two-trace amplifier, except that the beam is switched through four input signal channels. It provides the option to display one, two, three, or four signals on a chopped or alternate mode of operation.

Differential amplifier. A *differential amplifier* is one whose output signal is proportional to the algebraic difference between two input signals. A plug-in unit with this capability is shown in Fig. 7.21. With this unit it is possible to display difference signals as small as 10 μv while operating with a deflection factor of 10 μv/div. The figure-of-merit for the differential amplifier is called the common-mode-rejection ratio. The term "common mode" refers to signals that are identical with respect to both amplitude and time. Common-mode rejection refers to the ability of a differential amplifier to reject the common-mode signals of the two inputs and not display them on the screen. The common-mode-rejection ratio is the ratio of the amplitude of the common-mode input signal to the amplitude of the difference signal displayed on the CRT screen. A high ratio is desirable.

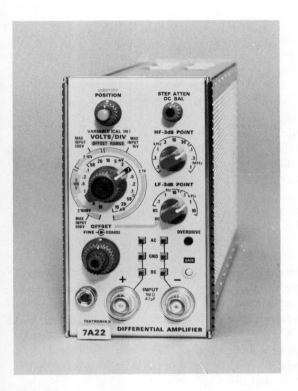

Fig. 7.21. Differential amplifier plug-in unit.

Operational amplifier.   The operational amplifier plug-in unit can be used to perform the operations of differentiation and integration. (Refer to Section 12.2 for a discussion of operational amplifiers.) In addition, it can be used to generate functions or perform linear or nonlinear amplification. The output of this unit is displayed on the CRT screen.

Other amplifier options.   There are other plug-in amplifiers available for special purposes, for example the dual-trace differential amplifier, the differential comparitor, and the transducer amplifier. Please refer to the manufacturer's information sheets for specifications and applications of any or all of the amplifiers introduced above.

Probes

The signal from the circuit being tested can be connected to the oscilloscope input with a pair of wires, one to the ground side of the signal source and the other to the signal terminal. At low frequencies almost any pair of wires will perform adequately if the insulation rating of the wire exceeds the voltage that will be applied to the wire. However, if the frequency of the signal is in the order of hundreds of kilohertz per second or higher, there is the possibility of measurement errors. Oscilloscope manufacturers provide probes, which are to be used to connect the signal to the oscilloscope. These probes are designed to match the input characteristics of the oscilloscope amplifiers and provide optimum performance.

The probes provide a convenient means of connecting onto a signal terminal or to touch a variety of electrical points in a circuit during a test. Each probe has an insulated handle that is designed to protect the user from electrical shocks. The probes are designed to either let the signal pass directly to the oscilloscope with no attenuation in amplitude or attenuate the signal by a factor of 10 or more before it enters the oscilloscope amplifier input. The latter probe is called a "times ten" or "× 10" probe. The × 10 probe can be used to measure voltages that are larger than the oscilloscope could normally display on the highest deflection factor setting. A × 1 probe should be used when measuring small voltages that require the smallest deflection factor setting. Other probes are available up to × 1000 ratings.

So far the only type of signal that has been discussed with respect to oscilloscopes is the voltage signal. Current can be measured by displaying the voltage across a resistor in series with the branch current in question. The actual current is equal to the voltage, as measured from the CRT screen, divided by the resistance. There may be occasions in which a resistor is not in the circuit or it is inconvenient to insert a resistor. Current probes are available that are designed for use with oscilloscopes. They have a tip that clips over the wire in which the desired current is flowing. A magnetic field is set up by the current which is sensed by the probe and converted into a voltage that the oscilloscope is capable of displaying. Sensitivities from 1-mA/div up to 1000-A/div are available in different probe models. Some current probes measure only ac currents, while others measure both ac and dc currents. The electric circuit that is being tested does not have to be broken by the insertion of a resistor when this probe is used; this is a very convenient feature.

Example 7.9   Transient display of sound generated by a small animal.   A zoology student is studying the sounds produced by small animals. She suspects that one particular species is capable of making sounds that are above the audible range for humans and decides to set up an experiment to detect these sounds. She then has the problem of figuring out what type of measurement system she should use and how to perform the experiment. One proposal for a system is shown in Fig. 7.22.

A general-purpose oscilloscope is used to display the signal picked up by a microphone. It is very likely that the signal level will be very low, so that a preamplifier matched to the impedance of the microphone must be used. The microphone must have a frequency response that is flat in the range of interest. One is chosen with a flat frequency response from 30 Hz to 140 kHz, in the hope that the frequency in question is in this range. The output of the preamplifier is connected

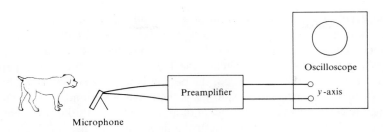

Microphone

Fig. 7.22. Measurement system for detecting signals above the audible range.

to the vertical input amplifier of the oscilloscope. This combination makes up the measurement system.

The microphone is placed near the animal and the time-base controls are set to provide a slow repetitive sweep with a time scale of 1 sec/div. The vertical amplifier control is set to a level where the general room noise causes the beam to be deflected by less than a division. If the background noise in the room is too large, a quieter place must be used in which to make the measurement. As the sweep moves across the screen, the observer must look to see if there are any deflections that might be produced by the animal but not heard by the observer. The observer has no idea when the animal may make the sound, so it may take quite a long time to ascertain whether or not such a sound is being produced. It may be necessary to increase the sensitivity and decrease the deflection factor of the oscilloscope, because the level of the sound may not be sufficient to produce an observable deflection at the first setting of the vertical amplifier controls. Another problem is that the duration of the sound may be so short that with a sweep rate of 1 sec/div the signal will not be visible. In the latter case the sweep speed will have to be increased.

Assume that the following happens. A small vertical displacement of the beam is noted but cannot be heard by the observer. The displacement looks just like a vertical line of almost no width. Once the signal is observed, the sweep speed should be increased, which will magnify the horizontal dimension of the wave. The wave will probably be somewhat sinusoidal in shape for a short period of time. One period of this oscillation can be measured along the time scale on the screen. (The frequency of a sine wave is the reciprocal of the period of the wave.) The animal may produce sporadic bursts of sine waves, as is typical of the waveform of the audible sound emitted by crickets.

The major limitation of the procedure described above is that the image of the signal is not retained on the screen. It is a transient presentation. This example shows the advantage of having a storage oscilloscope to retain the transient waveshapes for study. Furthermore, this example gives some clues as to the use of an oscilloscope but does not introduce the finer points of its operation.

Example 7.10   Detailed observation of a delayed reaction.   The reaction time and the character of the reaction of a human being to a light stimulus is to be determined. The problem is this. A light is located to the right of the person being tested. When he looks straight ahead, the light is just visible to the peripheral vision. If the light is switched on red, the person is to press a foot pedal hard and rapidly. If the light is orange, he is to press the pedal softly and slowly. The pedal is designed to respond like a brake pedal of an automobile. Initial study has shown that the delay between the turning on of the light and the onset of the response is relatively long compared to the duration of the response. What type of measurement system may be used?

One system is shown in Fig. 7.23. The switch that is used to turn on the light also provides a triggering voltage that is connected to the trigger input of the oscilloscope. The light and the trigger voltage come on at the same instant. A linear potentiometer is connected to a voltage source and the tap position is determined by the position of the pedal. This tap is connected to the vertical input of the oscilloscope. The farther down the pedal is pushed, the higher is the voltage delivered to the vertical input of the oscilloscope. The rate at which the pedal is pushed determines the rate at which the voltage at the tap changes. This voltage causes the beam of the CRT to move in direct proportion to the pedal position.

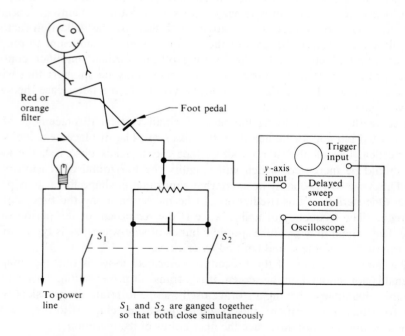

Fig. 7.23.   System for measuring delayed reaction.

The experiment may be done in two steps.

1. Set the sweep time on a relatively slow rate. Turn on the light and watch the beam move across the screen as a result of the triggering of the sweep. When the pedal is pushed in response to the light going on, a sharp rise of the beam will be observed. Very likely this rise will be almost a step-change in beam position. The time period between the beginning of the sweep and the step is the delay time. Very little detail of the rate of change of pedal position can be observed by means of the beam's step-change.

2. Knowing the delay time, it is possible to set a delay time on the oscilloscope. Arbitrarily pick a delay time, say three quarters of that measured. The sweep time can now be set at a higher rate than before. This will have a magnifying effect on the waveform observed and make it easier to ascertain the fine details of the rate at which the pedal is moved. Now repeat the sequence of turning on the light and observing the trace on the CRT screen. Instead of seeing a step-change this time, you should see a finite slope. This is the desired detail. Note that the total delay time is the sum of the delay time set on the oscilloscope and the delay time measured on the screen. Figure 7.24 shows an anticipated result.

The disadvantage of this system is that a transient response is being observed. A second proposal for the measurement system would be to use a split-screen storage oscilloscope. The rest of the system could be as in Fig. 7.23. With the storage oscilloscope it would be possible to retain the image of the pedal response on the screen. After one response has been obtained and stored, a second response could be induced by the same or a different colored light. This response could also be stored so that a comparison could be made between the two responses. Such responses could be correlated with alcohol content in the person's blood in a study to determine the effect of alcohol on reaction time and character.

7.10 ELECTRONIC COUNTERS

There are many situations in which the experimenter must count the number of events that occur, accurately measure the frequency of events, or measure the time

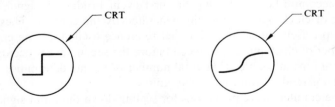

(a) Response with slow sweep rate   (b) Response with fast sweep rate

Fig. 7.24. Anticipated waveshapes for delayed-response measurement.

interval between two events. The *electronic counter* is an instrument designed to make these types of measurements as well as others. The counter may be fabricated in modules consisting of a main frame and snap-on or plug-in units. The main frame provides part of the electronics and the display panel. The numerical value of the function desired is shown in digital form on the display panel. This panel may produce numbers by electronically lighting up appropriate light-emitting diodes. There may also be provisions for direct connection of the digital output to a digital recorder that will print out a permanent record of the count. The snap-on or plug-in units provide the particular counter or timer characteristics needed. This type of construction allows for the expansion of measurement capabilities at relatively low cost.

The input to the counter must be an electrical signal related to the event being counted. The signal must change from a value below a specified threshold level to a value above this level for each event to be counted. This threshold level, or sensitivity, is given in the manufacturer's specifications for the counter. The sensitivity value is the minimum countable signal level. The input impedance of the counter and the output impedance of the source affect the level of voltage that appears at the input to the counter. (Refer to Sections 2.5 and 9.2 for a discussion of coupling problems such as this.)

The frequency of a signal is determined by counting the number of times the signal exceeds the threshold value during a specified unit of time called the gate time. The gate time is usually selectable and may have values of 0.1, 1, or 10 sec. In the auto position, the gate time is usually 1 sec. If there were 440 counts in 1 sec, a 440-Hz readout would appear on the display unit. If the same source was measured over a period of 10 sec and there were 4422 counts, the display unit would show 442.2 Hz.

The counter may be used to take the sum of the events that generate a signal exceeding the threshold value. The summation mode is started by manually turning on the gate with a start-stop switch and stopped by manually turning off the gate with the switch. There may be a provision for the gate to be turned on and off by an externally generated electrical gate signal. Thus you can control the time interval over which the count is added up.

The time interval between two events can be measured by some counters. This is accomplished by having the first event produce a signal that starts the counting of clock pulses internally generated by the counter. These clock pulses are very precisely timed by an internal reference oscillator. The counter registers the number of clock pulses produced before the second event occurs to produce a stop signal for the counter. The total number of counts determines the time interval, which is read out on the display unit.

Some counters have provisions for scaling down the input signal. This means that the counter divides the number of input counts by powers of 10, up to 10^9, for certain units. The scaled output is made available at a terminal on the unit.

7.11   REVIEW QUESTIONS AND PROBLEMS

7.1   A manufacturer of a D'Arsonval type meter states that the deviation of any readings will be ±3% of the full-scale reading. For example, if the full-scale reading is 10 V, the error may be ±0.3 V regardless of the indicator needle position. (a) For this meter, what range of voltages can be expected if the needle points to 9 V? (b) What range of voltages can be expected if the needle points to 2.4 V? (c) What is the percentage error (deviation between the indicated value and the actual value) of each of these readings if in both cases the needle is at its lowest position relative to the ±3% rating? Is the percentage error the same regardless of the voltage being read?

7.2   An experiment requires the measurement of a dc current that ranges from 4 to 11 mA. A dc ammeter with a 0 to 1 mA scale is available in the laboratory. The resistance of the meter is 20 Ω. The meter movement is rated to be accurate to within ±3% of full-scale reading. Modify this meter so that it can be used to measure the current required in this experiment. Draw the circuit diagram and show the values required of all the components that are added to the milliammeter. What tolerances are allowable for the components added to the milliammeter if the current readings are to be within ±5% of the actual value?

7.3   A measurement of a dc voltage must be made. A standard D'Arsonval meter movement with a one mA full-scale reading and internal resistance of 20 Ω is available. Modify this meter so a voltage of 4 V across the modified meter will cause full-scale deflection of the needle of the meter. Draw the circuit diagram and show all component values.

7.4   Design a series ohmmeter that can be used to measure resistances in the range from 500 to 1000 Ω. A zero- to 1-mA meter with an internal resistance of 20 Ω and standard flashlight batteries of 1.5 V each are available for use in this ohmmeter. Draw the circuit diagram and show all component values. Draw a picture of the meter scale and show where 500, 600, 700, 800, 900 and 1000 Ω should be indicated on the scale.

7.5   A zero- to 100-volt dc voltmeter is to be constructed using a zero to 1 mA dc meter movement and other appropriate components. Assume the meter is rated to be accurate to within ±5% of full-scale reading. Assume any resistors that are used have values which are within ±10% of their rated value. What is the maximum error in reading that could occur if the needle points to the midpoint on the scale when an unknown voltage is applied across the terminals of the voltmeter?

7.6   A circuit has been set up to measure the light intensity at the surface of a leaf. The output resistance (the internal resistance) of the circuit that produces the voltage being measured is found to be 50 kΩ. An electronic voltmeter with an input resistance of 10 MΩ is connected across the voltage source and a voltage of 100 mV is read. The voltmeter is disconnected. A chart recorder is connected across the voltage source so any slowly varying voltage can be displayed resulting from changes in light intensity. The chart recorder instruction manual indicates that the input resistance to the recorder is 100 kΩ. The chart recorder indicates only 66.7 mV for the same light intensity that was present when the voltmeter reading was taken. Why might these different readings occur?

7.7   Describe the functions of and the similarities between an X-Y recorder and a cathode-ray oscilloscope.

7.8   Describe the major differences between an X-Y recorder and a cathode-ray oscilloscope. Under what conditions would you use each of these instruments?

7.9   What function does the sweep circuit perform in a cathode-ray oscilloscope?

7.10 What do the terms, "free running," "internal trigger," and "external trigger" mean as related to a cathode-ray oscilloscope?

7.11 What effect does an improperly adjusted sweep synchronization control have on the picture seen on the screen of a cathode-ray oscilloscope?

7.12 Under what conditions would a storage oscilloscope be more desirable to use than a regular cathode-ray oscilloscope or an X-Y recorder?

7.13 What characteristics of a magnetic tape recorder should be considered by the entomologist who wants to get a faithful reproduction of the chirps of a cricket? Why are these characteristics important?

7.14 What are the major differences between a strip-chart recorder and an X-Y recorder?

8
biotelemetry

8.1 OBJECTIVES

The purpose of this chapter is to provide the reader with an overview of bio-telemetric measurement systems so that he can determine if a system of this type will be a useful tool in his research. The subject is very extensive and is given in detail in reference [27] by Mackay. He was one of the early pioneers of biotelemetric measurement systems and has spent much of his time engaged in developing and using these systems.

The chief advantage of using the biotelemetric measurement system is to avoid the disruption of the normal pattern of life of an animal while gathering data on its behavior, pulse rate, temperature, chemistry, or some other phenomena of interest. Data can be collected at some distance from the tested animal by use of an appropriate receiver. The experimenter need not be within sight of the animal being tested.

As was pointed out in Chapter 1, a biotelemetric measurement system consists of a transmitter, a transducer, a transmitting antenna, a receiving antenna, a receiver, and display devices. In some cases the receiver may be the display device. In many instances the transducer and the transmitter are placed inside the body of the experimental animal either through the mouth or by a surgical implant. In other cases the transmitter is external and is often fastened to the animal on a collarlike device. When the transmitter is external, there may or may not be a transducer involved in the system. When no transducer is used, the measurement system is often designed to be used as a tracking device. A signal is transmitted continuously so that the animal wearing the transmitter can be effectively tracked over large distances.

In the sections which follow, the various parts of the biotelemetric measurement system are introduced with indications of some of the things that can be done with such a system.

8.2 TRANSDUCERS AND SIGNAL GENERATION

A transducer, if used, is the first device in a biotelemetric system. This device produces an electrical signal that is related to the phenomena being measured. If one surveys the literature on transducers used in biotelemetric systems, he will find that they are usually developed or designed with specific applications in mind. Therefore, only those transducers which have relatively general applications will be discussed here. For information on other transducers, refer to Chapter 6. For the most part, transducers are used to measure one or more of the following parameters: pressure, temperature, chemical change, and movement.

Pressure

Several devices have been developed to record pressure. Some involve the displacement of a part of the transducer so that the electrical property of the transducer changes. Such a pressure transducer is designed so that when it is activated, a stable electrical circuit is changed. For example, when pressure is applied to the transducer, the inductance of the transducer is changed and thus the current flow through the inductor changes as a function of the pressure. If a force is exerted on a spring-loaded plunger which, when depressed, will push an iron rod through the center of or near an inductor or coil, the inductance will change. Thus physical displacement will modify an electrical circuit.

If one desires to measure the peristaltic movement within the intestine of a rabbit, the plunger type pressure transducer might be used. Since this would involve a measurement inside the animal body, the transducer or the transducer in combination with a transmitter could be inserted into a rabbit through the mouth. Changes in other electrical parameters may also be used to measure pressure.

Temperature

Some transducers used to measure temperature are well known and have been used for some time in the laboratory. They are the thermocouple, and more recently, the thermistor. These two devices can be manufactured in extremely small sizes. One of these two devices is often chosen as a transducer for the detection of temperature changes in an animal.

Another device used to detect temperature change may not be considered a true transducer because it is an integral part of a transmitter circuit. This device is a temperature-sensitive transistor. If a transistor of this type is used in a transmitter circuit, the change in its characteristics due to temperature change will cause the circuit performance to be altered in some way; for example, a change in the frequency generated by the circuit may occur. Once this circuit has been calibrated, temperature variations can be easily detected by measuring the frequency received from the circuit. We might regard this as an oscillatory transducer. For example, if a transmitter using a temperature-sensitive germanium transistor is designed to emit a pulse signal, there will be a distinctive time interval between each pulse for every temperature. An elapsed time between pulses will be known and can be correlated with a specific temperature before the transmitter is placed in the animal. The transmitter will be calibrated at this time. When temperature changes, the pulse rate or the time interval between pulses will change. The relation between the changes in temperature and in pulse rate may or may not be linear, but in either case, temperature may be determined by measuring pulse rate or the time interval between pulses.

Chemical Change

One of the major uses of the third type of transducer is to measure pH changes. Transducers to measure pH changes, like the thermocouple and thermistor, have been standard laboratory equipment for some time. A pH meter utilizes a glass electrode commonly filled with silver chloride. If this electrode is made small enough, it can be readily used as a pH transducer in a biotelemetric system. For example, if one desires to measure the pH changes in the stomach of a rabbit, a pH electrode attached to a transmitter might be designed so that the whole package is small enough for the rabbit to swallow.

Gases may also be detected by using other electrode transducers. For example, platinum wire may be used as a cathode to detect differences in oxygen levels within the blood.

The transducers discussed above are commonly used in telemetric measurement systems. Other transducers or modifications of the above have been designed for specific applications. Imagination fueled by need will produce many more. Transducers, like transmitters, are often custom designed for specific measurement problems.

8.3   TRANSMITTERS

There are nearly as many different types of transmitter designs as there are transducers. Therefore, only a basic type of transmitter and some modifications will be discussed in this chapter. For many applications in biotelemetric measurement systems, the transmitter must be extremely small. It must also be stable; that is, the transmitted frequency should not vary unless controlled by the transducer. In a frequency modulation system the frequency is continually varying in a specified way unless controlled by the transducer. In either case, the only thing that can cause variation in the operation of the circuit should be the transducer.

The transmitter is affixed to the test animal in one of three ways: externally on the animal, swallowed by the animal, and surgically implanted somewhere in the body of the test animal.

If the transmitter is to be swallowed or implanted, certain precautions must be taken. The transmitter must be sealed inside a material that will prevent body fluid or gastrointestinal chemicals from contacting the transmitter and destroying it. Animal tissue reactions to a foreign body which will result in the destruction of the transmitter must also be guarded against. Several methods have been attempted to prevent the transmitters from being destroyed. They involve the encapsulation of the transmitters with one or more of the following materials: a beeswax-paraffin mixture, teflon, silastic plastic, and a medical grade of silicone rubber material. The beeswax-paraffin coating will prevent moisture from reaching the transmitter, while teflon, silastic, or the medical-grade silicone rubber coating will prevent the transmitter from being chemically destroyed. The choice of the encapsulating material depends on the material's ability to withstand the degradation processes of the animal body tissues and the compatibility of the material with this tissue; an incompatible material will elicit tissue reaction, which will invalidate the experiment. Once the transmitter has been encapsulated with a satisfactory material, it then must be sterilized to eliminate pathogens. Zephiran chloride has been used as a successful sterilant. The sealed transmitter is usually soaked overnight in a Zephiran chloride solution of 1:1000. If the transmitter is designed to measure parameters inside the gastrointestinal tract, it is usually disguised in a food source so as to be swallowed by the animal. The surgical procedures required to implant the transmitter in other parts of the body are straightforward and will not be discussed here.

Before a transmitter is encapsulated, it should be tested for a sufficiently long time for the stability of its operation. When it has been encapsulated, it should be retested to ensure that the encapsulation process has not in any way changed the operation of the transmitter. If a defect is found after encapsulation, it may be feasible to remove the plastic and repair the transmitter. When it is time to remove an implanted transmitter from the animal, surgical procedures will again be required. The transmitter that is swallowed will usually pass through the gastrointestinal tract and be recovered.

Two transmitter circuits and their uses will indicate to the reader the simplicity of the basic circuits. These two circuits are reproduced from Reference 27. Let us assume that we wish to measure a temperature and would like to do this by generating a signal that is related to temperature. A blocking-oscillator transmitter will produce a signal that sounds like clicks on a standard AM radio. The rate at which the clicks occur is dependent on the temperature. Changes in the resistance of the thermistor will cause changes in the output signal from the transmitter. If the thermistor is calibrated at a specific temperature, a specific rate of clicks will be observed corresponding to that temperature. Deviations from the standard calibrated temperature will cause changes in the click rate noted at the receiver. The clicks can be timed with a stopwatch if they are slow enough or be counted with an electronic counter which is connected to the speaker of the radio. A usable transmitter for this job is shown in Fig. 8.1.

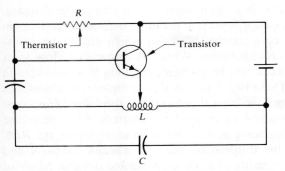

Fig. 8.1. A simple transmitter circuit for transmitting temperature data.

The components in combination, L, C, and $R_{\text{thermistor}}$ constitute an RLC circuit. When power is applied to the circuit, a radio signal is radiated from the coil L and may be received at a distance several feet away up to more than one hundred feet away, depending on the particular environment and the power output of the transmitter. The specific output that will be transmitted is determined by the values of L, C, and $R_{\text{thermistor}}$. If the value of one of the components, such as $R_{\text{thermistor}}$, is changed, the oscillations will change. The combination of R, L, and C occurs in almost all transmitters. The frequency that is generated by such a combination of components is called the resonant frequency of the transmitter.

It must now be clear that the basis of the transmitter is an RLC circuit of some type, and that any change in one or more of the devices in the RLC circuit will result in a frequency change. This phenomenon makes for a useful device in biotelemetric measurement systems. A transmitter similar to that in Fig. 8.1 can be used to measure pressure and also chemical changes so long as one of the three devices, inductor, capacitor, or resistor, is in some way changed by the pressure or chemical transducer. In Fig. 8.2 is a schematic diagram of another simple transmitter. This particular transmitter utilizes a transistor, a battery power supply, a capacitor, a coil tapped off center, and an iron core that is attached to a diaphragm.

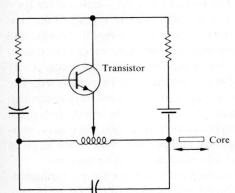

Fig. 8.2. A simple transmitter for measuring pressure.

As you will note, the *RLC* circuit is again shown in this transmitter diagram. It is sufficient to say that the transistor is used to maintain oscillatory currents in the tuned *LC* circuit. The iron core attached to a diaphragm makes this transmitter useful for detecting pressure differences. When the core comes close to or away from the coil, the tuned circuit will be changed, resulting in a modification of the frequency of oscillation. These two diagrams show simple transmitters, but many more sophisticated circuits have been developed for specialized functions.

In almost all cases of implanted or internal transmitters, frequencies are changed by changing or modifying some portions of or some devices in the *RLC* circuit. One can imagine that the transmitters used to measure chemical and physiological parameters are necessarily of more sophisticated designs. Many of these transmitters utilize some kinds of multivibrator circuit. Various types of multivibrators are defined in Chapter 12. Readers who are interested in multivibrator transmitters will find Reference 27 a good source of circuits and applications of these transmitters.

8.4 POWER SUPPLIES

All transmitters require some sort of power supply. Although there are some transmitters which use other radio signals or chemical reactions as sources of power, most transmitters in biotelemetric measurement systems utilize some sort of battery power source. The battery is chosen with the following considerations in mind. If the transmitter is to be located a few feet up to fifty feet away from the receiver, a low-voltage low-power battery will usually be adequate. However, if the transmitter is to be at a significant distance from the receiver, then a more powerful battery must be used. The distance for which a particular power supply and transmitter-receiver combination are effective must be determined experimentally.

A battery must also be chosen on the basis of the length of time for which the transmitter is to be attached to or will remain inside the test animal. The life of a battery depends on how it is constructed. The output voltage-vs.-time curves for a particular load current are shown in Fig. 8.3 for two different types of batteries.

The battery size should always be as small as possible, so that its volume and weight do not disturb the animal any more than is absolutely necessary. Unfortunately, this requirement points to very low-power batteries. Adequate power capabilities must be obtained if a successful experiment is to be performed. The battery must also be encapsulated in the materials that were previously described. Therefore, it must be carefully chosen with a specific use in mind. Reference should be made to tables showing various types of batteries, their chemistry, voltage, service capacity in mA/hr, weight in grams, and physical dimensions as given in Reference 27. The latest manufacturers' information should be sought.

Problems can occur in transmitters. In one particular experiment a transmitter was designed, built, and surgically implanted in a monkey to determine minute

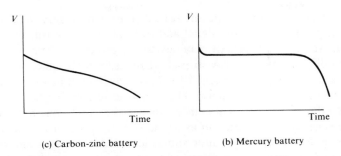

(c) Carbon-zinc battery   (b) Mercury battery

Fig. 8.3. Battery voltage-vs.-time curves for two different types of batteries.

temperature changes when the monkey ovulated. The monkey was housed in a cage with the receiving antenna built around it. The transmitter seemed to be functioning perfectly for a period of time after it was implanted. The surgery upset the monkey's normal cycle and she did not ovulate at the expected time. Before she did so the next time the transmitter had stopped functioning. The failure was either due to loss of power of the battery because of normal aging or due to a leak in the seals protecting the circuit components. Considerable time was lost in the experiment regardless of the reason for the failure. This type of problem should be avoided by using the best components and materials available and thoroughly testing them before implanting them in the animal.

8.5 ANTENNAS

We have briefly discussed transmitters and the power supplies necessary to operate them. There is one more component of the "transmitting station" that must be considered before we leave this particular subject. The signals generated in the transmitter must be relayed to a distant receiver. In communications systems this is usually done by antennas. Most of the radiated signals from a transmitter come from the coil. The coil, therefore, not only serves as a device in the resonant circuit but can also serve as an antenna. In many transmitter designs the coil serves as the transmitting antenna system. When a transmitter is attached to the exterior of an animal, a wire of a known length is attached to the coil and left exposed to the air. Since in most cases the external transmitter is used for tracking animals over long distances, as much signal as possible must be fed into the atmosphere. Most often the antenna wire is a loop which is fashioned into or connected to a collar. The length of the antenna wire is not chosen randomly; it is determined by the frequency of the transmitter. There are almost as many different antenna designs as there are transmitter designs. In most biotelemetric measurements the coil will be sufficient as an antenna system. If the reader desires more information on the design of sophisticated antennas, he should consult the *Antenna Manual* published by the American Radio Relay League [57].

We now have the signal in the air! It is, therefore, necessary to have some sort of display device to collect this signal and translate it into a form that will yield usable data. At least one basic display device is the receiver. The receiver utilizes a speaker to display the signal. A strip-chart recorder, an oscilloscope, or a magnetic-tape recorder may be attached to the receiver so that other displays and permanent records may be obtained. The signals generated by the transmitter and radiated into the air from the antenna are then picked up by the receiver antenna. Since there is usually no restriction as to the size of the receiver and the receiver antenna, these devices are often quite sophisticated. The receiver antenna must be designed with regard to the frequency of the transmitted signal. It may be much like a television receiver antenna, an array of bars of specified lengths and with specified spacing. On the other hand, the receiver antenna may be very simple. For example, if a transmitter is implanted in an animal that is to be confined within a laboratory, the antenna may be a coil of wire attached to the receiver antenna terminals. The antenna and receiver may then be placed in the vicinity of the test animal. The two coils, the one in the transmitter and the one attached to the receiver, will act like a transformer. This coil-antenna configuration is satisfactory only if the animal is immobilized or moves very slightly. If the transmitter coil and the coil-antenna attached to the receiver are not directly facing each other, loss of signal will result. One of the more practical antennas, both for transmission and for receiving purposes, is a loop of wire. The receiving loop of wire may be arranged to encircle the area in which the test animal is placed. This loop antenna will have directional properties such that it is more sensitive to radiation from one direction than from another direction. Unfortunately it is possible for the test animal to move, so that the antenna will not always be able to efficiently receive the transmitted signal.

For more information on antennas the reader should consult References 27 and 57.

8.6 RECEIVERS

The receiver used in biotelemetric measurement systems need not be sophisticated. For many measurements, when parameters are slowly varying, such as temperature, humidity, pH, pressure, and light, and when they are to be measured over relatively short distances, an inexpensive pocket transistor radio will be quite adequate. Usually, the transmitter used to generate a signal representing these parameters is constructed to transmit *pulse* signals. Such signals may be audibly displayed as beeps or clicks, and the pulse rate will determine the differences or variability in the parameter being measured. The transmitter can be constructed so that signals are transmitted on the AM band (530–1600 kHz) or the FM band (88–108 MHz) if the transmission is to be over very short distances. Some type of electronic counter or stopwatch can be used to measure the pulse rate. In choosing a receiver of this type, one should try out several before making a purchase. Receivers that are insensitive, that drift or do not have sharp signals should be rejected.

In recent years, Citizens Band receivers have been chosen as display devices. Again, the transmitter frequency must fall within the range of this receiver. Receivers may also be modified to operate over a range of frequencies by changing the coils and/or capacitors in the input section of the receiver. American Radio Relay League publications discuss such modifications. Reference 27 is also helpful in introducing the receiver to the reader.

In many instances, if a transmitted frequency is merely close to the frequency range of the receiver, the signal will be strong enough so that pulse counts can be made. If the receiver is very selective, it must be tuned carefully to the transmitted frequency. One of the major problems that may be encountered with a receiver is noise interference. If noise appears to be a problem, grounding of the receiver to a good earth ground may be enough to reduce the interference. If the problems of noise cannot be corrected by grounding, the reader should read about other methods of reducing the noise such as discussed in Chapters 10 and 11.

8.7 SIGNAL READOUT

The speaker built into a receiver provides one means of audibly displaying a signal. The investigator listens to the sound emitted by the speaker and records the data at the instant it is heard. For example, the presence or absence of a tone at a particular time may represent the information being sought. The time when the tone is noted is recorded. However, if data are to be collected over an extended period of time, the investigator could well use his time more efficiently doing other tasks than sitting before a speaker. Therefore, some permanent display device should be installed. Several of the display devices commonly used in measurement systems have been discussed in Chapter 7. For example, a strip-chart recorder may be used to permanently record the data that is being transmitted. The analog type of chart recorder gives specific values of the signal being received and displays a waveform of the signal. This type of presentation will be needed if the information is contained in the shape of the signal.

Some types of measurement systems do not use waveshape to convey the needed information. The information may be related to the presence or absence of a pulse. The particular shape of the pulse, then, is of little value. When this type of signal is used, an event-type recorder may be quite adequate for recording purposes. Every time a pulse is received, the pen will be activated and make a mark on the chart. When the pulse is not present, the pen rests at the zero position. If the chart speed is calibrated so that the time between the marks is known, the parameter of elapsed time between pulses can be measured.

A magnetic-tape recorder can also be used. In this case the signal recorded on the tape would be an audio signal. This information may then be used at a later time for transcribing the data or the signals from the tape to a chart recorder so that the information becomes visually available. The information could also be processed by an analog-to-digital converter and then fed into a digital computer for appropriate processing. Any of the display devices discussed in Chapter 7 may be used with the receiver output.

8.8 DISCUSSION

The idea of monitoring pH changes, temperature changes, and other parameters inside or on the animal to be studied has wide applications. In the foregoing discussion we have presented only an overview of the subject. The successful design of such a measurement system will require further in-depth study. However, the reader should not be deterred from entering this field of measurement. Reference 27 will provide much information on the theory and practical problems of biomedical telemetry. Important and inexpensive adjuncts to this book are publications by the American Radio Relay League (ARRL). These books are published primarily for the use of amateur radio operators. They present the material in a straightforward and simple manner making for easy understanding. It will be helpful for anyone venturing in this field to have some background in communications electronics. The ARRL publications will provide a satisfactory background in communications. Once the reader has gained a basic knowledge of communications electronics, he can proceed to the development of telemetry systems. Much data can be gained from such systems. Do not fear to experiment, because the results will be useful in research and will provide the investigator with a high degree of self-satisfaction.

circuit analysis

9.1 OBJECTIVES

Chapters 2 and 3 served as an introduction to the basic concepts of electrical-circuit analysis. The idea and usefulness of considering various phenomena in terms of electrical circuits were discussed at that time. Ohm's law was used to show how simple series and parallel circuits could be analyzed. But the intent of those chapters was not to help the reader become proficient at analyzing complicated circuits. Rather, it was to help the reader gain an intuitive feeling for what to expect, in general, from elementary combinations of power supplies, signal sources, and resistors. Sometimes this type of knowledge is sufficient helping the experimenter arrive at a desired conclusion without the need of doing a detailed circuit analysis or involved mathematical calculations. On the other hand, such an overview is often insufficient, and detailed numerical calculations must be done. The experimenter may need specific numerical data for the circuits that he must use to get at the specific scientific phenomena he is studying. In that case he must be able to work with more complicated circuits and develop an understanding of how they can be analyzed. Fortunately very few rules in addition to Ohm's law are required to analyze the more complicated circuits.

The objective of this chapter is to introduce the reader to the basic rules for circuit analysis required to handle most of the circuit problems that he may need to solve. The method of obtaining an equivalent voltage-source model, called *Thevenin's equivalent circuit,* as well as the method of obtaining an equivalent current-source model, called *Norton's equivalent circuit,* are given. Knowledge of these equivalent circuits will enable the experimenter to anticipate how various loads will affect the outputs from specific circuits. These basic concepts can then be used in analyzing more complicated circuits if the need arises.

Kirchhoff's current law and *voltage law* are the two most commonly used methods of analyzing electrical circuits. They are used with Ohm's law to enable the investigator to determine the various voltages and currents that will occur in the circuit. Applications of these laws are given together with detailed step-by-step procedures for using them.

9.2 EQUIVALENT MODELS USEFUL IN ANALYSIS PROBLEMS

Voltage-source Model: Thevenin's Equivalent Circuit

Whenever a load is connected to a circuit consisting of several parts in addition to a source, the experimenter must determine how the load voltage or current will vary as the load resistance changes. Thevenin's voltage-source model is a circuit consisting of an ideal voltage generator in series with a single impedance. This circuit can be used to help determine effects due to load resistance changes. This circuit is equivalent to the original circuit in that it will produce the same voltage and current to the load as would the original circuit. Its advantage in analysis work is that the voltage-source model contains only two components.

Consider the example given in problem 3.3. A voltage source was available which was too large for the particular application. A voltage divider was designed which could be used to produce the required voltage for a specific load resistance. What would happen if the load resistance were to vary instead of being constant? Let us assume that the load was a chemical solution whose resistance changed as the experiment progressed. What would be the voltage across the solution as the resistance of the solution changed? We can get a clue as to what might happen by looking at the circuit in Fig. 9.1 and then referring back to Fig. 3.5.

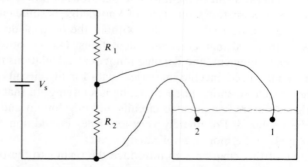

Fig. 9.1. Voltage-divider source driving a chemical solution.

The arguments in Chapter 3 indicated that the voltage across the load would change with the load resistance when the source had some internal resistance. The problem can be resolved by means of a model of the source as shown in Fig. 9.1 that is of the form of an ideal voltage source in series with an internal resistance, as shown in Fig. 3.5. More specifically, Fig. 9.2 shows what must be done.

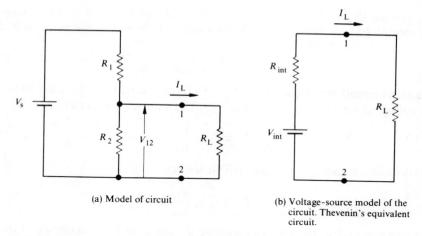

(a) Model of circuit

(b) Voltage-source model of the
circuit. Thevenin's equivalent
circuit.

Fig. 9.2. Two circuits that are to be made equivalent in their performance.

A number of assumptions should be stated at the outset. First, the chemical
solution may change from almost a short circuit into an open circuit. Second, the
resistors used in the voltage-divider circuit are constant and in particular do not
change with the current through them. Third, the source of voltage V_s is an ideal
one such that its voltage does not change even though the current flow from it
varies. Finally, the equivalent circuit must respond exactly as the voltage-divider
circuit would respond as the load resistance R_L changes.

Two limiting conditions will be used to determine the equivalent voltage-
source model, Thevenin's equivalent circuit:

1. The load between points 1 and 2, where it is connected to the circuit, is assumed to be an open circuit or infinite resistance.
2. The load between points 1 and 2 is assumed to be a short circuit or zero
   resistance.

Using these two conditions, we can obtain the equivalent internal voltage V_{int} and
resistance R_{int} of the voltage-divider source. The internal voltage is determined
as follows:

The open-circuit condition ($R_L = \infty$). The load current is zero: $I_L = 0$. Using
Eq. (3.45), we get the following for the voltage-divider circuit:

$$V_{12} = \frac{R_2}{R_1 + R_2} V_s.$$

For the voltage-source equivalent circuit we get

$$V_{12} = V_{int}.$$

The voltage V_{12} for the voltage-source-equivalent circuit must be made equal to the voltage V_{12} for the voltage-divider circuit. Thus the open-circuit voltage is

$$V_{oc} = V_{12} = \mathrm{V}_{int} = \frac{R_2}{R_1 + R_2} V_s. \tag{9.1}$$

The short-circuit condition ($R_L = 0$). The load current can be calculated. For the voltage-divider circuit we get $V_{12} = 0$. The short-circuit current is

$$I_{sc} = I_L = \frac{V_s}{R_1}. \tag{9.2}$$

For the voltage-source-equivalent circuit we get

$$I_{sc} = I_L = \frac{V_{int}}{R_{int}}.$$

The currents under this condition must be the same for the two circuits if the circuits are to be equivalent. Therefore,

$$\frac{V_s}{R_1} = \frac{V_{int}}{R_{int}}$$

and

$$R_{int} = R_1 \frac{V_{int}}{V_s}.$$

Substituting Eq. (9.1) into the above equation, we obtain

$$R_{int} = \left(\frac{R_1}{V_s} \right) \left(\frac{R_2}{R_1 + R_2} V_s \right)$$

$$= \frac{R_1 R_2}{R_1 + R_2}. \tag{9.3}$$

Note that R_{int} equals the value of a resistor R_1 in parallel with a resistor R_2. [See Eq. (3.21).] The voltage-equivalent model as shown in Fig. 9.3 is now complete and can be used to determine the variation in voltage across the chemical solution as the solution resistance changes.

Current-source Model: Norton's Equivalent Circuit

Sometimes a source is designed to act primarily as a current source such that its output current does not vary substantially with the load resistance. In such cases it is convenient to make a current-source model of the actual source. For example, let us make a current-source model of the voltage-divider source just discussed (Fig. 9.4).

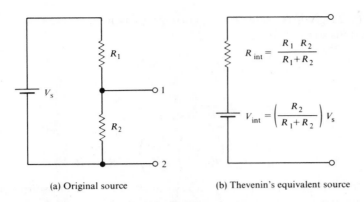

(a) Original source   (b) Thevenin's equivalent source

Fig. 9.3.   These two circuits will give equivalent performance when connected to the same loads.

Once again there are two limiting conditions that can be used to establish the equivalent circuit. If we let R_L be an open circuit, then the open-circuit voltage can be determined. If we let R_L be a short circuit, then the short-circuit current can be determined. Note that for the current-source equivalent circuit, the short-circuit current is just I_{int} and the open-circuit voltage is $I_{int}R_{int}$. Thus with these two conditions $I_{int}R_{int}$ can be determined.

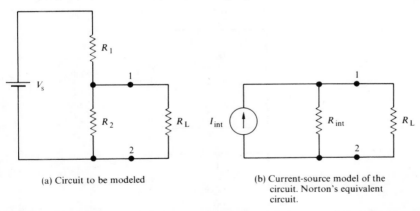

(a) Circuit to be modeled   (b) Current-source model of the circuit. Norton's equivalent circuit.

Fig. 9.4.   Two circuits to be made equivalent in performance when connected to the same load.

From the previous discussion we know that the open-circuit voltage for the voltage divider circuit is

$$V_{oc} = V_{int} = \frac{R_2}{R_1 + R_2} V_s. \tag{9.1}$$

Equation (9.2) gives the short-circuit current: $I_{sc} = V_S/R_1$.
For the current-source circuit,

$$I_{int} = I_{sc} = \frac{V_S}{R_1},$$

$$V_{oc} = R_{int} I_{int} = \frac{R_2}{R_1 + R_2} V_S,$$

$$R_{int} = \left(\frac{R_2}{R_1 + R_2} V_S\right)\left(\frac{R_1}{V_S}\right) = \frac{R_1 R_2}{R_1 + R_2}. \qquad (9.4)$$

Note that this equation for the internal resistance of the current-source model is exactly the same as that for the voltage-source model (Eq. 9.3). However, in Fig. 9.4 R_{int} is placed in parallel with the ideal current source I_{int}. In Fig. 9.3 R_{int} is placed in series with the ideal voltage source V_{int}. Thus the current-source model and the voltage-source model are very closely related. Once you have the appropriate values for one of these models, the values for the other model can be readily established.

A point to remember

A voltage- or current-source model can be made of a circuit by determining the open-circuit voltage and the short-circuit current for the circuit.

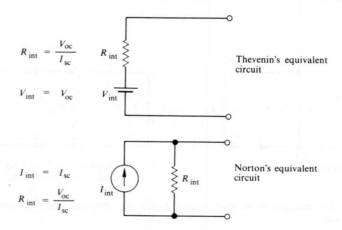

$R_{int} = \dfrac{V_{oc}}{I_{sc}}$ R_{int} Thevenin's equivalent circuit

$V_{int} = V_{oc}$ V_{int}

$I_{int} = I_{sc}$ Norton's equivalent circuit

$R_{int} = \dfrac{V_{oc}}{I_{sc}}$ I_{int} R_{int}

9.3 BASIC LAWS USED IN ANALYSIS PROBLEMS

Kirchhoff's Voltage Law: dc-Circuit Examples

The current- and voltage-source models discussed in the previous section are very helpful when there is a need to determine how a load will affect a source voltage or current. It may be necessary in a particular experiment to go further than this and calculate the voltage or current that should occur at a specific point in the circuit other than at the source. If this is necessary, two more laws must be introduced and discussed. These laws are called Kirchhoff's current and voltage laws. In conjunction with Ohm's law, these two laws will enable the experimenter to analyze both relatively simple circuits and very complicated circuits. In this section the voltage law will be discussed in detail.

Kirchhoff's voltage law.

The sum of the voltages around a closed loop is equal to zero:

$$\sum_{i=1}^{n} V_i = 0,$$

where n = number of components in series around the loop.

This law is very easy to apply once a polarity convention has been established and is carefully followed. The convention that will be used is shown in Fig. 9.5.

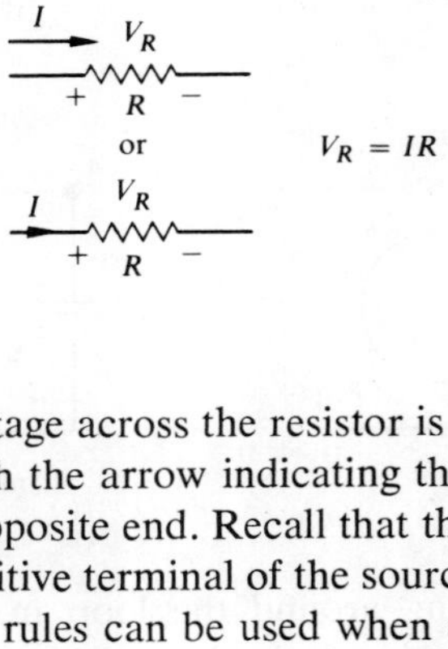

Fig. 9.5. Polarity conventions.

The voltage across the resistor is V_R and is positive at that end of the resistor toward which the arrow indicating the direction of current flow points and negative at the opposite end. Recall that the direction of current flow was defined to be from the positive terminal of the source to the negative terminal.

Specific rules can be used when applying the voltage law to a circuit.

1. Assume a direction of current flow in each circuit loop. It makes no difference which direction you assume it to flow. If you assume the wrong direction, the answer you will get at the end of your calculations will be negative. This negative sign indicates that you assumed the wrong direction initially when setting up the problem. Thus no damage is done by that assumption. This phenomenon will be demonstrated shortly.

2. Label the voltage across each resistor with a symbol, such as V_{R1}.

3. Label the polarity of the voltage across the resistor in accordance with the convention shown in Fig. 9.5.

4. Start at a particular point (of your choice) in the circuit and, while tracing through the circuit in a clockwise or counterclockwise direction, add the

voltages across the various resistors and the source. Be careful and use the first polarity sign you come to at each resistor or source. Trace through a complete loop and return to the starting point. Set this sum equal to zero.

5. Substitute the Ohm's law values for each of the V_i terms for the resistors.
6. Repeat steps 4 and 5 for each loop in the circuit.
7. Solve for the desired unknown currents.

Example 9.1   dc series circuit, voltage source.   As an example of this procedure, consider Fig. 9.6. Note the various steps that have been followed. Continuing with the analysis, we get the following.

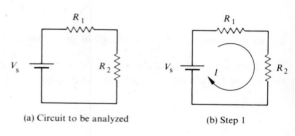

(a) Circuit to be analyzed   (b) Step 1

Fig. 9.6. Nomenclature for Kirchhoff's voltage law circuit diagram.

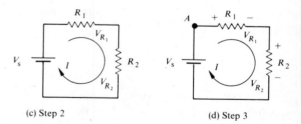

(c) Step 2   (d) Step 3

Step 4.   Starting at point A and going around the loop in a clockwise direction, we take the sum of the voltages across all the components and set it to zero:

$$\sum_i V_i = 0,$$
$$-V_{R_1} - V_{R_2} - V_s = 0.$$

Step 5.   Making the appropriate substitutions, we obtain

$$+IR_1 + IR_2 - V_s = 0.$$

Step 6.   Solving for I, we have

$$I = \frac{V_s}{R_1 + R_2}. \tag{9.5}$$

To see what would happen if we assumed different directions of current flow, see Fig. 9.7. Proceeding with the analysis, we get the following.

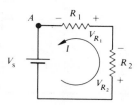

Fig. 9.7. Different directions of current flow.

Step 4. Starting at point A and going around the loop in a clockwise direction, we take the sum of the voltages across all the components and set it to zero:

$$\sum_i V_i = 0,$$
$$-V_{R_1} - V_{R_2} - V_s = 0.$$

Step 5. Making the substitutions, we obtain

$$-IR_1 - IR_2 - V_s = 0.$$

Step 6. Solve for I, we find that

$$I = -\frac{V_s}{R_1 + R_2}. \tag{9.6}$$

Note that Eq. (9.6) is exactly the same as Eq. (9.5) except for sign change. The negative sign in Eq. (9.6) indicates that the direction of current flow was wrongly assumed in Fig. 9.7. The current actually flows from the positive to the negative terminal, as first assumed in Fig. 9.6.

A point to remember

Any current-flow direction may be assumed when doing a loop analysis by Kirchhoff's voltage law if the basic sign conventions given in Fig. 9.5 are used.

Example 9.2 dc voltage-divider circuit. As a second example of the application of the voltage law, let us analyze the voltage-divider source circuit discussed in Sections 9.1 and 9.2. There are two loops in this circuit and the direction of current flow in each loop must be assumed and designated on the diagram. It is usually helpful to assume the same direction of current flow in both loops, as in Fig. 9.8. Proceeding with the analysis, we take the following steps.

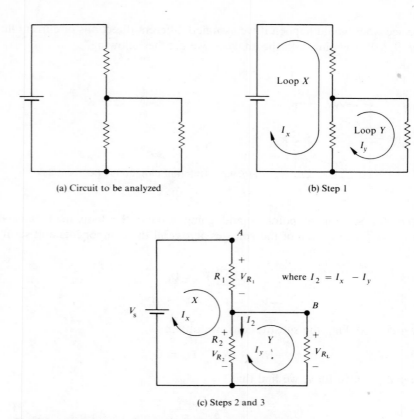

(a) Circuit to be analyzed

(b) Step 1

where $I_2 = I_x - I_y$

(c) Steps 2 and 3

Fig. 9.8. Steps 1, 2, and 3 of Kirchhoff's voltage law analysis.

Step 4. Starting from point A and going around the closed loop X in a clockwise direction, we take the sum of the voltages across all the components and set it to zero:

$$\sum_i V_i = 0,$$

$$+V_{R_1} + V_{R_2} - V_S = 0.$$

For loop Y and starting from point B, going in a clockwise direction, we have

$$\sum_i V_i = 0,$$

$$+V_{R_L} - V_{R_2} = 0.$$

Step 5. For loop X we have

$$V_{R_1} = I_X R_1, \quad V_{R_2} = I_2 R_2 = (I_X - I_Y) R_2,$$

and

$$+I_X R_1 + (I_X - I_Y) R_2 - V_S = 0.$$

For loop Y we have

$$+I_Y R_L - (I_X - I_Y) R_2 = 0.$$

Step 6. There are two equations that must be solved simultaneously, because there are two loops in this circuit. If I_Y is determined, the voltage across the load resistor can be determined. We have

$$V_{R_L} = I_Y R_L.$$

These two examples of applying the voltage law should serve to show the major problems that might occur when using this law to analyze a circuit. A more complex and useful circuit, a bridge circuit, will be analyzed in problem 9.6.

Kirchhoff's Current Law: dc-Circuit Examples

All circuits may be analyzed by means of Kirchhoff's voltage law as given above. Similarly all circuits may be analyzed by means of Kirchhoff's current law. Sometimes fewer equations are needed to analyze a circuit by the current law than by the voltage law. Thus it is helpful to know both laws and understand their application in circuit analysis.

Kirchhoff's current law

The sum of all of the currents entering a *node* is equal to zero. (This assumes that all currents at the node enter the node.)

$$\sum_{i=1}^{n} I_i = 0,$$

where n = number of parallel branches at the node.

This law is as easy to apply as the voltage law if proper conventions are established and carefully followed. The conventions that will be used are shown in Fig. 9.9.

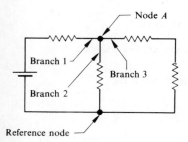

Fig. 9.9. Conventions for Kirchhoff's current law.

The specific rules for applying the current law to a circuit are the following:

1. Label the nodes, for example A, B, etc.
2. Pick a reference node to which you will refer all other voltages in the circuit.

3. Assume a direction of current flow through each of the components connected to the node. (Any direction may be assumed.)

4. Label the voltages at all of the nodes with respect to the reference node and assume polarities for these voltages.

5. Take the sum of all of the currents at the node, using Kirchhoff's current law. Associate a positive sign with currents flowing into the node.

6. Substitute the appropriate Ohm's law equation for each current term.

7. Repeat step 5 for every node other than the reference node.

8. Solve for the desired unknown.

Example 9.3   dc parallel circuits, current source.   As an example of this procedure, consider Fig. 9.10 and follow the steps to see how this method of analysis may be used when there are current sources in the circuit. The final steps in the analysis yield the following results.

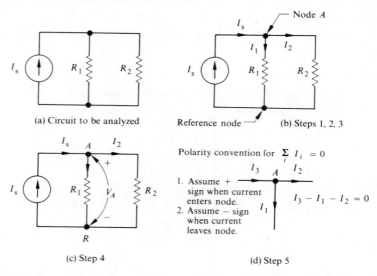

(a) Circuit to be analyzed

Reference node ⟶   (b) Steps 1, 2, 3

(c) Step 4

(d) Step 5

Fig. 9.10.   Steps 1 through 4 of the Kirchhoff's current law analysis.

Step 5.   Taking the sum of the currents at node A, we have

$$\sum_i I_i = 0,$$

$$+I_s - I_1 - I_2 = 0.$$

Step 6.   Using the polarity convention shown in Fig. 9.5 to determine the substitutions for the currents in the above equation, we obtain

$$+I_s - \frac{V_A}{R_1} \qquad I_2 = \frac{V_A}{R_2},$$

and therefore,

$$+I_\mathrm{s} - \frac{V_A}{R_1} - \frac{V_A}{R_2} = 0. \tag{9.7}$$

The voltage at node A with respect to the reference node can be determined by using Eq. (9.7). I_s, R_1, and R_2 are all assumed to be known quantities. Therefore,

$$-V_A\left(\frac{1}{R_1} + \frac{1}{R_2}\right) = -I_\mathrm{s},$$

$$V_A = \frac{I_\mathrm{s}}{1/R_1 + 1/R_2}.$$

As a further example, let us assume the direction of the current flow through the resistors to be opposite to that assumed in the previous example. See Fig. 9.11 and compare the following analysis with the previous analysis. Continuing with the analysis, we obtain the following.

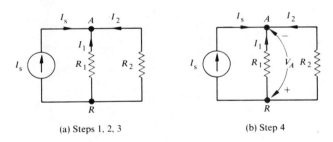

(a) Steps 1, 2, 3   (b) Step 4

Fig. 9.11. Steps 1 through 4 with different directions of current flow as compared to those in the previous example.

Step 5. Taking the sum of the currents at node A, we have

$$\sum_i I_i = 0,$$

$$+I_\mathrm{s} + I_1 + I_2 = 0.$$

Step 6. Substituting the appropriate Ohm's law equation for each current term, we obtain

$$I_\mathrm{s} + \frac{V_A}{R_1} + \frac{V_A}{R_2} = 0,$$

$$V_A = -\frac{I_\mathrm{s}}{1/R_1 + 1/R_2}.$$

The last equation is the same as Eq. (9.8) except for the negative sign. The negative sign indicates that the actual polarity of the voltage at node A is positive with respect to the reference node. See Fig. 9.10(c) for the polarity of V_A.

A point to remember

Any current-flow direction may be assumed when doing a nodal analysis by Kirchhoff's current law if the basic sign conventions given in Fig. 9.5 are used.

Example 9.4   dc voltage-divider circuit.   As a second example of the application of the current law, let us analyze the voltage-divider source circuit once again. This will show how the law is applied when voltage sources are in the circuit. Refer to Fig. 9.12. Continuing with the analysis, we obtain the following.

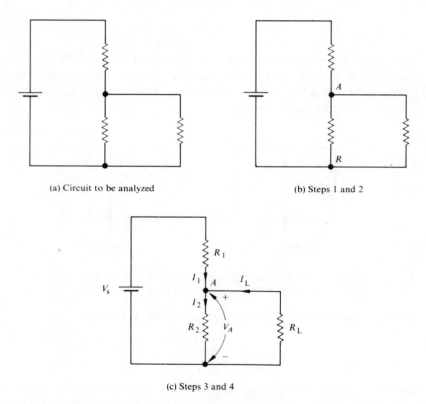

(a) Circuit to be analyzed   (b) Steps 1 and 2

(c) Steps 3 and 4

Fig. 9.12.   Steps 1 through 4 of a Kirchhoff's current law analysis.

Step 5.   Taking the sum of the currents at node A and assuming currents entering the node to have a positive sign and currents leaving the node to have a negative sign, we have

$$\sum_i I_i = 0,$$
$$+I_1 + I_L - I_2 = 0. \tag{9.9}$$

Step 6.   The substitutions for I_2 and I_L are easily made so long as the polarity conventions are followed:

$$I_2 = \frac{V_A}{R_2}, \quad I_L = -\frac{V_A}{R_L}.$$

The substitution for I_1 is not so obvious. Let us use Kirchhoff's voltage law to obtain the equation for I_1 (refer to Fig. 9.13). First, we solve for V_{R_1}. Starting at point A and going clockwise in a closed loop, we take the sum of the voltages across all the components in the loop:

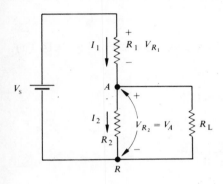

Fig. 9.13. Kirchhoff's voltage law applied to voltage-divider circuit.

$$\sum_i V_i = 0,$$

$$+V_A - V_S + V_{R_1} = 0,$$

so that

$$V_{R_1} = V_S - V_A.$$

Thus

$$I_1 = \frac{V_S - V_A}{R_1}. \tag{9.10}$$

Substitute this into Eq. (9.9) together with the values for I_2 and I_L:

$$\frac{V_S - V_A}{R_1} - \frac{V_A}{R_L} - \frac{V_A}{R_2} = 0. \tag{9.11}$$

Now V_A may be determined.

The most difficult part of applying the current law is to determine the appropriate substitution for the current in a branch that contains both a resistor and a voltage source in its loop. The procedure used above will always yield the correct result if correctly applied. Several different situations like this are shown in Fig. 9.14.

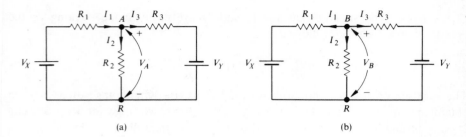

Fig. 9.14. Examples of substitutions for currents designated in Kirchhoff's current law equations.

The equations for the circuits in Fig. 9.14 are as follows. For Fig. 9.14 (a),

$$\sum_i I_i = 0,$$

$$+I_1 - I_2 - I_3 = 0,$$

where

$$I_1 = \frac{V_X - V_A}{R_1}, \quad I_2 = \frac{V_A}{R_2}, \quad I_3 = \frac{V_A + V_Y}{R_3}.$$

For Fig. 9.14 (b),

$$\sum_i I_i = 0,$$

$$-I_1 - I_2 - I_3 = 0,$$

where

$$I_1 = \frac{(-V_X + V_B)}{R_1}, \quad I_2 = \frac{V_B}{R_2}, \quad I_3 = \frac{V_Y + V_B}{R_3}.$$

The final equations for both sets of assumptions are the same since $V_A = V_B$. Therefore, any set of assumed directions and polarities may be used so long as the convention given in Fig. 9.5 is followed when the individual currents are determined.

9.4   ac-CIRCUIT ANALYSIS

In the previous sections the basic rules and laws necessary for solving ac circuits were discussed along with examples of dc circuits. In this section circuits with capacitors, inductors, and resistors will be discussed, and the similarities with dc-circuit analysis will be pointed out. Examples will be given to show how the basic Kirchhoff laws can be applied in ac-circuit analysis. This discussion will lead to the introduction of the rules required to make specific numerical calculations of ac-circuit performance.

Application of Ohm's and Kirchhoff's Laws

The modeling of an ac circuit is exactly the same as in the case of dc circuits. Resistors, capacitors, and inductors are shown in the appropriate places in the circuit. The circuit equations discussed in the previous sections are written in exactly the same way, except that the impedance equations for the capacitor and the inductor are slightly more complicated than those for resistance circuits. .

Example 9.5   RC filter circuit.   As the first example of ac-circuit analysis, consider the performance of an RC filter, such as the one discussed in Example 4.4 and shown again in Fig. 9.15. If specific numerical results are required, appropriate equations must be set up.

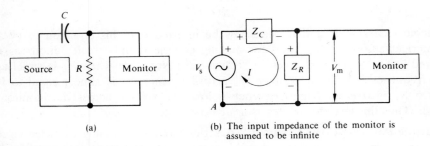

(a)

(b) The input impedance of the monitor is
assumed to be infinite

Fig. 9.15.   High-pass RC filter.

Note that a source drives a circuit consisting of a capacitor in series with a resistor which is in parallel with some type of monitoring circuit. This circuit may be modeled as shown in Fig. 9.15 (b), where a block labeled Z_C represents the capacitor and a block labeled Z_R represents the resistor. Assume for the moment that the monitor has infinite input resistance and thus will not have any effect on the current flowing from the source. Kirchhoff's voltage law can be used to determine the current flowing in the series circuit. The source is assumed to be an ac voltage. This means that its polarity changes alternating from positive to negative. In ac-circuit analysis we must assume a polarity at some fixed instant in time when we write the circuit equations. Recall from Chapter 4 that a phase difference may occur between the current and voltage in various parts of the circuit. The Kirchhoff equation for this circuit is as follows. Taking the sum of the voltages, start at point A and going clockwise, we have

$$\sum_i V_i = 0,$$

$$-V_\text{s} + IZ_C + IZ_R = 0. \tag{9.12}$$

Substituting the appropriate equations for Z_C and Z_R, we obtain

$$Z_C = \frac{-j}{2\pi f C} = \frac{-j}{\omega C}, \quad \text{where } \omega = 2\pi f, \tag{4.30}$$

$$-V_S + I\left(\frac{-j}{\omega C}\right) + IR = 0,$$

where V_S is an rms voltage value and j indicates a $+90°$ angle. Solving for current, we have

$$I = \frac{V_S}{-j/\omega C + R} = \frac{V_S}{-jX_C + R}$$

where

$$X_C = 1/\omega C. \tag{4.31}$$

The voltage V_M across the monitor is IZ_R and therefore

$$V_M = \frac{R}{-jX_C + R} V_S. \tag{9.13}$$

Specific values of R and X_C can now be inserted into this equation to obtain numerical answers. [The rules for making complex-number calculations as required in Eq. (9.13) are given in Section 9.5.] Note that when X_C is small and the frequency is high, the voltage V_M across the monitor is almost equal to V_S. When X_C is large and the frequency is low, the voltage across the monitor is small. Thus this circuit operates as a high-pass filter.

Example 9.6   Series RLC circuit.   A series circuit containing all three circuit elements (Fig. 9.16) can be analyzed in a manner similar to that used for the RC filter. The source for the circuit shown in Fig. 9.16 is an ac voltage. The Kirchhoff

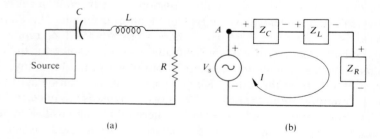

(a)   (b)

Fig. 9.16.   A series RLC circuit.

voltage law equation is similar to the one in the previous example, except that there is now a new term for the inductor:

$$\sum_i V_i = 0, \quad +IZ_C + IZ_L + IZ_R - V_S = 0,$$

$$I = \frac{V_S}{Z_C + Z_L + Z_R} = \frac{V_S}{-j/\omega C + j\omega L + R} = \frac{V_S}{R + j(X_L - X_C)}. \tag{9.14}$$

Equation (9.14) provides some interesting information on the performance of this circuit. If X_L equals X_C, the current that flows in the circuit will be determined only by the source voltage and the resistance, the capacitor and the inductor having nullified each other. If X_L is much larger than either X_C or R, it will have a dominant effect on the current flow and the current will be relatively small. This occurs when the frequency is quite large. If X_C is much larger than either X_L or R, it will have a dominant effect and the current will once again be small. This occurs when the frequency is very low. Thus this circuit impedes the flow of current at low and high frequencies and allows it to flow at some middle-level frequencies. Hence it is a simple band-pass filter.

Example 9.7   Parallel RLC circuit.   Parallel ac circuits are readily analyzed by means of Kirchhoff's current law, as shown by the following example (Fig. 9.17). The variable of interest in this circuit may be the current flow from the source.

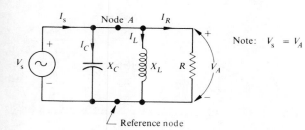

Fig. 9.17. A parallel *RLC* circuit.

This current can be determined by carefully applying Kirchhoff's current law. Here node A is the top line of the circuit. The only currents that must be assigned directions are those in each branch connected to the node. There are four branches; hence only four currents need to be defined. Taking the sum of the currents at node A, we have

$$\sum_i I_i = 0,$$

$$I_S - I_C - I_L - I_R = 0,$$

where

$$I_C = \frac{V_S}{Z_C}, \quad I_L = \frac{V_S}{Z_L}, \quad I_R = \frac{V_S}{R}$$

and V_S = the rms value of the source voltage. Solving for the source current I_S we obtain

$$I_S = I_C + I_L + I_R$$

$$= \frac{V_S}{Z_C} + \frac{V_S}{Z_L} + \frac{V_S}{R}$$

$$= \left(\frac{1}{-jX_C} + \frac{1}{jX_L} + \frac{1}{R} \right) V_S. \qquad (9.15)$$

A study of Eq. (9.15) reveals the following performance of this circuit. When either X_C or X_L is small, the current from the source is very large. This situation occurs at very high and very low frequencies. At some intermediate frequency X_C and X_L will be equal and the current will be dependent only on the source voltage and the resistor. This circuit has the characteristics of a band-rejection filter; it rejects or impedes the flow of current at the frequency where X_C equals X_L.

Example 9.8   Series-parallel RLC filter circuit.   Consider next a series-parallel circuit that may be used as a filter (Fig. 9.18). The output voltage of this filter will be taken across the resistor. Since a nodal analysis by means of Kirchhoff's current law will yield the unknown voltages directly, this method may be used to determine the output voltage. The equations for the currents at node A are as follows:

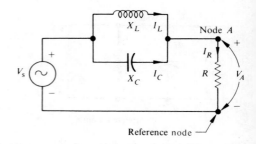

Fig. 9.18.   Series-parallel *RLC* circuit.

$$\sum_i I_i = 0,$$

$$+I_L + I_C - I_R = 0,$$

where

$$I_L = \frac{V_\mathrm{s} - V_A}{Z_L}, \quad I_C = \frac{V_\mathrm{s} - V_A}{Z_C}, \quad I_R = \frac{V_A}{R},$$

yielding

$$V_A = \frac{R V_\mathrm{s}}{R + Z_C Z_L / (Z_C + Z_L)}.$$

Let $Z_\mathrm{p} = Z_C Z_L / (Z_C + Z_L)$. Then

$$V_A = \frac{R}{R + Z_\mathrm{p}} V_\mathrm{s}. \tag{4.16}$$

For Z_p substitute

$$Z_\mathrm{p} = \frac{(-jX_C)\,(jX_L)}{jX_L - jX_C} = \frac{X_C X_L}{j(X_L - X_C)}.$$

Note that Z_p can take on values from zero to infinity and thus, according to Eq. (4.16), the voltage V_A at the output ranges from zero to V_S. Once again we note that a filtering action occurs. This combination of an inductor and a capacitor in parallel is commonly called a *parallel resonant circuit*. It is said to be at resonance when the inductive reactance equals the capacitive reactance. Under this condition the impedance of the parallel circuit is infinite when ideal components are used.

Comparing the parallel resonant circuit with the series LC circuit, the second example in this section, we note an important difference. At one specific frequency, depending on L and C, the series circuit offers zero impedance to the flow of current. This series combination of L and C is called a *series resonant circuit* and is said to be at resonance when the inductive reactance equals the capacitive reactance. Thus we have two basic filtering circuits: the parallel resonant circuit and the series resonant circuit. One circuit will act as an infinite impedance at a specified frequency and the other will act as a short circuit at a specified frequency.

Points to remember

1. Kirchhoff's laws may be applied to ac circuits when appropriate impedance terms are given for capacitors and inductors.

2. Parallel resonant circuits have high impedance over a narrow band of frequencies and relatively low impedance at other frequencies.

3. Series resonant circuits have low impedance over a narrow band of frequencies and relatively high impedances at other frequencies.

9.5   RULES FOR COMPLEX-NUMBER CALCULATIONS

It can be seen that the application of Kirchhoff's laws to ac circuits is exactly the same as it was for dc circuits. The only additional problem comes when the resulting equations involving a j term are to be evaluated. The j term refers to a $90°$ angle and is an imaginary number. Mathematicians commonly use the symbol i to represent imaginary terms, but this symbol is not used for this purpose in electrical work because the i is reserved for current. All of the rules normally used to handle complex-number problems may be used in calculating numerical answers in ac-analysis problems. The basic rules needed are given below.

Operations Involving the Rectangular Form of Impedance

Let impedance $Z_1 = a_1 + ja_2$ and impedance $Z_2 = b_1 + jb_2$. These are called the rectangular form of impedance, where $j = \sqrt{-1}$ and $j^2 = -1$.

Addition law

$$\begin{aligned} Z_1 + Z_2 &= (a_1 + ja_2) + (b_1 + jb_2) \\ &= (a_1 + b_1) + j(a_2 + b_2). \end{aligned} \tag{9.16}$$

Multiplication law

$$Z_1 Z_2 = (a_1 + ja_2)(b_1 + jb_2)$$
$$= (a_1 b_1 - a_2 b_2) + j(a_2 b_1 + a_1 b_2). \tag{9.17}$$

Operations Involving the Polar Form of Impedance

The polar form of an impedance includes an amplitude term and an angle term. The amplitude of Z_1 where Z_1 is as defined above is

$$|Z_1| = |a_1 + ja_2| = \sqrt{a_1{}^2 + a_2{}^2}$$
$$= A.$$

The amplitude of Z_2, where Z_2 is as defined above, is

$$|Z_2| = |b_1 + jb_2| = \sqrt{b_1{}^2 + b_2{}^2}$$
$$= B.$$

The angle of Z_1 is $\qquad \theta_{Z_1} = \theta_A, \qquad$ where

$$\tan \theta_A = \frac{a_2}{a_1} \quad \text{and} \quad \theta_A = \tan^{-1}\left(\frac{a_2}{a_1}\right).$$

The angle of Z_2 is $\qquad \theta_{Z_2} = \theta_B \qquad$ where

$$\tan \theta_B = \frac{b_2}{b_1} \quad \text{and} \quad \theta_B = \tan^{-1}\left(\frac{b_2}{b_1}\right).$$

The general form for impedance in polar form is

$$Z_1 = |Z_1| \angle \theta_{Z_1}$$

Multiplication is defined by

$$Z_1 Z_2 = (|Z_1| \angle \theta_{Z_1})(|Z_2| \angle \theta_{Z_2})$$
$$= A B \angle (\theta_A + \theta_B). \tag{9.18}$$

Division is defined by

$$\frac{Z_1}{Z_2} \frac{|Z_1| \angle \theta_{Z_1}}{|Z_2| \angle \theta_{Z_2}}$$

$$= \frac{A}{B} \angle (\theta_A - \theta_B). \tag{9.19}$$

Complex-number Notation for Impedance: RL Circuit

$$Z = Z_L + R = jX_L + R.$$

The amplitude of Z is $|Z| = \sqrt{X_L{}^2 + R^2}.$

The R term in the impedance equation for Z represents the x-axis or "real" component of the impedance. The X_L term in the impedance equation represents the y-axis or "imaginary" component of the impedance. The amplitude of Z, $|Z|$, is the graphical sum of the two components.

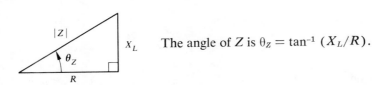 The angle of Z is $\theta_Z = \tan^{-1}(X_L/R)$.

The accompanying triangle is called the impedance triangle and shows the angle and amplitude of the impedance. Note the angle is positive for a resistor-inductor circuit.

Complex-number Notation for Impedances: RC Circuit

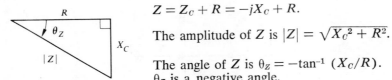

$Z = Z_C + R = -jX_C + R.$

The amplitude of Z is $|Z| = \sqrt{X_C^2 + R^2}.$

The angle of Z is $\theta_Z = -\tan^{-1}(X_C/R).$
θ_Z is a negative angle.

This impedance can also be represented by a triangle. In this circuit the y-axis component $Z_C = -jX_C$ is a negative quantity. The X_C side of the triangle is drawn in the negative y-direction. The angle of the impedance of this circuit is negative.

Complex-number Notation for Impedances: RLC Circuit

The series circuit

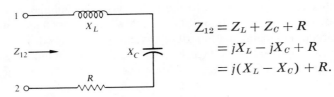

$Z_{12} = Z_L + Z_C + R$
$\quad = jX_L - jX_C + R$
$\quad = j(X_L - X_C) + R.$

Showing Z graphically, we get the following.

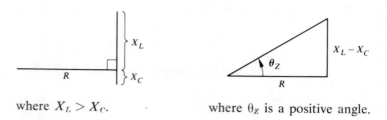

where $X_L > X_C$.   where θ_Z is a positive angle.

The parallel circuit.   The calculation of the impedance of a parallel circuit containing a resistor, an inductor, and a capacitor is slightly more complicated than in the case of the series circuit shown. This impedance can be determined by using Eq. (4.19):

$$Z_{12} = \frac{1}{1/R + 1/Z_C + 1/Z_L} = \frac{1}{1/R + 1/-jX_C + 1/jX_L}$$

$$= \frac{1}{1/R + j(1/X_C - 1/X_L)}, \qquad \text{where } j^2 = -1.$$

When adding complex numbers, use rectangular forms of the numbers. When multiplying or dividing complex numbers, it may be easiest to use the polar forms of the numbers.

9.6   CONCLUSIONS

Ohm's law and Kirchhoff's laws can be applied to any combination of resistors, capacitors, inductors, voltage sources, and current sources. A proper convention concerning current flow in relation to the polarity of the voltage across a component must be used. Any direction of current flow can be assumed for a loop or branch of a circuit so long as the polarity convention is followed. If the final calculated value for a current or voltage is negative, then the assumed direction of flow or the assumed polarity of voltage is the opposite of the actual one.

When numerical values of current or voltage are required in a circuit involving ac sources, resistors, capacitors, and inductors, the rules for manipulating
complex numbers must be followed. The initial equations obtained by using Ohm's
law and Kirchhoff's laws must be written in rectangular form. Sometimes it is
more convenient to use the polar notation for impedances. In such cases it is
possible to translate the expressions in rectangular form into the polar form.

9.7 PROBLEMS WITH SOLUTIONS

Problem 9.1 In Section 9.1 we obtained a voltage-equivalent model, the Thevenin
equivalent circuit, for a voltage-divider source. Assume that the following values
are given for the various components shown in Fig. P9.1. Verify that the two circuits give the same voltage between points 1 and 2 when the load resistance R_L is
2000 Ω.

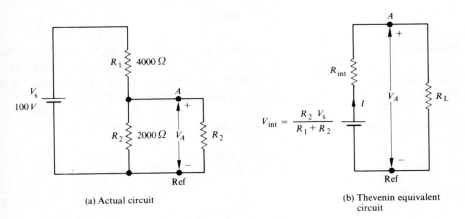

(a) Actual circuit

(b) Thevenin equivalent
circuit

Fig. P9.1. Circuits to be verified.

Solution. Solve for V_A using the original circuit. Start with Eq. (9.11):

$$\frac{V_S - V_A}{R_1} - \frac{V_A}{R_L} - \frac{V_A}{R_2} = 0, \tag{9.11}$$

$$V_A \left(\frac{1}{R_1} + \frac{1}{R_L} + \frac{1}{R_2} \right) = \frac{V_S}{R_1},$$

$$V_A = \frac{V_S}{R_1} \left(\frac{1}{1/R_1 + 1/R_L + 1/R_2} \right)$$

$$= \frac{100}{4000} \left(\frac{1}{1/4000 + 1/2000 + 1/2000} \right) = 20 \text{ V}.$$

Solve for V_A, using the Thevenin voltage-equivalent circuit:

$$V_A = IR_L, \quad I = \frac{V_{int}}{R_{int} + R_L}$$

$$V_A = \frac{R_L}{R_{int} + R_L} V_{int},$$

$$R_{int} = \frac{R_1 R_2}{R_1 + R_2} = \frac{(4000)(2000)}{4000 + 2000} = \frac{4000}{3}, \quad (9.3)$$

$$V_{int} = \frac{R_2}{R_1 + R_2} V_S = \frac{2000}{4000 + 2000} (100) = \frac{100}{3}.$$

Substituting these values into the equation for V_A, we have

$$V_A = \frac{2000}{4000/3 + 2000} (100/3) = 20 \text{ V}.$$

Problem 9.2 Assume that an experimenter has a 12-V storage battery and he needs an 8-V source that will stay within ±0.1 V of 8 V when the load resistance is increased from 2000 Ω to 4000 Ω. What values should be used for R_1 and R_2 in Fig. P9.2(a) if this voltage divider is connected across the battery?

Solution. Equation (3.45) will serve as a good starting point:

$$V_L = \frac{R_p}{R_1 + R_p} V_b, \quad \text{where} \quad R_p = \frac{R_2 R_L}{R_2 + R_L}. \quad (3.45)$$

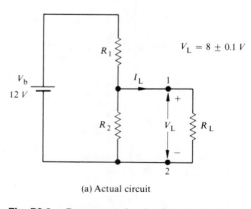

(a) Actual circuit

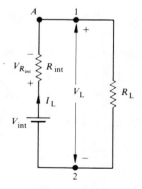

(b) Thevenin equivalent circuit

Fig. P9.2. Power supply circuit to be designed.

Using the Thevenin equivalent circuit (Fig. P9.2(b)) and the allowed upper and lower output voltages, we can determine the required values of R_1 and R_2. First, we use Kirchhoff's voltage law. Starting at point A and going around clockwise, we obtain the following equation:

$$+V_L - V_{int} + V_{R\,int} = 0,$$
$$+V_L - V_{int} + I_L R_{int} = 0.$$

Condition 1. $R_L = 2000\ \Omega$. For given R_{int} and V_{int} this load resistance will yield the lowest allowed output voltage: $V_{L1} = 7.9$ V. Under this condition, the current is $I_{L1} = 7.9/2000 = 3.95 \times 10^{-3}$ A.

Condition 2. $R_L = 4000\ \Omega$. For the same values of R_{int} and V_{int} as assumed above, this load resistance will give the highest allowed output voltage: $V_{L2} = 8.1$ V. Under this condition the load current is $I_{L2} = 8.1/4000 = 2.03 \times 10^{-3}$ A.

Using these two conditions, we can make two different substitutions into the Kirchhoff's voltage law equation to get two independent equations. By these two equations the two unknowns, R_{int} and V_{int}, can be determined:

$$7.9 - V_{int} + 3.95 \times 10^{-3} R_{int} = 0,$$
$$8.1 - V_{int} + 2.03 \times 10^{-3} R_{int} = 0,$$

so that

$$R_{int} = 104\ \Omega, \qquad V_{int} = 8.31\ \text{V}.$$

Now we solve for the voltage-divider resistor values:

$$V_{int} = \frac{R_2}{R_1 + R_2} V_b, \tag{9.1}$$

$$8.31 = \frac{R_2}{R_1 + R_2}\ (12)$$

$$\frac{R_2}{R_1 + R_2} = 0.692,$$

$$R_{int} = \frac{R_1 R_2}{R_1 + R_2}, \tag{9.4}$$

$$104 = 0.692\ R_1,$$

$$R_1 = 150\ \Omega, \qquad R_2 = 337\ \Omega.$$

Problem 9.3 A technician is asked to design a current source to deliver a current of 1 mA $\pm$ 0.1 mA into a chemical solution which has a resistance that varies from 2000 Ω to 4000 Ω during a particular experiment. He suggests the circuit shown in Fig. P9.3. What is the Norton equivalent circuit of this source? Will the circuit meet the specifications?

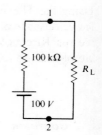

Fig. P9.3. Suggested circuit for a current source driving a load with a varying resistance.

Solution. Solve for the Norton current-source-equivalent circuit for the source. The open-circuit voltage between points 1 and 2, V_{oc}, is 100 V. The short-circuit current between points 1 and 2, I_{sc}, is easily determined:

$$I_{sc} = \frac{100 \text{ V}}{100 \text{ k}\Omega} = 1 \text{ mA}.$$

Using the open-circuit voltage and the short-circuit current, we can find the value of R_{int}:

$$R_{int} = \frac{V_{oc}}{I_{sc}} = \frac{100 \text{ V}}{1 \times 10^{-3} \text{ A}} = 100 \text{ k}\Omega.$$

The equivalent circuit is thus as shown in Fig. P9.3s1.

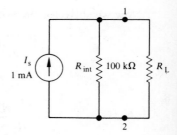

Fig. P9.3s1. Norton equivalent circuit for the current source circuit suggested by the technician.

Using Kirchhoff's current law, we can check to see how the current through the load will vary as the load resistance varies (Fig. P9.3s2):

$$\sum_i I_i = 0,$$

$$+I_S - I_i - I_L = 0,$$

where $I_i = V_A/R_{int}$, $I_L = V_A/R_L$,

$$+I_S - \frac{V_A}{R_{int}} - \frac{V_A}{R_L} = 0.$$

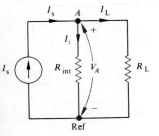

Fig. P9.3s2. Direction and polarity assumptions made for the current law analysis.

Therefore,

$$V_A = \frac{I_S}{1/R_{int} + 1/R_L}$$

and

$$I_L = \frac{V_A}{R_L} = \frac{I_S}{R_L/R_{int} + 1}.$$

When $R_L = 2000\ \Omega$,

$$I_L = \frac{1 \times 10^{-3}}{(2 \times 10^{+3})/(1 \times 10^5) + 1} = 0.98\ \text{mA}.$$

When $R_L = 4000\ \Omega$,

$$I_L = \frac{1 \times 10^{-3}}{(4 \times 10^{+3})/(1 \times 10^5) + 1} = 0.96\ \text{mA}.$$

Thus this circuit will meet the given specifications. Note that R_L is small with respect to R_{int}. This will always be true when the circuit shown in Fig. P9.3 is used as a current source.

Problem 9.4 The growth characteristic of a certain culture is to be investigated under two different conditions of humidity while the temperature is maintained at a specified value. The scientist has decided to use two temperature-controlled growth chambers set to the same temperature but having different humidities. A primary culture has been produced that is to be split into halves and then placed in the two chambers. The scientist wishes to monitor the temperature directly above each of the cultures and record these temperatures on two chart recorders together with the temperature difference between the two chambers. In searching the literature he found that he could use a thermistor, a temperature-sensitive resistor, in a relatively simple circuit to monitor the temperature. The circuit is shown in Fig. P9.4.

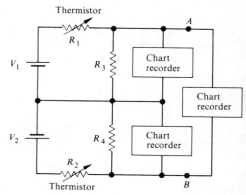

Fig. P9.4. Suggested circuit for monitoring the temperatures of two different environments.

Initially he assumed that he would have ideal chart recorders with infinite input resistances. He obtained a calibration curve for the thermistors which tells how the thermistor resistance varies with temperature. What are the relationships between the various components and the voltages that will be applied to the chart recorders?

Solution. First, we use Kirchhoff's voltage law to solve for the voltages across R_3 and R_4. It should be apparent that as the thermistor resistance R_1 varies, the voltage across R_3 will vary. Similarly, the voltage across R_4 will vary with the thermistor resistance R_2. Following the steps used in solving voltage law problems, we can obtain the following calculations.

Note that this circuit could be redrawn as shown in Fig. P9.4s1 so that there

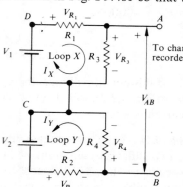

Fig. P9.4s1. The circuit to be analyzed.

are two independent circuits connected by only one wire. Variation in component values in circuit X have no effect on circuit Y, and vice versa.

Consider loop X. Starting at point D and going clockwise around loop X and taking the sum of the voltages across all the components, we obtain

$$\sum_i V_1 = 0.$$

$$+V_{R_1} + V_{R_3} - V_1 = 0.$$

But

$$V_{R_1} = I_X R_1, \quad V_{R_3} = I_X R_3,$$
$$+I_X R_1 + I_X R_3 - V_1 = 0,$$

and

$$I_X = \frac{V_1}{R_1 + R_3},$$

which yield

$$V_{R_3} = \frac{R_3}{R_1 + R_3} V_1.$$

Consider loop Y. Starting at point C and going counterclockwise around loop Y and taking the sum of the voltages across all the components, we have

$$\sum_i = 0,$$
$$-V_2 + V_{R_2} + V_{R_4} = 0.$$

But

$$V_{R_2} = I_Y R_2, \quad V_{R_4} = I_Y R_4$$
$$-V_2 + I_Y R_2 + I_Y R_4 = 0,$$

which yield

$$I_Y = \frac{V_2}{R_2 + R_4}, \quad V_{R_4} = \frac{R_4}{R_2 + R_4} V_2.$$

Now we can determine the voltage that is to represent the difference between the temperature in the two chambers. An inspection of Fig. P9.4s1 shows that the voltage between points A and B is the difference between the voltage across R_3 and the voltage across R_4. Since the latter two voltages are related to the temperatures of the two chambers, V_{AB} is the voltage needed to represent the temperature difference between the two chambers.

Once again we use the voltage law to determine V_{AB}. Starting at A and going clockwise around and taking the sum of the voltage across all the components, we have

$$+V_{AB} + V_{R_4} - V_{R_3} = 0,$$
$$V_{AB} = V_{R_3} - V_{R_4}.$$

The sign of the voltage V_{AB} will be determined by the magnitudes of V_{R_3} and V_{R_4}.

If $R_3 = R_4$, $V_1 = V_2$, and the thermistors R_1 and R_2 have identical characteristics, then the difference voltage V_{AB} will be zero if the two chambers are at the same temperature. As the temperature changes in one of the chambers with respect to the other chamber, the voltage at point A with respect to point B may be either positive or negative. The specific polarity at A with respect to point B depends on whether V_{R_3} is greater or less than V_{R_4}. With the calibration data given for the thermistors and the equations given above, it is possible to calibrate the temperature difference between the two chambers in terms of V_{AB}. Recall that ideal chart recorders were assumed for this problem. Errors can occur, some of which will be discussed in the following problem.

Problem 9.5   Since the last problem was worked out under the assumption that ideal chart recorders with infinite input resistances were used, it is important to consider what would happen if the recorder used to measure the temperature-difference voltage was not ideal. We assume that the same circuit as shown in Fig. P9.4 is used and that only the temperature-difference voltage is needed. We shall modify this circuit to include the input resistance of the chart recorder, as shown in Fig. P9.5s1.

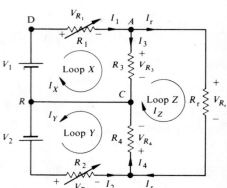

Fig. P9.5s1.   Circuit modified to include the chart recorder resistance R_r.

This circuit is considerably more difficult to analyze than the one in problem 9.4. Kirchhoff's voltage law can be used to solve for the voltage across the chart recorder input resistance R_r.

Consider loop X. Starting at point D and going clockwise around and taking the sum of the voltages across all the components, we have

$$\sum_i V_i = 0,$$

$$+V_{R_1} + V_{R_3} - V_1 = 0.$$

The branch currents and the loop currents are related in the following way:

$$I_1 = I_X, \quad I_3 = I_X - I_Z.$$

But

$$V_{R_1} = I_1 R_1 = I_X R_1, \quad V_{R_3} = I_3 R_3 = (I_X - I_Z) R_3,$$

which yield

$$+I_X R_1 + (I_X - I_Z) R_3 - V_1 = 0. \tag{*}$$

Consider loop Y. Starting at point C and going clockwise and taking the sum of the voltages across the several components, we obtain

$$\sum_i V_i = 0,$$

$$-V_{R_4} - V_{R_2} + V_2 = 0.$$

The branch currents and the loop currents are related in the following way:

$$I_2 = I_Y, \quad I_4 = I_Z + I_Y.$$

But

$$V_{R_2} = I_2 R_2 = I_Y R_2, \quad V_{R_4} = I_4 R_4 = (I_Z + I_Y) R_4,$$

which yield

$$-(I_Z + I_Y) R_4 - I_Y R_2 + V_2 = 0. \tag{*}$$

Consider loop Z. Starting at point A and going clockwise around and taking the sum of the voltages across all the components, we have

$$\sum_i V_i = 0,$$

$$+V_{R_r} + V_{R_4} - V_{R_3} = 0.$$

The branch currents and the loop currents have the following relations:

$$I_3 = I_X - I_Z, \quad I_4 = I_Z + I_Y, \quad I_Z = I_r.$$

But

$$V_{R_4} = I_4 R_4 = (I_Z + I_Y) R_4,$$

$$V_{R_3} = I_3 R_3 = (I_X - I_Z) R_3,$$

$$V_{R_r} = I_r R_r = I_Z R_r,$$

which yield

$$+I_Z R_r + (I_Z + I_Y) R_4 - (I_X - I_Z) R_3 = 0. \tag{*}$$

Three simultaneous equations are required to solve for the current through the chart recorder. They are designated by (*). The voltage across the recorder input is the product of the current through the recorder and the input resistance of the recorder.

As an example of how Kirchhoff's current law can be applied to this circuit, we give the following calculations. (Refer to Fig. P9.5s2. R is the reference node.)

Note that the currents at nodes A and B are labeled independently. The fact that the current through R_r is called I_5 at A and I_6 at B is of no consequence even though they are shown to be in opposite directions. When the V/R relations are

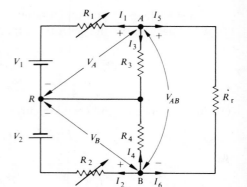

Fig. P9.5s2. Circuit assumptions for Kirchhoff's current law analysis.

substituted for the I's, these discrepancies will disappear, as we shall presently see.
Consider node A. We have

$$\sum_i I_i = 0,$$

$$-I_1 - I_3 - I_5 = 0,$$

$$-\frac{(V_A - V_1)}{R_1} - \frac{V_A}{R_3} - \frac{(V_A - V_B)}{R_r} = 0,$$

Consider node B. We have

$$\sum_i I_i = 0,$$

$$-I_2 - I_4 - I_6 = 0,$$

$$-\frac{(V_B - V_2)}{R_2} - \frac{V_B}{R_4} - \frac{(V_B - V_A)}{R_r} = 0.$$

Only two equations are necessary to solve for the unknown voltages when
the current law is used, whereas three equations are necessary when using the
voltage law. There is thus a saving in effort to obtain the final values. The voltage
V_{AB} from node A to node B is readily obtained:

$$V_{AB} = V_A - V_B.$$

Problem 9.6   The scientist has now decided to use the same voltage source for all
the temperature-detecting circuits discussed in problem 9.5. He has decided that
the temperature difference between the two chambers is the only information that
he must record. How will the use of only one battery affect the analysis of the
circuit? Can he use a storage battery, whose voltage may drop a little over the
period of the experiment, without adversely affecting the results?

Solution.   If only one battery is used, we must redraw the circuit and observe
that it becomes what is commonly called a bridge circuit (Fig. P9.6). We use
Kirchhoff's current law to solve for the voltages at points A and B.

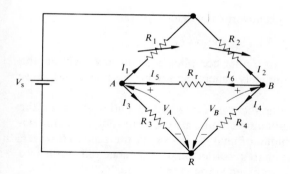

Fig. P9.6. Bridge circuit for measuring the temperature difference between two chambers.

Consider node A. We have

$$\sum_i I_i = 0,$$

$$-I_1 - I_3 - I_5 = 0,$$

$$-\frac{(V_A - V_S)}{R_1} - \frac{V_A}{R_3} - \frac{(V_A - V_B)}{R_r} = 0,$$

$$V_A \left(\frac{1}{R_1} + \frac{1}{R_3} + \frac{1}{R_r} \right) - \frac{V_B}{R_r} = \frac{V_S}{R_1}.$$

Consider node B. We have

$$\sum_i I_i = 0,$$

$$-I_2 - I_6 - I_4 = 0,$$

$$-\frac{(V_B - V_S)}{R_2} - \frac{(V_B - V_A)}{R_r} - \frac{V_B}{R_4} = 0,$$

$$-\frac{V_A}{R_r} + V_B \left(\frac{1}{R_2} + \frac{1}{R_4} + \frac{1}{R_r} \right) = \frac{V_S}{R_2}.$$

Solving the final equations for node A and node B yields the solutions for V_A and V_B:

$$V_A = \frac{\dfrac{1}{R_2} + \dfrac{R_r}{R_1} \left(\dfrac{1}{R_2} + \dfrac{1}{R_4} + \dfrac{1}{R_r} \right)}{R_r \left(\dfrac{1}{R_1} + \dfrac{1}{R_3} + \dfrac{1}{R_r} \right) \left(\dfrac{1}{R_2} + \dfrac{1}{R_4} + \dfrac{1}{R_r} \right) - \dfrac{1}{R_r}} V_S = X V_S,$$

$$V_B = \frac{\dfrac{1}{R_1} + \dfrac{R_r}{R_2} \left(\dfrac{1}{R_1} + \dfrac{1}{R_3} + \dfrac{1}{R_r} \right)}{R_r \left(\dfrac{1}{R_2} + \dfrac{1}{R_4} + \dfrac{1}{R_r} \right) \left(\dfrac{1}{R_1} + \dfrac{1}{R_3} + \dfrac{1}{R_r} \right) - \dfrac{1}{R_r}} V_S = Y V_S.$$

The voltage across the recorder V_{AB} is now readily determined:

$$V_{AB} = V_A - V_B = XV_S - YV_S = (X-Y)V_S.$$

The equations for V_A and V_B are rather complicated, but they will give the desired results. This solution is completely general so it can be applied whenever a bridge circuit is to be analyzed.

The question was asked regarding the use of one battery and its effect on the analysis of the circuit. Actually one-battery circuits are easier to solve for than two-battery circuits, although the technique of analysis is exactly the same. However, in this example the addition of the chart recorder input resistance did result in a solution that involved many terms in the equations for V_A and V_B.

A second question was asked regarding the effect of changes in the battery voltage on the chart recorder input voltage. Unfortunately the equation for V_{AB} above indicates that the difference voltage is directly proportional to the battery voltage. Therefore, any variations in the battery voltage could be misread as an indication of temperature change in the two chambers. A further complication can be seen. The temperature difference is determined by the quantity $X-Y$. If this difference is small, it can be easily masked by a small change in the battery voltage. In addition, note that as the temperature changes in the chambers, the thermistor resistances R_2 and R_1 will change. The equations for V_A and V_B will give some indication as to how sensitive the X and Y terms are to temperature changes. To investigate this problem, let us establish the following conditions. Let $R_r = \infty$, $R_3 = R_4 = R$. Then

$$V_A = \frac{1}{1 + R_1/R} V_S, \quad V_B = \frac{1}{1 + R_2/R} V_S.$$

Case 1. Let the nominal values R_1 and R_2 be R when the temperature of the two chambers are set at the desired value. Then

$$V_A = 0.5 \, V_S, \qquad V_B = 0.5 \, V_S, \qquad V_{AB} = 0.$$

Case 2. Let $R_1 = 0.95 R$ and $R_2 = R$, indicating that the temperature in one of the chambers has changed from the specified value. Then

$$V_A = \frac{1}{1 + 0.95} V_S = 0.5128 \, V_S, \quad V_B = 0.5 \, V_S, \quad V_{AB} = 0.0128 \, V_S.$$

Table P9.5 shows what would happen if R_1 were to continue changing while R_2 stayed constant for different values of R_2 relative to R_3 and R_4.

Note that for the values chosen, the largest output voltage between points A and B occurs when the thermistors R_1 and R_2 have the same nominal values as the other two resistors. In each case a change in R_1 from 95% to 90% of R_2 causes the output voltage to approximately double. A study such as this will help the circuit designer determine optimum values of the components he should choose for this bridge circuit.

TABLE 9.5
Effects of changing thermistor by 5% and 10% in bridge circuit

R_1	R_2	$V_A - V_B$	
R	R	0	
$0.95R$	R	$0.0128V_S$	} Ratio $= 2.05$
$0.9R$	R	$0.0263V_S$	
$0.1R$	$0.1R$	0	
$0.095R$	$0.1R$	$0.00415V_S$	} Ratio $= 2.01$
$0.09R$	$0.1R$	$0.00834V_S$	
$10R$	$10R$	0	
$9.5R$	$10R$	$0.00433V_S$	} Ratio $= 2.1$
$9R$	$10R$	$0.00909V_S$	
$100R$	$100R$	0	
$95R$	$100R$	$0.000516V_S$	} Ratio $= 2.11$
$90R$	$100R$	$0.001088V_S$	

Problem 9.7 A black box containing an *RC* filter is in a biologist's laboratory. The circuit diagram indicates that the circuit is as shown in Fig. P9.7. The biologist wants to know how this filter will respond to sinusoidal voltages of 100 Hz and 200 Hz applied across its input. The output is to be monitored on an ac voltmeter that will respond accurately to frequencies between 5 Hz and 5 MHz. The input impedance of the voltmeter is 100 kΩ for the range between 5 Hz and 500 kHz.

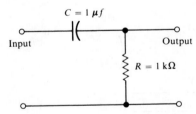

Fig. P9.7.   RC filter.

Solution. Consider the loading effect of the voltmeter on the filter. Will the voltmeter have any appreciable effect on the operation of the filter? The voltmeter will be placed in parallel with the resistor. (See Fig. P9.7s1.) Calculate the parallel combination of the resistor and the input impedance of the voltmeter and see if the impedance across the output terminals of the filter changes when the voltmeter is connected to the filter.

We use Eq. (4.19) for parallel impedances:

$$Z_{eq} = \cfrac{1}{\sum_i (1/Z_i)} = \cfrac{1}{1/Z_R + 1/Z_V} = \cfrac{1}{1/1000 + 1/Z_V}.$$

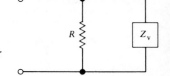

Fig. P9.7s1. Voltmeter connected in parallel with the filter output.

The statement of the problem does not tell us what the angle of the voltmeter impedance is. The amplitude is given to be 100 kΩ. Using this information, we can make a valid approximation:

$$Z_{eq} = \frac{1}{10^{-3} + 1/10^5 \angle \theta} = \frac{1}{10^{-3} + 10^{-5} \angle -\theta}.$$

The 10^{-5} term is much smaller than the 10^{-3} term. We can assume that ignoring this small term will not cause very much error. Therefore, we conclude that the voltmeter will probably not affect the filter appreciably.

Now we analyze the circuit without the voltmeter being connected across the filter output. Since this circuit is the same as that in Fig. 9.15, Eq. (9.13) may be used to determine the output voltage:

$$V_M = \frac{R}{R - jXc} V_s \qquad (9.13)$$

$$= \frac{1}{1 - j\left(\dfrac{X_c}{R}\right)} V_s = \frac{1}{1 - j\left(\dfrac{1}{2\pi fCR}\right)} V_s$$

$$= \frac{1}{1 - j\left(\dfrac{1}{2\pi(10^{-6})(10^3)f}\right)} V_s$$

$$= \frac{1}{1 - j\left(\dfrac{1}{2\pi(10^{-3})f}\right)} V_s.$$

When the frequency is very low, f is small, the term involving j and f will be very large and V_M will be small. In the limit, when f is zero, V_M is zero. The capacitor will not pass a direct current. When the frequency is very large, the term involving j and f will be very small and V_M will approach V_s. In the limit when f is infinite, $V_M = V_s$. This general tendency is shown in Fig. 4.14.

We can calculate the specific response of this circuit to a frequency of 100 Hz.

$$V_M = \cfrac{1}{1 - j\left(\cfrac{1}{2\pi(10^{-3})(100)}\right)} V_S$$

$$= \frac{1}{1 - j(1.59)} V_S = \frac{1}{1.88 \angle -57.8°} V_S$$

$$V_M = 0.532 \angle 57.8° V_S.$$

The specific response of this circuit to a frequency of 200 Hz is

$$V_M = \cfrac{1}{1 - j\left(\cfrac{1}{2\pi(10^{-3})(200)}\right)} V_S$$

$$= \frac{1}{1 - j(0.797)} V_S = \frac{1}{1.278 \angle -38.6°} V_S$$

$$= 0.783 \angle 38.6° V_S.$$

Problem 9.8   In a particular experiment noise in the form of an unwanted sinusoidal voltage of 120 Hz is observed on a cathode-ray oscilloscope. The scientist wants to filter out this particular frequency while passing frequencies between zero and 10 Hz and frequencies between 1 kHz and 2 kHz. He is told that a circuit like that shown in Fig. P9.8 can be used for this purpose. He wants to know how this circuit will respond to frequencies in the three critical ranges.

Solution.   Equation (4.16) can be used in the analysis of this circuit:

$$V_{out} = \frac{1}{1 + Z_1/Z_2} V_S \tag{4.16}$$

$$Z_p = \frac{X_C X_L}{j(X_L - X_C)}.$$

We let $Z_1 = Z_p$, $Z_2 = R$. Then

$$V_{out} = \cfrac{1}{1 + \cfrac{X_C X_L}{[j(X_L - X_C)/R]}} V_S.$$

Note that if $X_L - X_C$ is zero, the denominator is infinite and the output voltage goes to zero. Therefore, at a frequency of 120 Hz, which is to be rejected, X_L must equal X_C. At low frequencies and at high frequencies, the Z_p term should become small if the output voltage is to approach the source voltage. Expanding the equation for Z_p will show the relationship involving frequency:

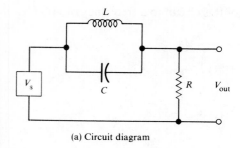

(a) Circuit diagram

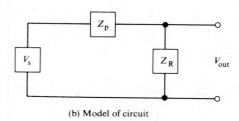

(b) Model of circuit

Fig. P9.8. Filter circuit to be analyzed.

$$Z_p = \frac{\omega L/\omega C}{j(\omega L - 1/\omega C)} = \frac{L/C}{j(2\pi fL - 1/2\pi fC)}. \tag{9.20}$$

From Eq. (9.20) we can see that when $f = 0$, $Z_p = 0$. When f is infinite, $Z_p = 0$. Equation (4.16) shows that for these last two conditions, the output voltage will equal the source voltage; thus the circuit will begin to approach the characteristics stated in this problem.

We pick a standard value for the inductance L; say, $L = 1$ henry. We can determine the value of C such that Z_p is infinite when $f = 120$ Hz:

$$2\pi fL = \frac{1}{2\pi fC},$$

$$C = \frac{L}{4\pi^2 f^2 L} = 1.76 \times 10^{-6} \text{ F} = 1.76 \ \mu\text{F},$$

where F stands for farads. Then we can determine the value of Z_p for the frequencies specified in the statement of the problem (Table P9.8.1). Equation (9.21) shows that the important ratio is Z_p/R:

$$V_{\text{out}} = \frac{1}{1 + Z_p/R} V_s. \tag{9.21}$$

The last important step in the solution is to determine what value R should have in order that the circuit will perform adequately. If the ratio Z_p/R is small compared to 1, the output voltage will be almost equal to the source voltage. Table P9.8.2 shows the output voltage for two values of R. If R is 1000 Ω or more,

TABLE P9.8.1

f (Hz)	Z_p (Ω)
0	0
10	$+j\,(62.8)$
120	∞
1 k	$-j\,(91.8)$
2 k	$-j\,(45.4)$
∞	0

the output voltage at the specified frequencies will be essentially equal to the source voltage. Thus this circuit will have the desired filtering characteristics.

TABLE P9.8.2

R (Ω)	f (Hz)	V_{out}
100	10	$0.847V_S$
100	120	0
100	1 k	$0.735V_S$
100	2 k	$0.91V_S$
1000	10	$0.997V_S$
1000	120	0
1000	1 k	$0.996V_S$
1000	2 k	$0.999V_S$

9.8 REVIEW QUESTIONS AND PROBLEMS

9.1 A voltage divider circuit has been designed to provide a voltage less than the dc power supply voltage. Determine the voltage V_{12} that will be present when a load resistance, R_L, of 1 k Ω is connected between points 1 and 2. First, determine the Thevenin equivalent of the voltage divider circuit without the load resistance connected between 1 and 2. Second, calculate V_{12} when the load resistance is connected between points 1 and 2. Third, check your answer by another method using Fig. R9.1.

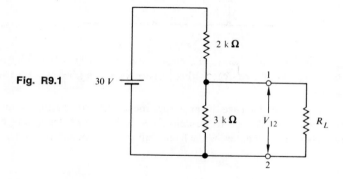

Fig. R9.1

9.2 Using the voltage divider circuit in review problem 9.1, determine the variation in voltage V_{12} as a function of the load resistance, R_L, connected between points 1 and 2. Draw a curve of your results.

9.3 A regulated dc power supply has an output voltage of 10 V. It has a maximum output current rating of 100 mA. In a particular set of experiments a dc voltage of 4 V is to be applied across a load that has a resistance that ranges from 100 to 400 Ω. What values should be used for the two resistors needed in the voltage divider required to provide this voltage? What factors affect the voltage variation that may occur across the load?

9.4 What are the major differences between a Thevenin equivalent circuit and a Norton equivalent circuit?

9.5 State, in words, Kirchhoff's voltage and current laws.

9.6 Write a Kirchhoff voltage law equation for the circuit in Fig. R9.2.

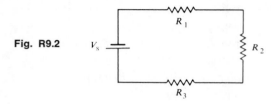

Fig. R9.2

9.7 What are the unknown variables in a Kirchhoff's voltage law equation?

9.8 What are the unknown variables in a Kirchhoff's current law equation?

9.9 Write the Kirchhoff's voltage law equations for the circuit in Fig. R9.3.

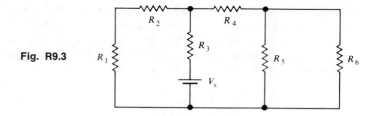

Fig. R9.3

9.10 Calculate the current that flows in the circuit shown in Fig. R9.4. The power rating for R_3 is 0.5 W ($P = I^2R$). Is this resistor operating below, at, or above its power rating?

9.11 A heated chamber is to be used in an experiment. Two different amounts of power, 100 W and 200 W, are to be delivered to the heater depending on the time of day. Assume the heater has a fixed value of resistance of 40 Ω. (This

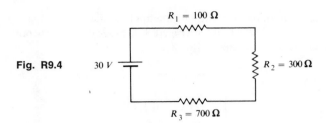

Fig. R9.4

is not usually true but it makes the problem easier to solve.) The source voltage is 60 Hz 120 V rms. Design a series circuit that can be used to produce these two heater powers. (Hint: Use a resistor or resistors in series with the heater.) Is this an efficient system?

9.12 For the circuit in Fig. R9.5:
    (a) Determine the voltage V_{12} using Kirchhoff's voltage law.
    (b) Determine the current flowing through the source.
    (c) Determine the power delivered by the source.
    (d) Determine the voltage V_{34}.

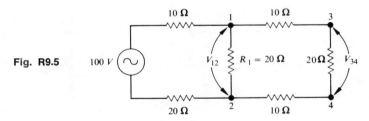

Fig. R9.5

9.13 What is the Thevenin equivalent of the circuit in Fig. R9.5 as seen looking into terminals 1 and 2 if R_1 is disconnected from the circuit? Using this Thevenin equivalent circuit, determine the voltage V_{12} and compare it with that calculated in the previous problem.

9.14 If R_1 is a variable resistor in the circuit in Fig. R9.5, do you see any advantages in calculating V_{12} for various values of R_1 via the Thevenin equivalent circuit method as compared to using the straightforward approach of the Kirchhoff's voltage law approach? Justify why you think your answer is valid.

9.15 Set up the Kirchhoff's current law equation required to solve for the voltage V_{12} for the circuit in Fig. R9.6.

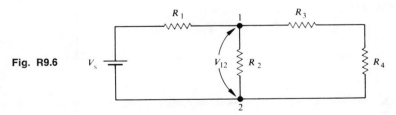

Fig. R9.6

9.16   Use the Kirchhoff current law method to find the voltage at the output of the voltage divider circuit in Fig. R9.7. Solve for the current flowing through R_L and the power dissipated in R_L.

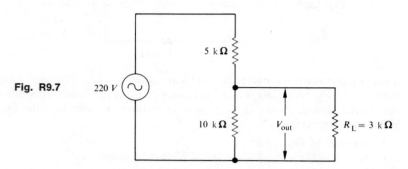

Fig. R9.7

9.17   Set up the two equations required to determine the two unknown node voltages, V_{14} and V_{34}, in Fig. R9.8.

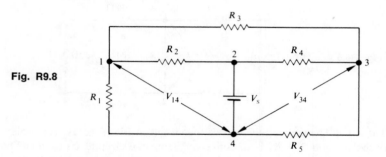

Fig. R9.8

9.18   Using the Kirchhoff current law analysis method as a procedure, determine the power rating required for the resistor R_x in Fig. R9.9.

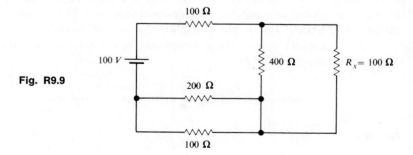

Fig. R9.9

9.19   Determine the voltage V_{12} for the circuit with the two power sources in Fig. R9.10.

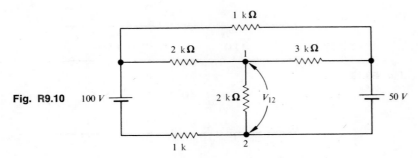

Fig. R9.10

9.20 The network in Fig. R9.11 is required as part of a measurement system. The current that is to flow through R_0 is to be 1 mA. What dc voltage, V_s, is needed at the source? What current will be drawn from the source?

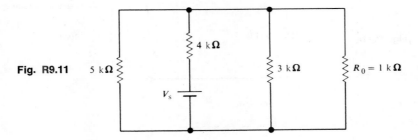

Fig. R9.11

9.21 Determine the voltage variation that will occur between points 1 and 2 of the circuit in Fig. R9.12 if the source voltage, V_s, varies ±3 V from a center value of 30 V. What change in power dissipated in R_0 will occur as a result of the source voltage variation?

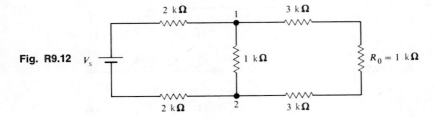

Fig. R9.12

9.22 An ideal current source is connected to a test circuit shown in Fig. R9.13. How much current will flow through R_x?

9.23 An ideal current source is to be approximated by the circuit shown in Fig. R9.14. (a) What should the power rating of resistor R_s be? (b) How much current will flow through the specimen that is modeled as having resistance R_x? (c) If R_x varies from 50 to 300 Ω, what variation in source current will occur? Will the source actually act as an ideal current source?

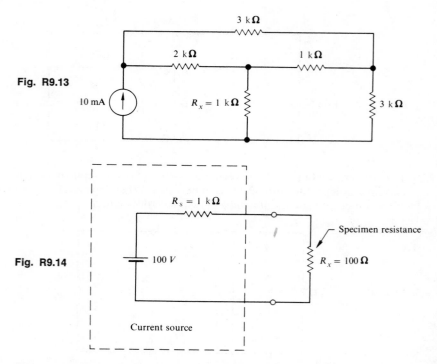

Fig. R9.13

Fig. R9.14

9.24 Determine the value of current that flows through R_n, the null detector resistance, in the bridge circuit shown in Fig. R9.15. If R_x varies from 500 to 2000 Ω, what change in the current through R_n will be noted. (This question simulates what might occur if a bridge circuit becomes unbalanced. Recall that at balance, the current through the null detector would be zero.)

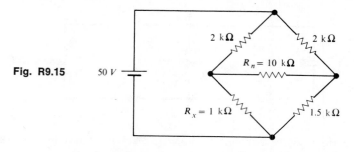

Fig. R9.15

9.25 Convert the following complex numbers to polar form:

(a) $Z = 3 + j4$ (f) $Z = 120 + j5$
(b) $Z = 25 + j25$ (g) $Z = 75 + j90$
(c) $Z = 30 - j20$ (h) $Z = 6 - j5$
(d) $Z = 37 - j20$ (i) $Z = 14 - j19$
(e) $Z = 9 - j3$ (j) $Z = 32 - j20$

9.26   Convert the following complex numbers to rectangular form.
    (a) $Z = 10 \ \underline{/25°}$ (f) $Z = 307 \ \underline{/-17°}$
    (b) $Z = 32 \ \underline{/-45°}$ (g) $Z = 141 \ \underline{/62°}$
    (c) $Z = 45 \ \underline{/75°}$ (h) $Z = 87 \ \underline{/-34°}$
    (d) $Z = 7 \ \underline{/-30°}$ (i) $Z = 14 \ \underline{/-53°}$
    (e) $Z = 100 \ \underline{/60°}$ (j) $Z = 28 \ \underline{/64°}$

9.27   Determine the impedance of a one-microfarad capacitor at each of these frequencies. $f = $ 100 Hz, 500 Hz, 1 kHz, 50 kHz.

9.28   Determine the impedance of a 0.02 microfarad capacitor at these frequencies. $f = $ 100 Hz, 500 Hz, 1 kHz, 50 kHz.

9.29   Determine the reactance of a one-henry inductor at each of these frequencies. $f = $ 100 Hz, 500 Hz, 1 kHz, 50 kHz.

9.30   Determine the total impedance of the circuit in Fig. R9.16. Give your answer in both polar and rectangular form.

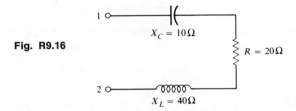

Fig. R9.16

9.31   Determine the total impedance of the circuit in Fig. R9.17. What conclusions can you make?

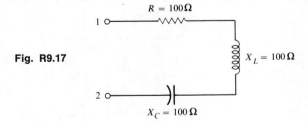

Fig. R9.17

9.32   Determine the general equation for the impedance of the circuit in Fig. R9.18.

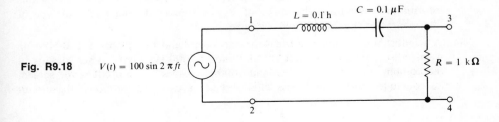

Fig. R9.18 $V(t) = 100 \sin 2 \pi f t$

9.33 At what frequency will the capacitive reactance equal the inductive reactance in the circuit of Fig. R9.18? At that frequency, what is the voltage across the resistor?

9.34 For the circuit in Fig. R9.18, determine the current that will flow as a function of frequency.

9.35 Using the circuit in Fig. R9.18, determine the voltage across the resistor as a function of frequency. Plot your results. What type of filter circuit is this: low pass, band pass, band reject, or high pass?

9.36 Determine the impedance Z_{12} for the circuit in Fig. R9.19.

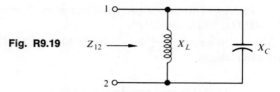

Fig. R9.19 $Z_{12} \longrightarrow$ X_L X_C

9.37 Determine the impedance Z_{12} for the circuit in Fig. R9.20. What conclusions can you make?

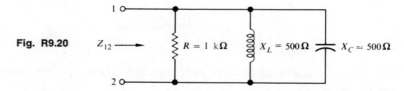

Fig. R9.20 $Z_{12} \longrightarrow$ $R = 1 \text{ k}\Omega$ $X_L = 500 \Omega$ $X_C = 500 \Omega$

9.38 Determine the general equation for the impedance Z_{12} for the circuit in Fig. R9.21.

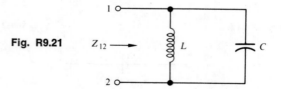

Fig. R9.21 $Z_{12} \longrightarrow$ L C

9.39 Determine the general equation for the impedance Z_{12} of the circuit in Fig. R9.22 and then determine the source current vs. frequency curve. Using this information, determine the curve of V_R vs. frequency. What general type of filter characteristic does this circuit have?

9.40 A scientist made some electrical measurements and found that a 120-Hz sine wave noise voltage was masking the desired 1000-Hz signal. After looking at the combination of the 120-Hz and 1000-Hz waves on an oscilloscope screen, he concluded that a high-pass filter should be used. He proposed the circuit

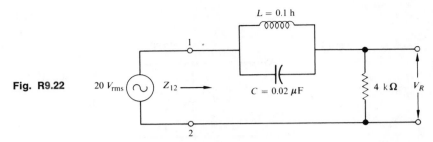

Fig. R9.22 $20\ V_{\text{rms}}$ $Z_{12} \longrightarrow$ $L = 0.1\ \text{h}$ $C = 0.02\ \mu\text{F}$ $4\ \text{k}\Omega$ V_R

in Fig. R9.23 but was unable to determine the proper value for the capacitor. Which of the following values of capacitance would be the most appropriate and why? $C = 0.04\,\mu\text{F}$, $C = 0.53\,\mu\text{F}$, $C = 1.2\,\mu\text{F}$. Assume that the signal source has a very low internal impedance and the oscilloscope has a one megohm input resistance.

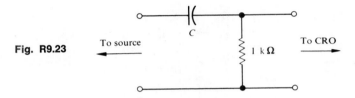

Fig. R9.23   To source C $1\ \text{k}\Omega$ To CRO

9.41   Noise in the upper audio frequency range, 10 kHz to 20 kHz, is interfering with an electrical measurement. A low-pass filter has been designed and is available for use in blocking out this noise and to pass the desired 10-Hz signal. The circuit to be used is shown in Fig. R9.24. What is its transfer function characteristic? Does it look like this filter will be capable of doing this filtering job?

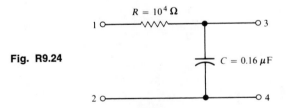

Fig. R9.24 $R = 10^4\ \Omega$ 1   3 $C = 0.16\ \mu\text{F}$ 2   4

9.42   Assume the filter circuit in Fig. R9.24 is connected into a measuring circuit that has the component values shown in Fig. R9.25. Determine the curve of V_o/V_s vs. frequency. Does this curve have the same shape as the transfer function curve for the circuit in Fig. R9.24? Discuss your findings after comparing these two curves.

9.43   Determine the voltage across the output terminals 1 and 2 of the circuit in Fig. R9.26.

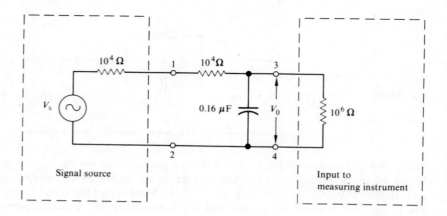

Fig. R9.25

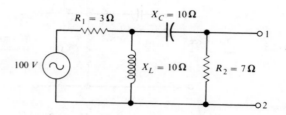

Fig. R9.26

10
noise in
measuring systems

10.1 OBJECTIVES

With advancing knowledge the signals that scientists desire to measure get smaller and smaller every year. If the environment between the test specimen and the display unit were quiet, it would be possible to detect signals of any level. All that would be needed is an amplifier that will give the amplification required to make the signal visible on the type of display unit being used. Unfortunately, the environment is invariably noisy and noise plagues scientists whenever they want to measure small signals.

As a result of this noise, the scientist is forced to ask one major question. What is the smallest signal I can measure with acceptable accuracy? This question in turn leads her or him to several other questions.

1. What does the noise do to the display of signals that I wish to see?
2. What is the source of that noise that causes interference?
3. How high is the noise level?
4. What are the frequencies contained in the noise and how do they compare with the frequencies of the desired signal?
5. What is the likelihood of very large noise peaks that will completely mask the desired signal?

These questions were not posed in the previous chapters. The basic building blocks discussed so far are used when the scientist is measuring signals that are not significantly affected by noise. The study of noise problems, however, is an essential part of a scientist's electrical background.

Noise is defined as *any voltage or current that is unwanted in a circuit*. It is any extraneous disturbance tending to interfere with the normal reception of a desired signal. Noise is always present with the signal, so it is only a question of how large it is relative to the signal amplitude. If the noise amplitude is one-hundredth of the amplitude of the signal, there will be no difficulty in determining the presence and the shape of the signal waveform. When the amplitude of the noise is equal to that of the signal, it is sometimes quite difficult to learn much about the characteristics of the signal.

Noise that causes difficulties in experiments is usually one of the following types:

1. Noise derived from the 60-Hz power line supply.

2. Noise derived from random sources not related to the power line or desired signal source.

The effects of noise on the display of signals, the sources of noise, and the methods of characterizing noise are discussed in this chapter. This discussion will help the reader anticipate problems that may occur when he tries to measure small electrical signals.

10.2   NOISE ENTERS THE SYSTEM

Frequently the rms voltage or current of a signal given by a voltmeter or ammeter will yield little useful information to the experimenter. Instead, the waveshape of the signal will contain the information needed on the important characteristics of the organism being investigated. In this case a cathode-ray oscilloscope or a chart recorder may be used to display the measured waveform. If the signal to be measured is small (in the order of millivolts or microvolts) the noise present in the system may mask the signal. The noise that causes the problem may enter the circuit in several places, as shown in Fig. 10.1.

Noise may enter at any point in the circuit and combine with the signal from the test animal to the display unit. The effect that this noise will have on the display of the signal may be the same regardless of where the noise enters the measuring system. However, the method by which we can reduce the noise to the lowest possible level depends on the type of noise and the way it gets mixed with the signal. Methods of processing noisy signals will be discussed in Chapter 11.

The noise indicated in Fig. 10.1 may be caused by the 60-Hz power line or by a source of *random noise* that is not related to the power line or the desired signal source. Examples of these sources of noise are easily recognized. Almost all laboratories are supplied with 60-Hz power, which produces magnetic fields whenever current is flowing in the power line. These fields may induce a 60-Hz voltage in the measuring-circuit wires that are nearby and thus combine with the desired signal. It may also be coupled to the system by a stray capacitance between the power wires and the system. If the desired signal happens to be only several microvolts in amplitude, an amplifier will have to be used to increase the signal level to an observable amplitude for the display devices.

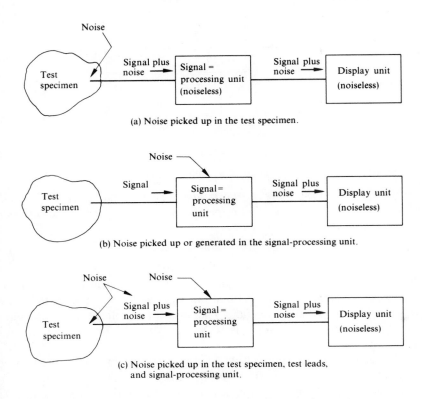

Fig. 10.1.   Points at which noise may enter the measuring system.

Assume for the moment that it is possible to eliminate all of the 60-Hz noise in the system and any other extraneous noise that combines with the signal at the test point in the specimen. Are there still problems which remain? Unfortunately all amplifiers generate random noise. Amplifiers use either vacuum tubes or transistors and resistors, and each of these components is an inherent source of random noise. This random noise will combine with the desired signal to produce a composite electrical signal which is displayed to the observer.

It will be worthwhile to determine the relative importance of noises introduced at different stages of an amplifier. The noise that is generated at the input to the first stage of an amplifier will usually prove to be the most troublesome. Figure 10.2 shows a block diagram of an amplifier. Let us assume that the amplifier stages are noiseless and introduce noise at specific points in the amplifier for purposes of explanation.

For the first test, assume that a noise voltage of 10 μV rms is applied at the input, between points 1 and 5, along with a sine wave of 10 μV rms. What effect will this noise have on the signal at the output? Before answering the question it will prove helpful to define a figure-of-merit term relating signal to noise. This

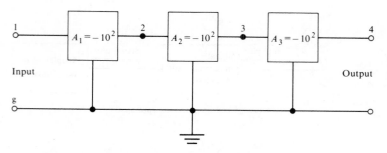

Fig. 10.2. Block diagram of a typical multistage amplifier.

figure of merit is called the *signal-to-noise ratio, (SNR)*, and is defined to be *the ratio of the rms value of the signal at a specific point in a circuit to the rms value of the noise at that point in the circuit:*

$$\text{SNR} = \frac{\text{rms value of signal}}{\text{rms value of noise}}. \tag{10.1}$$

(Sometimes the SNR is assumed to be the ratio of signal power to noise power.) In this example the signal-to-noise ratio at the input to the amplifier is 1, because both voltages are 10 μV in amplitude. The sine wave voltage at the output is 10 V rms and the noise at the output is 10 V rms. Thus the SNR at the output of the amplifier is also 1.

For the second test, assume that we feed in a 10-μV rms sine wave between points 1 and 5 while feeding in a 10-μV rms noise between points 2 and 5. The sine wave will be multiplied by 10^6, yielding 10 V rms at the output. The noise voltage will be multiplied by only 10^4, yielding 0.1 V rms at the output. In this second test, the output SNR will be 100. This example points out the important fact that the noise that is generated or induced at or near the input to an amplifier will mask the desired signal much more than will noise that is generated or induced near the output of the amplifier.

A point to remember

The noise characteristics of the input stage of an amplifier must be minimized if the SNR at the output is to be relatively large. The other stages of the amplifier are not so critical in terms of their contribution to noise at the output.

10.3   EFFECTS OF NOISE ON THE DISPLAY OF SIGNALS

How serious are the detrimental effects of broadband noise† on a sine wave can be appreciated after you have studied the following waveforms observed with the aid of a cathode-ray oscilloscope.

---

† Broadband noise is noise containing many frequencies spread over a wide band of frequencies.

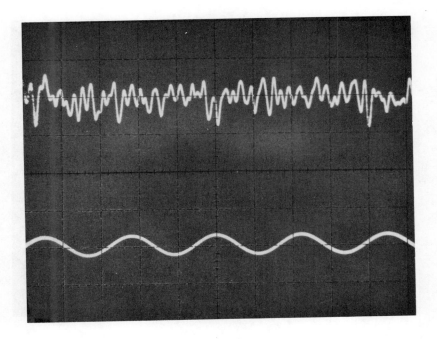

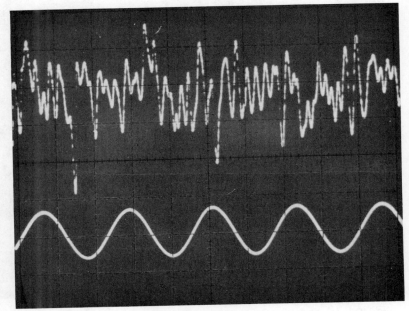

Fig. 10.3. (a) and (b) Oscillograms of signals and noise.

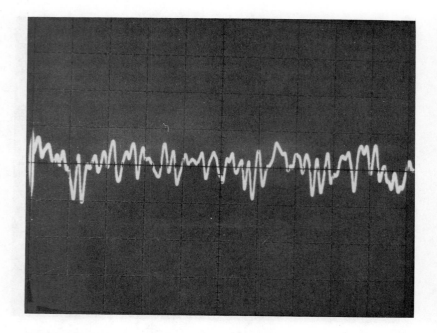

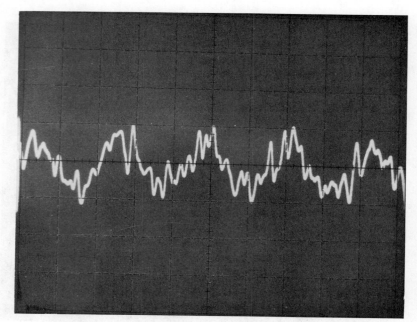

Fig. 10.3. (c) and (d) Oscillograms of signals and noise.

In part (a) of Fig. 10.3 you will see a sine wave of the same rms value as that of a broadband noise. The noise contains frequencies of significant amplitude up to about 50 kHz. In part (b) the two waves of part (a) are superimposed on each other. Thus the SNR for this combination is 1. Part (c) shows a sine wave that has been added to noise so that the SNR is now 0.5. Note that the presence of the sine wave is not obvious from a study of this oscillogram. At this point it becomes apparent that some type of processing of the combined signal and noise must be done if the signal is to be detected. In part (d) the signal-to-noise ratio is increased to 3 and the signal is now evident from the shape of the waveform.

The spectral characteristics of the noise used when obtaining the oscillograms of Fig. 10.3 are shown in Fig. 10.4. Note that a continuous range of frequencies up to about 20 kHz are present with approximately equal amplitude. Frequencies higher than 20 kHz are also generated, but they are not of the same amplitude, having been limited by the circuitry in the noise generator.

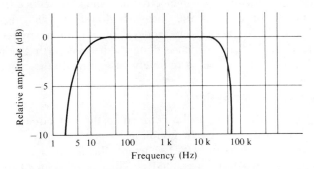

Fig. 10.4. Spectral characteristics of the noise used in the examples shown in Fig. 10.3.

10.4   NOISE EXTERNAL TO THE MEASUREMENT SYSTEM

The noise that causes trouble in a measurement system may be produced by a source that is many feet or miles away from the test specimen, as in the case of lightning. As previously mentioned, the 60-Hz power line quite often can cause problems. But this is only one type of environmental noise that the experimenter must contend with. Any device near the location of the experiment that produces sparking, such as electric motors with commutators, can cause electrical noise that will be picked up by the measuring circuit and combined with the signal. Fluorescent lights or other flickering lights may cause electrical disturbances. Structural vibration may cause parts of a circuit to move with respect to one another and thus cause varying electrical potentials to be induced in the test circuit. Similarly temperature variations may cause circuit performance to change and, in effect, produce very low-frequency variations, on the order of small fractions of a cycle per second, which can be classified as noise.

Electrostatic Coupling to the System

Electrostatic disturbances can be coupled into the test circuit through the stray capacitance that always exists between components. Figure 10.5 shows the way stray capacitance couples noise signals into the test circuit. All along the system there will be stray capacitance distributed between the wire from the noise source and the test specimen, the connection wires and the measuring instruments. Thus there is a complete circuit from the source of noise, through the stray capacitance, to the measuring system, to ground, and back to the other side of the noise source. This type of interference can be reduced by reducing the stray capacitance to a minimum. This may be done in several ways. Move the experimental equipment and test organism as far away as possible from the source of noise and associated wires. Use an electrostatic shield to reduce the capacitance between the noise source and the measuring system. That is, confine the organism and associated probes, electrodes, etc. within a copper screen cage which serves as the shield and which is connected to an earth ground. All of the apparatus is then usually controlled remotely from outside the cage.

Magnetic Coupling into the System

A second way in which noise can be coupled to the test circuit is by magnetic fields. Figure 10.6 shows a magnetic coupling.

A noise current, such as the 60-Hz current, flowing in a wire in the vicinity of the test circuit will have an associated varying magnetic field around it. This varying field will induce a noise voltage into the test specimen and the connecting wires and thus cause problems. The noise introduced this way can be reduced by

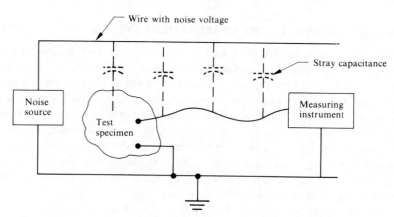

Fig. 10.5. Introduction of noise to test circuit by stray capacitance.

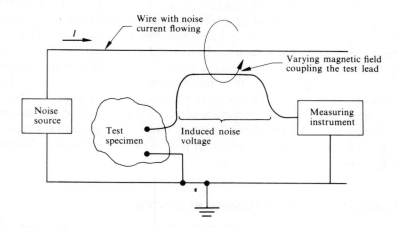

Fig. 10.6. Introduction of noise to test circuit by magnetic coupling.

moving the test organism as far away as possible from wires carrying the noise currents. However, this is not always possible in a relatively small laboratory because the power line wires are usually located so as to provide convenient access to electric power. The best magnetic coupling occurs when the wires are close together and are parallel to each other. If the wires can be arranged at right angles to each other, the magnetic coupling will be minimized. Twisting together the pair of wires carrying the noise current will reduce the magnetic field noise coupled into the measurement system.

The use of shielded wire for the connection between the test specimen and the measuring instrument is a very common and recommended practice. Two types of shielded wire are shown in Fig. 10.7.

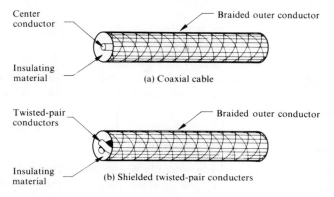

Fig. 10.7. Two types of shielded wire used for reducing noise.

In addition to the use of shielded wire to reduce the effects of externally generated noise, it is usually helpful to make the connecting leads as short as possible to minimize both the stray capacitance to noise sources and the conductor length in which noise voltage can be induced magnetically.

The references cited in Appendix 4 should be consulted if the reader experiences severe noise problems that are obviously caused by sources of noise external to the experiment. The sources of these noises are quite often very difficult to track down, and the reduction of the coupling to these sources can be an exasperating task. An experiment may be relatively noiseless on one part of a laboratory bench but when reoriented or moved to another location become so affected by noise as to lose all its value.

10.5   NOISE WITHIN THE MEASUREMENT SYSTEM

When the experimenter applies sufficient skill and care to the design of the physical layout of his measurement system, he can eliminate most of the extraneous noise coupled into his system. When the noise from sources external to his system has been minimized, he is still faced with another source of noise: from the components he must use in his measurement circuits. Resistors produce noise. Vacuum tubes produce noise. Transistors produce noise. The noise generated by these components will determine the limit of signal-detection sensitivity that can be achieved by the measurement system. As indicated in Section 10.2, the noise generated at the input to the measurement circuit is the most detrimental.

The noise generated by the resistors, vacuum tubes, and transistors is generally random. Random noise may be defined as a disturbing fluctuation which cannot be precisely predicted for any specific moment. One cannot say, with assurance, what the random-noise voltage or current will be at the next instant. Random noise is a nondeterministic function as compared to a 60-Hz sine wave noise. A sine wave is a deterministic function and can be specified by the following equation:

$$f(t) = A \sin 2\pi f t$$

where f is frequency, t is time, and A is a constant.

With this equation it is possible to determine the value of the 60-Hz noise at any time in the future. This kind of prediction is not possible for random noise such as shown in Fig. 10.3.

Thermal Noise

The random noise generated by commonly encountered electrical components is called *fluctuation noise*. This type of noise may be further subdivided into *thermal noise* and *shot noise*. Thermal noise or *Johnson noise*, as it is often called, s caused by the random motion of free electrons in a conducting medium. The amount of motion is determined by the temperature of the medium. It is always present in a circuit and usually establishes the lower noise limit in the circuit. The random motion of the electrons produces many different frequencies. In fact, it produces all the frequencies over a very wide band of frequencies up to approximately 10^{13} Hz. This means that thermal noise will affect any measurement in which the signal voltage is in the nanovolt or microvolt range regardless of the frequency.

Shot Noise

Shot noise is caused by the random motion of charged carriers. In a vacuum tube the emission of electrons from the cathode occurs randomly and this action produces noise in the electron stream because the flow of electrons is not uniform with time. A similar random action takes place as charged carriers move through semiconductor materials. The average number of charged carriers moving past a point over a relatively extended period may be a constant, but during very small increments of time the number moving past a point may vary widely; thus the current contains a component of noise due to the random rates at which the carriers pass that point. In diode tubes this noise is directly proportional to the average flow of current. In amplifying tubes this type of noise is usually lower in triode tubes than in pentode tubes. Shot noise produces frequencies in the range from near dc to somewhere above 50 MHz.

The frequency spectra of both thermal noise and shot noise are essentially flat, which means that all frequencies are generated at about the same amplitude of voltage or current. In addition to these noises, another type of noise also appears in both tubes and transistors and is predominant in the low-frequency range: the *flicker noise*. Flicker noise is caused by slow changes in the materials used in cathodes and transistors. It has significant amplitudes for frequencies between about 1 kHz and dc. It is sometimes called $1/f$ noise because the slope of its frequency spectrum is proportional to $1/f$. This noise increases its amplitude at the lower frequencies and is a major limiting factor when measuring small dc voltages or ac voltages below 10 Hz. Near dc it appears to give the measuring system a slow drifting characteristic.

10.6 CHARACTERISTICS OF RANDOM NOISE

The detailed calculation of specific values of random noise that can be expected in various circuits is beyond the scope of this book. However, there are two characteristics of noise which are helpful to know when planning experiments involving the measurement of small electrical signals. These characteristics pertain to the frequencies and the amplitudes of noise that can be expected.

Power Density Spectrum

A common way of describing the frequencies present in a noise wave is the *power density spectrum.* The general shape of the power density spectrum for thermal noise is shown in Fig. 10.8. This spectrum gives the relative amounts of power that can be found in any frequency band of interest. For example, the power in the frequency range between f_1 and f_2 is given to be equal to the area under this portion of the curve. This curve is described by the following equation that reveals the importance of temperature and resistance:

$$P(f) = 4kTR, \tag{10.2}$$

where $P(f)$ is the power density in V^2-sec, k is Boltzmann's constant, 1.38×10^{-23} joule/°K, T is temperature in degrees Kelvin, and R is resistance in ohms.

Thermal noise in resistors, as described by Eq. (10.2), is commonly called *white noise,* because it contains all frequencies with equal amplitude over the entire range of frequencies commonly used in electrical circuits. The equation is considered to be valid for frequencies up to approximately 10^{13} Hz. Open-circuit rms noise voltage in a small range of frequencies is given by Eq. (10.3):

$$V_{rms} = \sqrt{P(f)\Delta f} \tag{10.3}$$

where $P(f)$ is the power density spectrum and Δf is a small range of frequencies.

An inspection of Eqs. (10.2) and (10.3) will lead to the following important ideas:

Points to remember

1. The rms noise voltage produced by a resistor will increase as the resistance increases.

2. The rms noise voltage output of a resistor will increase as the temperature increases.

3. The rms noise voltage output of a resistor will increase as the bandwidth of noise accepted by the measurement circuit increases.

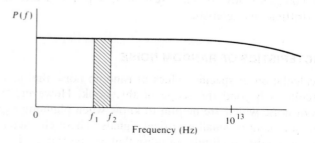

Fig. 10.8. Power-density spectrum for thermal noise.

If thermal noise is limiting the sensitivity of the measuring system, the resistance that is producing the noise should be lowered, the temperature should be reduced, and some means of limiting the frequency band of noise should be employed. This band may be limited by means of a filter that will pass only the frequencies that are contained in the desired signal and reject all other frequencies generated by the noise source.

Amplitude Probability Density Functions

One last characteristic of random noise should be described. It is the *probability density function* (pdf) of the noise voltage or current. An example is shown in Fig. 10.9. The probability density function for random noise is usually normal or *gaussian* in shape, as shown in Fig. 10.9. The curve gives an indication of what voltage amplitudes can be expected at any instant. The rms value of the noise gives only very general information about the amount of noise. It does not give any indication of how large the sharp impulses of noise might be or the likelihood that they will occur. But the probability density function of the noise voltage or current will give some help. From this density function it is possible to determine the probability that the noise voltage will fall between any two values V_1 and V_2.

$$\text{Probability } (V_1 \leqslant V \leqslant V_2)$$
$$= \text{Area under the pdf curve from } V_1 \text{ to } V_2. \tag{10.4}$$

Probability density function information about random noise is usually not available to the experimenter. However, an estimate of the pdf curve can be made if a true rms reading of the noise can be obtained. Fortunately, the rms value of the random noise is equal to the standard deviation σ of the normal-distribution curve. Thus, if the experimenter can get a measurement of rms voltage of the noise which he suspects is random, he can predict the specific shape of the pdf and make some estimates about the significance of peak noise voltages.

Suppose, for example, that a biologist wants to measure a signal voltage that he suspected to be in the order of 10 μV. His amplifiers in the laboratory do not have a sufficient amplification to enable him to display this signal. He purchases a

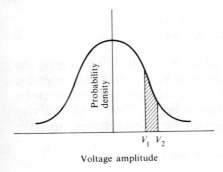

Voltage amplitude

Fig. 10.9. Typical probability density function for random-noise current or voltage.

solid-state amplifier with an amplification of 1000 in the mode of operation he is going to use. He needs to know how much noise is generated by this amplifier. Having a true rms-reading voltmeter available, he connects the voltmeter to the output of the solid-state amplifier and obtains a measurement of 10 mV of noise when the amplifier is not connected to a source. He then short-circuits the input to the amplifier and finds that he still has 10 mV of noise at the output of the amplifier. Since the amplification is 1000, the equivalent noise voltage at the input is 10 μV rms. (This is not an uncommon value of equivalent input noise voltage). He has

$$\text{Equivalent input noise voltage} = \frac{\text{Output noise voltage}}{\text{Amplification}}. \qquad (10.5)$$

He then makes the assumption that the noise is caused by thermal or shot effects and is random. This means that the probability density function of voltage has a gaussian curve shape in which the standard deviation σ is 10 μV (Fig. 10.10).†

With this information in hand he can say that 68.3% of the time the noise voltage will be within ± 10 μV and 31.7% of the time it will exceed ± 10 μV. The $\pm 2\sigma$ limits for this curve enclose 95.4% of the total area of the curve, which means that 95.4% of the time the noise voltage will be within ± 20 μV, and 4.6% of the time the noise voltage will exceed 20 μV and there will be significant noise peaks up to about 30 μV or the 3σ limits of the gaussian curve. The noise voltage will not exceed ± 30 μV more than about 0.3% of the time.

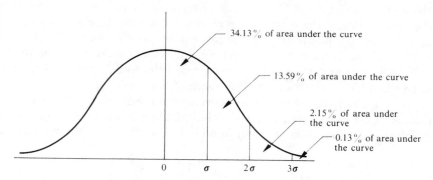

34.13% of area under the curve

13.59% of area under the curve

2.15% of area under the curve

0.13% of area under the curve

0   σ 2σ 3σ

Fig. 10.10.   Relation between σ and areas of a gaussian curve.

The biologist is now able to speculate about how well he can display the desired signal in the presence of the noise generated by the solid-state amplifier. Unfortunately the noise voltage is comparable to the expected signal voltage for a significant percentage of the total time in this example. Thus it will be very difficult to distinguish between the noise voltages and the signal voltages, especially

† Refer to a table for the gaussian or normal-distribution curve areas.

if the signal voltage will reach its peak value only a small percentage of the total time. In this case it is doubtful that the signal could be distinguished unless it has some periodic characteristics. Even then, it is very likely that the noise will mask the signal characteristics sought by the biologist.

What is the biologist to do in such a situation? He should find an amplifier with a lower equivalent-noise voltage at the input if that is possible. He may have some guesses as to the frequencies that are contained in the signal and thus be able to reduce the noise frequencies outside the signal band. In so doing, however, he may filter out some of the signals that he does not know exist and thus fail in his efforts to discover the desired characteristics of the specimen.

A point to remember

Knowledge of the rms value of random noise will help the scientist estimate the probability density function of the noise. With this function he can estimate the likelihood that the noise voltage will exceed specified limits.

10.7   ESTIMATING NOISE VOLTAGE VALUES

The following examples are all based on limited theoretical relations. They provide a starting point for thinking about the amount of noise that will be generated by the measuring circuit. Unfortunately limited theoretical relations and real life do not always agree, especially when low-level noise problems are being considered. For example, two resistors of the same resistance value may actually generate quite different amounts of noise due to the difference of composition. Two transistors of the same type number and similar amplification characteristics may have quite different noise characteristics. Components must be carefully chosen when the experimenter is assembling his equipment. The theoretical values given in the examples to follow give only an indication of the magnitude of noise voltage that can be expected from typical components. Many devices may give considerably more noise than predicted. Rarely will similar circuits produce less noise than those estimated in the following examples.

The first two examples given below indicate that connecting the noise source to the measuring circuit will have an effect on the noise voltage actually delivered to the input of the measuring circuit.

Example 10.1   Thermal noise and coupling with filtering. Assume that a source contains a resistor R_s of 10^6 Ω. This source drives a measuring circuit which looks like a load R_L to the source. This load appears to be a 10^3 Ω ideal noiseless resistance. The temperature is 300 °K. Also the measuring circuit acts as a filter at the input. The system is shown in Fig. 10.11.

The band-limiting characteristics of this load cannot be realized in fact, but it can be approximated. The noise voltage appearing across the output terminals 1 and 2 can be calculated and is 40.7 nV (nanovolts). The $\pm 2\sigma$ limits for this

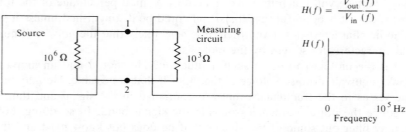

(a) Circuit with noisy source

(b) Band-limiting characteristics of the load

$$H(f) = \frac{V_{out}(f)}{V_{in}(f)}$$

Fig. 10.11.   Resistor noise source connected to a band-limiting measuring circuit.

random noise is ± 81.4 nV. Ninety-five percent of the time the noise voltage will be within ± 81.4 nV.

Example 10.2   Thermal noise and coupling with filtering.   What would happen if the source resistance R_s that generated the thermal noise as described in Example 10.1 was reduced to 10^4 Ω? Would the output noise voltage increase or decrease? According to Eq. (10.2), $P(f)$ would decrease by a factor 10^2, leading us to suspect that the noise voltage across points 1 and 2 would decrease. However, this would not happen. The coupling of the noise generated by the source resistor to the measuring circuit would increase and counteract the decrease in generated noise. In this example with $R_s = 10^4$ Ω the noise voltage produced between points 1 and 2 of the circuit shown in Fig. 10.11 would increase to 370 nV, so that the noise voltage would be within ± 0.74 μV during 95% of the time. Therefore, it is important once again to remember that the coupling between a source and a measuring circuit will have a significant effect on the results of the experiment.

A point to remember

The amount of noise power developed across a load depends on the relative sizes of the source resistance and the load resistance.

The next examples will show the effect of thermal noise in relatively simple circuits.

Example 10.3   Thermal noise plus signal.   Let us once again use the circuit described in Example 10.2 and assume that the source generates an open-circuit sine wave of 1 μV rms in the pass band of the load. The equivalent circuit will then be as shown in Fig. 10.12. The voltage at the output of this circuit due to the signal can be easily calculated by using Eq. (4.16). The signal voltage between points 1 and 2 will be 90.8 nV. From Example 10.2 we have the noise voltage

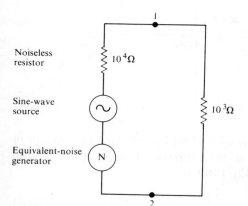

Fig. 10.12.   Equivalent circuit to be used in SNR check.

due to the source resistance between points 1 and 2 as 370 nV. Using Eq. (10.1), we can obtain the signal-to-noise ratio between points 1 and 2:

$$\text{SNR}_{1\text{-}2} = 0.245.$$

The output noise voltage is significantly larger than the output signal voltage. A signal-to-noise ratio of 10 or more would have been more desirable. However, as this example shows, it may not be possible to obtain these high ratios without processing the composite signal in an appropriate manner. Some useful methods of processing noisy signals will be discussed in Chapter 11.

Example 10.4   Thermal noise at input of voltmeter with stray shunt capacitance.   The examples given above indicate the important effect of coupling on the noise introduced to the input of a measuring circuit. As another example, let us consider the effect of an input circuit which has a noisy resistor in parallel with a stray shunt capacitance. The circuit may be as shown in Fig. 10.13 and may represent the input circuit of a voltmeter.

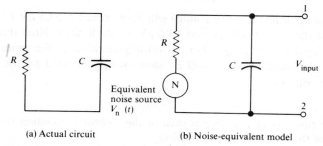

(a) Actual circuit   (b) Noise-equivalent model

Fig. 10.13.   Input circuit of a voltmeter.

Thermal noise generated by the input resistor will develop across the input capacitance. The input resistance and capacitance will act as a filter whose trans-

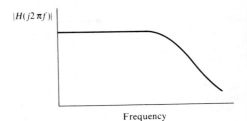

Fig. 10.14. Transfer characteristics of RC filter.

fer characteristics are as shown in Fig. 10.14.† This filter will limit the amount of noise that can develop across the input to the voltmeter. The voltage developed between points 1 and 2 is given by the Eq. (10.6):

$$V_{\text{out, rms}} = \frac{kT}{C},\tag{10.6}$$

where k is Boltzmann's constant, 1.38×10^{-16} erg/°K, T is temperature, and C is capacitance. It is interesting to note that the source resistance does not appear in this equation and thus has no effect on the noise voltage between points 1 and 2.

What is the noise voltage generated by the input resistance between points 1 and 2 for typical component values that might be found in a vacuum-tube voltmeter, where $R = 10^6$ Ω, $C = 100$ pf (picofarads), $T = 300°$ K? For these values the input noise is

$$V_{\text{input rms}} = 6.43 \ \mu\text{V}.$$

During 32% of the time the noise voltage will exceed $\pm 6.43 \ \mu\text{V}$ ($\pm 1\sigma$ limits); 4.6% of the time the noise voltage will exceed 12.86 μV ($\pm 2\sigma$ limits). If the shunt capacitance across the input of the voltmeter is reduced to 10 pf while the other values are kept constant, the input noise voltage will increase so that

$$V_{\text{input rms}} = 20.3 \ \mu\text{V}.$$

During 32% of the time the noise voltage will then exceed $\pm 20.3 \ \mu$V ($\pm 1\sigma$ limits), while 4.6% of the time it will exceed 40.6 μV ($\pm 2\sigma$ limits). Note that these last two voltages are due only to the thermal noise generated by the input resistor of the voltmeter. In addition, there will be shot noise generated by the amplifying devices in the voltmeter.

---

† The transfer function of the filter is used in the following equation for calculating the rms value of the output noise from a filter:

$$V_{\text{out,rms}} = \left[\int_0^\infty P_{\text{in}}(f) \ |H(j2\pi f)|^2 \ df \right]^{1/2},$$

where $P_{\text{in}}(f)$ is the power density spectrum of the noise at the input to the filter and $|H(j2\pi f)|$ is the amplitude of the complex transfer function of the filter.

Example 10.5 Shot noise estimate for triode tube. The theoretical value of shot noise generated by a triode tube and delivered to the next stage of an amplifier can be predicted. A typical triode amplifier might have the following components:

$$\text{triode mutual conductance } g_{\text{m}} = 5 \times 10^{-3} \text{ mhos,}$$
$$\text{triode dynamic plate resistance } r_{\text{P}} = 10^4 \ \Omega,$$
$$\text{dynamic plate load resistance } R_{\text{L}} = 10^4 \ \Omega.$$

The stray shunt capacitance across the output of the amplifier might be $C = 100$ pf. Assuming that no noise is generated by the input resistor to this amplifier, the output noise due to the shot effect will be 50.8 μV. The noise will exceed 101.6 μV ($\pm 2\sigma$ limits) 4.6% of the time.

A point to remember

It is quite likely that many general-purpose amplifiers will generate equivalent input noise voltages ranging from somewhat less than a microvolt to several hundred microvolts.

10.8 CONCLUSIONS

Whenever measurements are to be made of voltages in the microvolt or nanovolt range, maybe even in the millivolt range, noise problems can be expected. The sources of noise may be external to the measuring system or they may be generated by the measuring system itself. If the noise is external to the system, it may be possible to isolate the system from the noise source and eliminate the trouble. Electrostatic shielding and shielded cables may help, as well as changing the orientation of the measuring system on the bench.

Magnetic coupling of noise into a circuit can be minimized by placing the measuring system wires picking up this noise at right angles to the wires that carry the noise currents.

Noise that is generated by the measuring system itself establishes the lower limit of signal levels that can be readily identified. It is not uncommon to have equivalent input noise voltages of 10 μV. The input stages of amplification are the most important and should be made as noiseless as possible and isolated from sources of noise.

10.9 REVIEW QUESTIONS AND PROBLEMS

10.1 Define the term "noise" as it is used when discussing the performance of electrical circuits.

10.2 At what point in a circuit or measuring system can noise enter the circuit? What point is considered to be the most critical entry point?

10.3 What is meant by the term "Signal-to-Noise Ratio"? Is it usually desirable to have this ratio be large, unity, or small? Justify your answer.

10.4   Noise enters the circuit in Fig. R10.1 through the operation of some noisy devices in amplifier 2. The equivalent input noise at point 2 is 1 mV rms. What must the signal voltage at the input be if the signal-to-noise ratio at the output is to be 10?

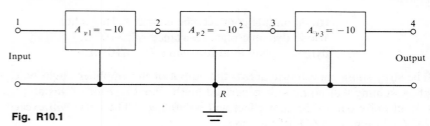

Fig. R10.1

$$Av_1 = \frac{V_{2R}}{V_{1R}}, \; Av_2 = \frac{V_{3R}}{V_{2R}}, \; Av_3 = \frac{V_{4R}}{V_{3R}}$$

10.5   Assume that the rms output noise voltage of the combined amplifier in Fig. R10.1 is 5 V. What is the equivalent input noise voltage? What is meant by the term "equivalent input noise voltage"? What must the rms signal voltage at the input be if the signal-to-noise ratio at the output is to be 15?

10.6   All amplifiers generate noise. Which stage of the amplifier is the most critical in terms of noise problems? Why?

10.7   How can electrical noise be coupled into a measurement system?

10.8   What methods can be used to reduce the amount of noise that is coupled into a measurement system?

10.9   Someone has brought you a jumble of miscellaneous types of wires. How can you tell the differences among an ordinary pair of wires, a coaxial cable, and a shielded cable?

10.10   What is the difference between random noise and periodic noise? What would you look for if you were trying to determine which of these two different types of noise was displayed on a cathode-ray oscilloscope screen?

10.11   What type of component can produce thermal noise?

10.12   What band of frequencies of noise do thermal sources produce?

10.13   Under what conditions will thermal noise cause problems in a measurement system?

10.14   What is white noise?

10.15   What is a typical shape of a probability-density-function curve of the amplitude of the noise produced by a random noise source? What is the value of knowing this curve?

10.16   A random noise source produced noise in a measurement system. The scientist running the tests used a true rms-reading voltmeter to measure the random noise at the output. It read 2 volts. What useful information can be derived from this measurement?

11
measuring
small signals in
the presence of noise

11.1 OBJECTIVES

The problems of making electrical measurements of small voltages or currents are two-fold. The first problem is to detect the presence of any signal that might be related to the phenomena being studied. The second problem is to get reliable data from the amplitude and waveshape of the signal once the signal has been detected. It may be possible to ascertain the presence of a signal, even though it is difficult to get any specific quantitative data on it.

The aphid experiment discussed in Chapter 1 serves as a good example of the problems that may be encountered. All that was desired initially was a reliable detection of a signal indicating that the aphid was or was not pushing the stylets into the leaf. The waveshape and the specific amplitude of the signal were not important at that stage of the investigation. Once signals were recorded which indicated that the aphid was performing the expected act, a second question had to be answered. Did the electric current that had passed through the aphid during the measurement alter the aphid's natural actions? It was helpful at this point to get a quantitative measurement of the current passing through the aphid's body and the voltage associated with this current. Needless to say, these currents and voltages had to be very small so as not to upset the aphid's normal feeding activity. Noise due to stray electrical pick-up was a severe problem initially and masked the desired signal much of the time. Good measurement techniques along with trial-and-error efforts were required to solve the noise problems.

We must try to reduce the coupling between sources of noise and the measurement system at the onset of an experiment so that noise will not enter the measurement system and combine with the desired signal. After this has been done as well as possible, there are methods for reducing to the lowest possible value the noise in the system derived from the 60-Hz power source. Then the last step is to reduce the effects of random noise picked up or generated by the measurement system. In this chapter these three major areas of signal detection and measurement will be discussed.

The term *signal* is used for different things depending on the circumstances. Sometimes it is used in connection with the electrical voltage which contains the useful information, and sometimes it is used when the electrical voltage is only noise and contains no useful information. In this chapter the following terminology will be used.

Signal is that portion of the voltage or current wave that contains the useful and desired information. The signal portion of the wave is given the symbol $s(t)$.

Noise is that portion of the voltage or current wave that does not contain any desired information and tends to obliterate or mask the signal. The noise portion of the wave is given the symbol $n(t)$.

Composite signal is the sum of the signal and the noise portions of the voltage or current wave. It is given the symbol $c(t)$:

$$c(t) = s(t) + n(t).$$

11.2   REDUCING THE COUPLING BETWEEN NOISE SOURCE AND MEASURING SYSTEM

Electrostatic Coupling

As indicated in Chapter 10, electrostatic coupling occurs when there is a relatively large amount of stray capacitance between a source of noise and the measuring system. Some means must be found to reduce this stray capacitance. One of the methods is to use an electrostatic shield, which may take one of two forms. It may be a metal box or a metal screen that is built around the system. The box or screen should be connected to the ground, as shown in Fig. 11.1. Note that with the shield connected to the ground, the noise currents are shunted around the test system through C_1 rather than passing through the test system as in Fig. 10.2. There is no need for the power line current to flow to another load; only the line voltage need be present to cause noise currents to flow in the test circuit.

If a screen is used, there will not be perfect shielding and therefore some noise currents may still get into the test system by way of C_3: the better the shield, the smaller is the value of C_3. Equation (4.31) indicates that as frequency increases, the capacitive reactance will decrease. Thus the coupling action through the stray capacitance will increase as the frequency increases. Any noise source that has high-frequency components is more likely to be capacitively coupled into the measuring system than a source with primarily low frequencies. The detrimental effect of noise coupled in this way is somewhat dependent on the frequencies of the signal being measured. If the test signal has frequencies close to those of the noise capacitively coupled into the system, then noise will be a serious prob-

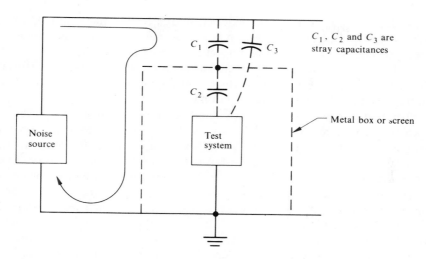

Fig. 11.1. Electrostatic screens used to reduce the effects of noise coupling through stray capacitance.

lem and electrostatic shielding should be tried as a means of reducing it. Also the physical placement of the equipment on the bench may affect this coupling. Move the experiment as far away from the source of noise as is possible.

Magnetic Coupling

Extraneous magnetic fields due to power line currents are almost always present in laboratories. This is very unfortunate because the magnetic fields induce noise voltages in the test specimen, in the wires connecting the specimen to the instruments, and in the instruments, as was shown in Fig. 10.6. These line currents are not always pure sine waves; harmonics of the 60-Hz line frequency are usually present. The dominant frequency will be 60 Hz mixed with 120 Hz and higher harmonics. The amplitude of the higher harmonics will usually be significantly smaller than that of the 60-Hz component.

Magnetic coupling is at a maximum when the two wires involved are parallel to each other and are close together. Therefore, this type of coupling can be reduced by moving the two wires as far apart as possible and placing them at right angles to each other. However, if the power line wire is fastened to the wall or table, it may be impossible to move it. The placement of the test specimen and apparatus will have to be experimented with to determine the physical layout that will give the minimum amount of 60-Hz and related noise pickup. Unfortunately this is a trial-and-error process, as is the case with electrostatic coupling.

Magnetic shielding may be accomplished by placing a ferromagnetic material around critical components in measuring instruments. For example, the cathode-ray tube in a cathode-ray oscilloscope may be covered with a magnetic shield so that the electron beam will not be deflected by the earth's magnetic field or any noise magnetic fields. Components such as transformers that carry audiofrequency low-level signals may have massive magnetic shielding around them to reduce the coupling between the noise magnetic field and the turns of wire on the transformer. Such shielding is essential whenever there are strong noise magnetic fields and when the signal to be measured is very small.

When building test equipment, it is standard practice to place the power supply, which is connected to the 60-Hz line, as far as possible from the low-level signal input point to the equipment. As indicated in Chapter 10, the input stage of amplification is the critical stage so far as noise intrusion is concerned. Every effort should be made to keep power line wires away from this part of the circuit. For example, a low-voltage transformer may be used to operate a microscope-illuminating system. If this transformer is located near a sensitive amplifier, 60-Hz noise may be induced into the amplifier circuitry and produce noise at the output of the amplifier. If vacuum tubes are used, the filament wires should be twisted so as to cancel out the magnetic fields set up by the currents in the two wires.

Grounding Problems

Noise problems can be caused by improperly arranging the ground connections to which the various parts of the circuit are connected. As indicated in Fig. 11.2, it is general practice to have many different circuits connected to a common point. Ideally all the points in these circuits designated by a grounding symbol should be at exactly the same potential. In practice the connection between these various points is made by some type of conductor. This conductor should have zero resistance if all of these points are to be at the same potential regardless of the current that may flow through the ground conductor from the various circuits. This condition can only be approximated in the actual hardware.

Problems due to the resistance of the grounding circuit may occur in the following way (Fig. 11.2a). In an actual circuit the conductor between points a, b, c, d, and e has some resistance. Currents from various parts of the circuit may flow through this conductor and produce a voltage $V = IR$. This voltage will then serve as a noise voltage V_{ab} which is introduced into the circuit of the transistor $T1$ and passed onto the display unit. As the resistance of this conductor increases, the noise voltage generated will increase.

Sometimes the grounding conductor forms a closed loop through which noise currents will flow. These currents may be caused by magnetic fields which couple into this conductor and induce a voltage in the loop. The induced voltage will cause noise currents to flow in the loop and in the signal circuit. Thus noise will be fed into the signal portion of the circuit. This action can also occur even when a shield is used to reduce the effects of high-frequency magnetic fields if multiple connections are made to the shield. Currents that flow through the shield

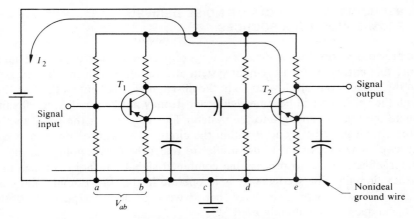

(a) $V_{ab} = IR$ voltage is produced by I_2. This voltage is fed into T_1 as a noise voltage.

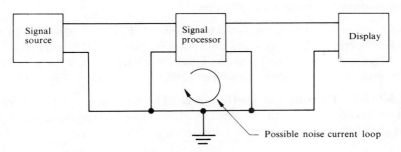

(b) Source of possible noise current loop problems.

Fig. 11.2. Grounding circuits and instruments.

will have voltages associated with them. These voltages can be coupled into the main circuit in the way shown in Fig. 11.2(b) if more than one connection is made between the test circuit and the shield. Similar effects will occur if there is capacitive coupling between the noise source and shield. These grounding problems are most severe in those portions of the circuit where the signal level is very small. Special care should be taken in the construction of these portions of the circuit.

Grounding problems can be reduced by observing the following practices:

1. Use a ground conductor with as low a resistance as possible.
2. Use as few ground connection points to the ground conductor as possible.
3. Eliminate all closed loops in the ground conductor.
4. Connect shields to the ground conductor at only one point.

11.3   REDUCING THE EFFECTS OF NOISE DERIVED FROM 60-Hz POWER SOURCES

In the previous sections we emphasized ways of preventing or reducing the amount of noise that enters the measurement system and combine with the desired signal. When the signal levels are low enough, the 60-Hz noise that enters the test circuit through the shielding will become significant. It may not be possible to effectively eliminate the stray coupling into the system. This means that the noise that gets into the circuit must be reduced within the circuit. This can be done in two different ways. The first way is to use a filter to reject the 60-Hz noise and pass the signal. In effect, this is to process the combined signal and noise voltage in the frequency domain. The second way is to operate in the time domain and cancel out the noise wave with a similarly shaped wave of opposite polarity. Both of these techniques are commonly used.

Frequency-domain Techniques: Filtering

Various types of filters were discussed in Chapter 4. Filters are designed to reject or block out certain frequencies and pass other frequencies. There are four major types of filters: *low-pass, band-pass, high-pass, band-rejection*. Typical frequency transfer characteristics of these four types of filters are shown in Fig. 11.3.

Example 11.1   Filtering out 60-Hz noise.   The particular type of filter that should be used depends on the frequencies of the noise and the frequencies of the desired signal. As the first example let us assume that the noise is a pure 60-Hz

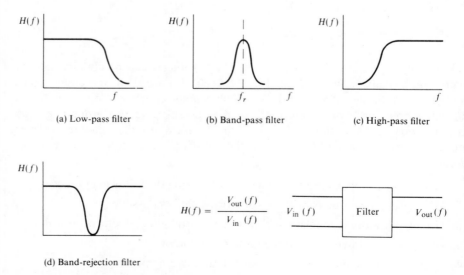

(a) Low-pass filter   (b) Band-pass filter   (c) High-pass filter

(d) Band-rejection filter

$$H(f) = \frac{V_{out}(f)}{V_{in}(f)}$$

Fig. 11.3.   Major types of filter transfer functions.

voltage and the desired signal contains only one frequency, 600 Hz. See Fig. 11.4, which also shows the characteristic of a high-pass filter that might be used to reduce the level of the noise. It is evident that the filter will reduce the level of the noise from a value equal to the signal voltage to $X\%$ of the signal voltage.

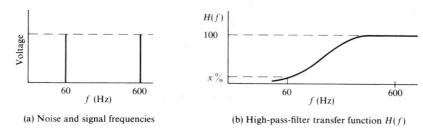

(a) Noise and signal frequencies   (b) High-pass-filter transfer function $H(f)$

Fig. 11.4. Frequencies in composite voltage and high-pass filter transfer function.

How much can the noise voltage be lowered relative to the signal voltage in this example? Consider the use of a simple RC high-pass filter as shown in Fig. 11.5. Assume that the load connected to the output terminals of the filter has infinite input impedance. The transfer function for this filter can be determined by means of Eqs. (4.16) and (4.30). From Fig. 11.5(b) we see that the output voltage of the signal is nine-tenths of the input signal voltage. The signal-to-noise ratio at the input of the filter is 1. The signal-to-noise ratio at the output of the filter is 0.9/0.2 or 4.5.

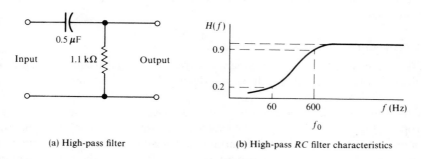

(a) High-pass filter   (b) High-pass RC filter characteristics

Fig. 11.5. RC high-pass filter characteristics.

Figure 11.6 shows the input and output waveforms for this example. Significant improvement has been made even though the noise is still present. If the desired signal was 6000 Hz and the noise was a 60-Hz sine wave, a high-pass filter with different values of R and C could be designed. Assume once again that the f_1 frequency point on the curve, where $H(f) = 0.9$, equals 6000 Hz. The 60-Hz frequency point would be further down on the curve than it was in the

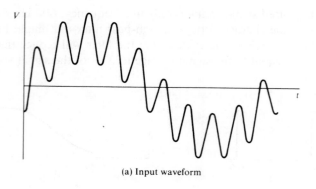

(a) Input waveform

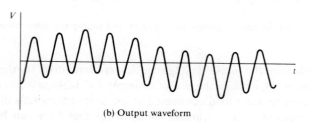

(b) Output waveform

Fig. 11.6. Waveforms for filtered composite signal.

previous example. It would be at the point where $H(f)$ is approximately equal to 0.02. At the output of this filter the noise would be significantly lower than it was in the previous example.

A point to remember

The farther apart the noise frequency is from the signal frequency, the more effective a particular filter will be in reducing the noise voltage.

Some waveform distortion will occur if the phase characteristic of the filter is not proper (Fig. 11.7). Note that in (a) the signal contains two frequencies, a fundamental component and a third harmonic. The sum of these two components gives a wave that approaches a square wave. In part (b) the third-harmonic component is shifted $180°$ from what it was in (a). The sum of these two waves is not the same as the composite wave in (a). The amplitudes of the two components are the same in both examples. A filter could cause a phase shift and an amplitude change in one of the components such that a distortion in waveshape is produced.

A low-pass filter (Fig. P4.2s1(a)) has a transfer function with almost constant amplitude and phase-shift characteristics below f_1 (Fig. 11.8). Above f_1 both of these characteristics change.

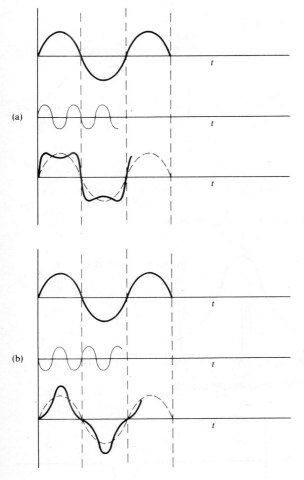

(a)

(b)

Fig. 11.7. Waveform distortion caused by filtering that produces improper phase shifts.

The band-pass filter is used when the noise is spread over a range of frequencies encompassing the signal frequencies, as shown in Fig. 11.9. A desirable filter transfer function is one similar to that superimposed on the frequency spectrum of the composite voltage.

Sometimes the signal has frequencies over a wide band and the noise consists of a single frequency. In this case a band-rejection filter is needed to reduce the noise while passing the desired signal. Figure 11.10 shows the $H(f)$ characteristic of this type of filter. This filter is most effective at retaining the true signal waveshape when f_{low} and f_{high} are as close together as possible and $H(f)_r$ is as low as possible. The filter may be expensive and difficult to produce. As the noise frequencies become closer and closer to the signal frequency, it becomes more and

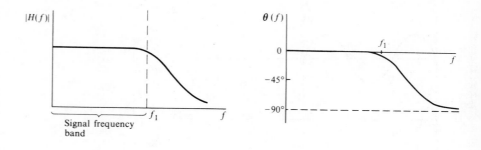

(a) Amplitude of filter transfer function

(b) Transfer characteristics for a low-pass RC filter

Fig. 11.8.   Transfer characteristics for a low-pass RC filter.

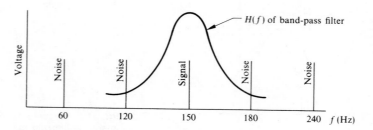

Fig. 11.9.   Broadband noise and narrowband filter.

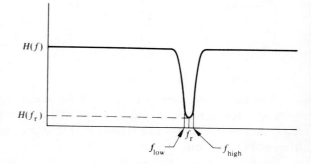

Fig. 11.10.   Transfer characteristics of a band-rejection filter.

more difficult to effectively reduce the noise by filtering. It is expensive and difficult to build filters that have very sharp transitions in their transfer characteristic curves; hence the importance of trying to prevent the noise from coupling into the circuit in the first place.

Time-domain Techniques: Canceling Out Noise

A noise voltage may be reduced to zero if there is some way of adding to the noise voltage a voltage of the same amplitude and waveshape but of opposite sign. This time-domain cancellation can be accomplished by using any device that will add two voltages together with proper phasing. A differential amplifier is commonly used for this purpose. This device is designed to take the difference between the voltages applied at its two inputs. In other words, the amplifier performs a subtracting operation. If the two input voltages are equal at all times, the output voltage will be zero at all times. See Fig. 11.11 for an example of this process. Here wave 1 is considered to be a 60-Hz noise voltage and is applied to input 1. Wave 2 is produced, in effect, by the differential amplifier when wave 1 is applied to input 2. The graphical sum of these two waves is zero, at every instant in time.

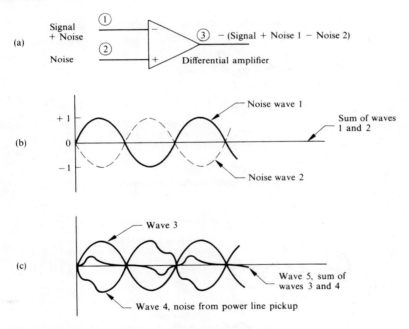

Fig. 11.11.   Time-domain cancellation of noise voltages.

The noise waves shown in Fig. 11.11(b) are mirror images of each other. This situation will probably not occur in practice. The waves shown in Fig. 11.11(c) are similar to those seen in the laboratory. Wave 4 represents the noise induced in the measuring circuit by the power-line current. Wave 3 shows the undistorted line voltage. The sum of these two voltages is a voltage which is lower in amplitude than the original noise voltage (wave 4). Thus the addition of an appropriate amount of line voltage results in a reduced amount of noise at the output of the differential amplifier. It is important to note in both (b) and (c) that the phasing of the noise voltage and the voltage used to cancel out part or all of the noise must be as shown in order to have maximum effect.

Example 11.2 Effects of phase shift on time-domain cancellation of noise. Figure 11.12 shows the undesirable effect of using improper phasing when attempting to cancel out 60-Hz noise that has distorted a signal. In Fig. 11.12(a) proper phasing is used. In Fig. 11.12(b) an improper phasing is used and the noise is increased. Sometimes the voltage for input 2 of the differential amplifier can be obtained by connecting a wire to terminal 2 and laying it near the other test leads and the test specimen where the noise voltage is being picked up. In this way one may be able to get the appropriate waveshape and phasing of the noise. The posi-

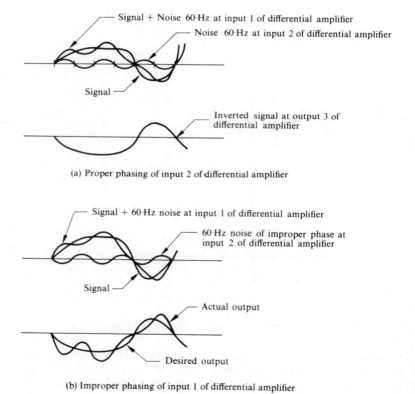

Fig. 11.12. The effect of improper phasing when attempting to cancel out noise.

tion of the wire will affect the amplitude of the noise voltage fed into terminal 2. This is a trial-and-error process that works in some cases.

The frequency-domain and time-domain techniques described above are used to help produce a signal waveform with minimum distortion. They are used when the experimenter needs to accurately measure the amplitude and shape of the signal being investigated.

11.4 REDUCING THE EFFECTS OF RANDOM NOISE

Random noise is more difficult to eliminate than the 60-Hz related noise derived from the power line because random-noise waveshapes are continually changing. The waves have no characteristic periodicity. Nevertheless, both frequency-domain techniques and time-domain techniques can be used to reduce the effects of random noise.

Frequency-domain Techniques: Filtering

The discussion of filtering in Section 11.3 is also applicable to the problem of rejecting random noise. However, this application is more difficult. Noise generated by the power line generally has its strongest interference at 60 Hz, 120 Hz, and 180 Hz. The higher harmonics are not usually very large in amplitude. This interference band is relatively narrow and at the low end of the frequency band. Random noise usually has a continuous band of frequencies up to 10^{13} Hz with fairly constant amplitude. Recall Section 10.5 where it was indicated that the power density spectrum for thermal noise is constant for the range of practical interest. Thus the noise will always be present with the signal, and simple filtering may not be able to improve the signal-to-noise ratio in the signal frequency band. The filter will also affect the signal as well as the noise, unless selective filtering is done as shown in Fig. 11.13 with filter transfer function 1. It may be difficult to build this type of filter to achieve the proper relative amplitudes and phase relationships between the various signal frequency components. A filter with transfer function 2 will reduce the noise outside the signal band but will not reduce the noise between the frequency components.

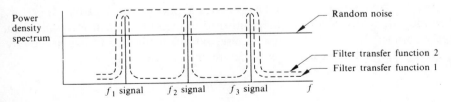

Fig. 11.13. Selective filtering to reduce noise within the band containing the signal frequencies.

Time-domain Techniques: Sampling

Random noise has certain statistical properties which suggest other means of reducing the noise. Quite often the circuits that generate noise produce noise voltages with zero average value. This means that there is *no* dc component in the noise voltage. If there is a dc voltage, it can be eliminated by putting a coupling capacitor in the circuit to block out the dc component. Of course, this cannot be done if the signal contains a dc component. When no dc component is present in the noise, the noise voltage will be positive as much as it is negative. This fact can be utilized in detecting the waveform of the signal in the presence of noise.

Sampling techniques have been devised to produce good signal waveforms even when a large amount of noise is present (Fig. 11.14). Assume that the signal buried in noise is periodic and that there is a means of looking at the combined signal and noise every time the signal reaches its peak positive value. If all of the sample signal voltages s_i are added together, the result will be some relatively large positive voltage:

$$V_s = \sum_{i=1}^{N} s_i = Ns, \tag{11.1}$$

where N = total number of samples, s = the peak value of the signal, and s_i = individual signal voltage sample values.

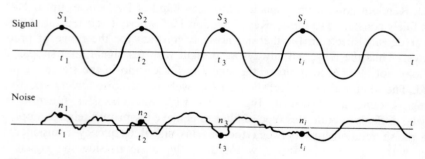

Fig. 11.14. Sampling signal and noise to reproduce signal waveform.

Part of the noise samples will be positive and part will be negative. Therefore, when they are added together, the positive values tend to be canceled out by the negative values. If all of the sampled noise voltages n_i are added together, the resultant voltage will be near zero if there are enough samples:

$$V_n = \sum_{i=1}^{N} n_i, \tag{11.2}$$

where n_i = individual noise voltage sample values, N = total number of samples. If the average value of the noise is zero and the number of samples is large enough, the noise summation should approach zero while the signal summation becomes quite large.

If the sampling procedure is done at many points within a period of the signal waveform, say 10 sampling points, the signal waveform can be defined by this procedure. Figure 11.15 shows what a sampled output waveform might look like if a sine wave was buried in noise and was to be detected.

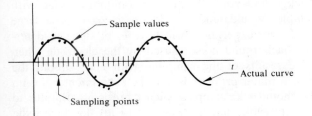

Fig. 11.15. Output of a sampling waveform detector.

One of the sampling points may fall on the zero-crossing points of the signal being detected. If this happens the summation voltage due to the signal component of the wave will be zero. Then the observer will not know whether the zero-summation voltage is due to a signal that happens to have zero-crossings at the sampling points or is due to random noise. This uncertainty will cause no problem if there are enough other sample points so that the wave can be defined. The sampling procedure described above is effective when the period and the phase of the detected signal are known—a usual situation which does hold in many experiments in which a stimulus is applied to a specimen. If this information about period and phase is not available, then the samples could be taken at the wrong times and there would be a very high probability that both the signal and the noise portions of the wave would add up to zero and yield no helpful information to the experimenter.

An estimate of the value of the actual signal voltage at any point in its cycle can be obtained by averaging the sample values at that particular point. This can be done by dividing the sample sum by the total number N of samples at that point. The measurements are done on the composite signal and therefore the average value is given by Eq. (11.3):

$$\bar{c}_i = \frac{1}{N} \sum_{i=1}^{N} c_i = \frac{1}{N} \left(\sum_{i=1}^{N} s_i + \sum_{i=1}^{N} n_i \right), \qquad (11.3)$$

where $\bar{c}_i$ stands for the average of composite signal. Several examples should serve to indicate the types of experiments where this method of sampling could be used.

Example 11.3 Response vs. stimulus. Suppose a frog is being stimulated by the periodical flashing of a small light at some distance away from one of its eyes.

The experimenter wants to measure the electrical voltages that might be produced somewhere in the frog's body on account of the stimulus. The experimenter knows the period and the timing of the stimulus. He proposes to connect an electrode to the frog and monitor the voltages that might appear. If the light is very faint, he is not sure he will get a response above the background noise level. The averaging technique specified by Eq. (11.3) can be used to determine the actual voltage at the electrode. He can take sample readings at various times relative to the time of light flashes. The background noise might be a random voltage with no dc value and thus its samples would tend to add up to zero for a large number of samples. A trial-and-error experiment will have to be done to determine the characteristics of the background noise caused by the electrode when there is no light stimulus. The results of the sampling with and without the light stimulus can be compared. A major problem is that the experimenter has no basis for determining when he should take samples when there is no stimulus to provide a reference point. It is possible that there is a very low-level periodic signal in the absence of external stimulus. This signal might be enhanced by the stimulus but would not be picked up if it had a different period than that of the stimulus. This is just one difficulty which may be encountered in an experiment.

Example 11.4   Obtaining Synchronization. Suppose that a physiologist wants to study the waveshapes of an electrical signal that occurs in the brain when an animal is walking or running on a treadmill. He may be particularly interested in the waveshape related to the time when the animal's left front paw hits the treadmill. A transducer must be used to provide some type of signal whenever the paw hits the treadmill. A second transducer must be used to make contact with the point where the brain signal wave is to be measured. The running action of the animal may produce considerable electrical noises and thus signal-averaging may have to be used to enhance the signal.

The sampling process described in Example 11.3 may be implemented by means of an analog computer having special circuits to generate gating signals and time delays. The sampling can be accomplished by multiplying the composite wave by a gating wave that is synchronized with the stimulus. A gating wave is a time-varying function that has a zero-value at all times when the wave being processed is not to be looked at. It may have a value of 1 when the wave being processed is to be looked at. In Fig. 11.16 this process is shown with two different gating waves that will produce samples 1 and 2. When $g_1(t)$ is 1, the product of $g_1(t)$ and $c(t)$ is just $c(t)$. At all other times this product is zero, as shown in the upper part of the $f_s(t)$ wave. When using gating wave 1 there is a time delay $t_d = t_1$ with respect to the positive zero-crossing point of the sine wave. When using gating wave 2 there is a time delay $t_d = t_2$. As t_d assumes different values, the sample averages will begin to form the shape of the signal wave being sampled.

This sampling process can be accomplished by connecting the analog computer as shown in Fig. 11.17. The system operates in this way: The stimulus

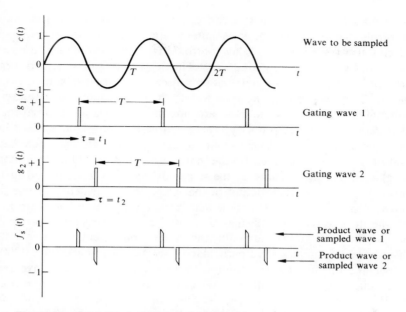

Fig. 11.16.   Sampling by using gating signals.

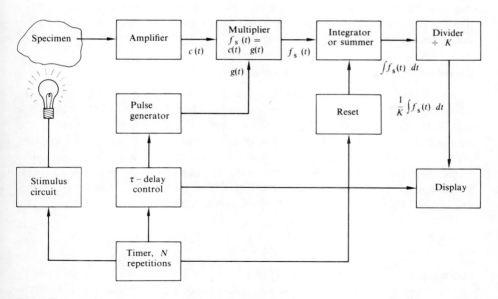

Fig. 11.17.   Connections for an analog computer used to take sample readings and averages.

circuit provides the stimulus that is desired for the particular experiment. The timer controls the length of time the stimulus circuit shall be in operation. The timer circuit also activates the τ-delay control circuit that is to be set to give the appropriate delay time for the gating wave. The delay circuit then triggers a pulse generator which puts out one short gating pulse every time the stimulus is on.

The specimen will respond in some way to the stimulus and its output is fed into the amplifier. The signal and noise are amplified to the level required for the multiplier circuit to operate properly. There is a certain threshold limit of input voltage below which most multipliers will not operate satisfactorily. The composite signal $c(t)$ is then multiplied by the gating wave $g(t)$, yielding the sampled wave $f_s(t)$. The integrator sums up the sampled waves for a set period of time determined by the timer. The output of the integrator is divided by some fixed constant K, depending on the experimenter's choice for appropriate scaling, and fed into the display unit. The display unit can be a chart recorder or an X-Y recorder with the time-axis controlled by the τ-delay control circuit.

The number of samples for a particular value of τ might be 1000, 10000, or more depending on the number required to cause the noise voltage average to become significantly lower than the signal voltage average. When an appropriate number of samples have been taken, the timer operates the reset circuit of the integrator and causes the delay control to advance to the next value of τ to be used.

The display of the sample averages will give an approximation of the actual shape of the signal. This faithfulness of reproduction will depend on the number of samples N taken at each value of τ and the number of delay times used within one period of the signal.

Time-domain Techniques: Autocorrelation

The sampling technique just described is a useful method of determining the waveshape of the signal in the presence of noise when the period of the waveshape is known. *Autocorrelation* is a technique used to detect a periodic wave in the presence of noise. It differs from sampling in that the autocorrelator does not always give an indication of the shape of the signal wave. Autocorrelation can be used only to detect the presence of the periodic wave and its period. It is a process whereby a wave is compared with itself as it is displaced by τ units of time. It is an average characteristic and is described mathematically by Eq. (11.5):

$$R_{11}(\tau) = \lim_{T \to \infty} \frac{1}{2T} \int_{-T}^{T} f_1(t) \, f_2(t + \tau) \, dt, \qquad (11.5)$$

where $f_1(t)$ is the composite signal, $f_1(t + \tau)$ is the composite signal delayed by τ units of time, and $R_{11}(\tau)$ is the autocorrelation. In a real situation, it is not possible to average over an infinite time period, as indicated in Eq. (11.5). Reliable detection of a very small signal buried in noise can be made only when longer and longer averaging periods are used. Long averaging periods tend to eliminate the effects of random noise present in the composite signal. On the other hand, long averaging periods are a disadvantage insofar as they mean that it must take seconds, minutes, or hours to detect the signal, depending on the severity of the noise and the periodicity of the signal being sought. Since in this case an average-value characteristic is being sought, a low-pass filter designed to reject almost all frequencies above dc can be used to do the averaging. Hence the correlator may be constructed with the blocks shown in Fig. 11.18.

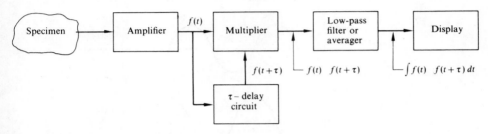

Fig. 11.18.   Block diagram for one type of autocorrelator.

The signal from the specimen is amplified along with any noise that may be combined with the signal at the input to the amplifier or generated by the amplifier. This composite signal is multiplied to a delayed replica of it. The resultant product waves are shown in the example pictured in Fig. 11.19 for several different values of delay.

If the delay between the two inputs to the multiplier is zero, $f_a(t)$ results. Note that this wave is entirely above the zero level and therefore has some average or dc value that is positive and may be detected at the output of a low-pass filter. When the delay equals $T/4$, the product wave is $f_b(t)$, the product wave centers about zero, and thus the average value is zero. When the delay equals $T/2$, the product wave is $f_c(t)$, which is just the inversion of $f_a(t)$. If this process were continued for all values of delay, a periodic wave would be displayed at the output with the same period as that of the signal being sought. This output is shown in Fig. 11.20 together with the output wave when the input signal is a square wave. Note that the period of the output waveshape is the same as that of the input signal, even though the output waveshape may be different.

The autocorrelator output for random noise will have a shape similar to that in Fig. 11.21(a). It will tend to drop off to zero for large values of τ, whereas the output for the periodic wave is periodic. Figure 11.21(b) shows the periodic output for a rectangular periodic-pulse input, and Fig. 11.21(c) shows the autocorrelator output when the composite signal into the autocorrelator is the sum of random noise and rectangular periodic pulses.

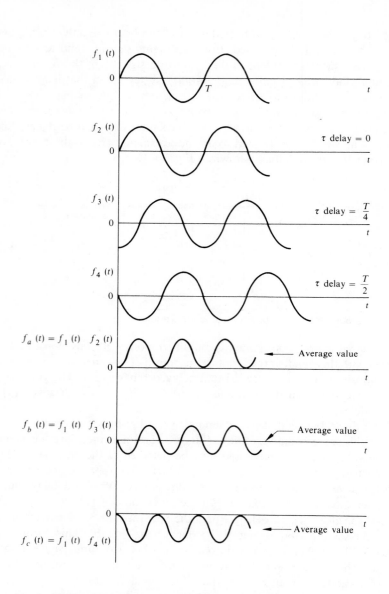

Fig. 11.19. Product waves for different values of delay.

A point to remember

An autocorrelator can be used to detect a periodic signal in the presence of a large amount of noise. The output of the autocorrelator will give the period of the signal but not the waveshape.

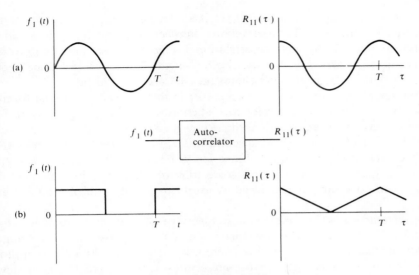

Fig. 11.20. Typical correlator outputs for periodic input waves.

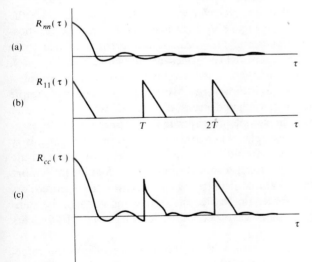

Fig. 11.21. Autocorrelator outputs for composite signal inputs.

Time-domain Techniques: Cross-correlation

Cross-correlation is another method of detecting a very small periodic signal in the presence of noise. It is an average characteristic defined by Eq. (11.6):

$$R_{12}(\tau) = \lim_{T \to \infty} \frac{1}{2T} \int_{-T}^{T} f_1(t)\, f_2(t + \tau)\, dt, \qquad (11.6)$$

where $f_1(t)$ is the composite signal, $f_2(t)$ is a reference signal of the same period as the signal being sought but delayed by τ units of time, and $R_{12}(\tau)$ is the cross-correlation. Note that in a cross-correlation a reference signal must be provided that has the same period as the signal being sought. To use this technique, therefore, some knowledge of the signal must be available or obtained.

The sampling technique described earlier in this chapter is a special form of cross-correlation in which the reference function is called a gating wave. In Fig. 11.16 the wave to be sampled is multiplied by gating wave 1, which produces the product wave $f_1(t) \, f_2(t + \tau)$, as specified in Eq. (11.6). If this product wave is averaged over a very long period of time for each value of the τ-delay, the output as a function of τ will be the cross-correlation of the composite wave and the gating wave. Thus sampling followed by averaging is one form of cross-correlation.

An example of this sample-and-average type of cross-correlation is shown in Fig. 11.22. A square-wave signal has been added to broadband noise with an rms voltage that is twice that of the square wave. The noise has a gaussian probability density function. The signal-to-noise ratio is 0.5. Figure 11.22(a) shows the waveshape as it is displayed on an oscilloscope. Note that this signal together with noise wave is severely distorted as compared to the square-wave signal.

The composite wave is sampled at eight different times during one period of the square wave. Figure 11.22(b) shows eight single samples taken from the composite wave of square wave signal plus noise. The mean-square-error is 7.1 for these sample values compared to the square-wave values at the same sample times. Figure 11.22(c), (d), and (e) show the results of taking 4, 16, and 32 samples, respectively, at each sample time and finding the average value for each sample time. Note that the mean-square-error has decreased to 0.127 when 32 samples are taken at each sample time. The sample averages tend to approach the square-wave values when the number of samples taken at each sample time becomes very large. Thirty-two samples at each sample time are insufficient for an accurate definition of this wave, which has a signal-to-noise ratio of 0.5. Significantly more samples will be needed for this example if better wave definition is required. As the rms noise voltage becomes greater than twice the signal rms voltage, the sample size required to define the square wave becomes even larger ([22] Chapters 11 and 12).

In this example of detecting a square wave in the presence of noise, a reference wave with the same period as that of the square wave is required. In effect, the reference wave is a periodic wave of very narrow pulses, such as the gating waves shown in Fig. 11.16. If each pulse is of very short duration compared with the period of the signal being studied, the output of the cross-correlator as a function of τ will closely represent the actual signal wave when the averaging time is long (many samples). If the reference wave has the same period as the signal but is not of a narrow pulse shape, then the output of the cross-correlator will not indicate the waveshape of the signal.

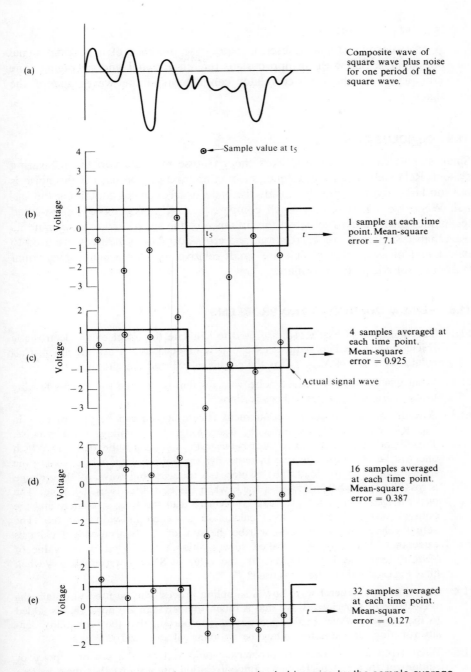

Fig. 11.22. Enhancement of a square wave buried in noise by the sample-average type of cross-correlation.

A point to remember

A cross-correlator can be used to detect the presence of a periodic signal buried in noise. With an appropriate reference signal and averaging time (sample size), the cross-correlator can determine the waveshape of the signal.

11.5 CONCLUSIONS

Small signals can be measured even though noise may get into the measuring system. Relatively simple techniques such as filtering can be used if the noise is not too large and falls mostly outside the band of frequencies containing the signal. When the signal is very small compared to the noise, more sophisticated techniques must be used to detect the presence of the signal and to determine its waveshape. Sampling, autocorrelation, and cross-correlation methods are used to detect and measure signals that are small relative to noise when conventional filters are not adequate or available.

11.6 REVIEW QUESTIONS AND PROBLEMS

11.1 The diagrams in Fig. R11.1 are used to simulate the effect of an electrostatic shield that is used to reduce noise that is induced into a test specimen. Calculate the value of $V_{induced}$ for the circuit in (a) and the circuit in (c).

11.2 What can be done to reduce noise voltages that occur due to currents flowing through grounding wires and connections?

11.3 Assume that a particular measurement system source can be simulated as in Fig. R11.2(a): voltage $v_s(t)$ is the desired signal and voltage $v_n(t)$ is noise. Two filters are available to connect between the source and the load. (a) Which one will be the most effective in removing the noise voltage while passing the signal voltage to the load? (b) Sketch the time-varying wave of the voltage across the load when no filter is used; when the best filter is used. (Note: The two voltages, $v_s(t)$ and $v_n(t)$ can be connected to the filter separately and the output voltage across the load calculated for each individual source. The actual voltage across the load will be the sum of the two individual voltages calculated. This process is called superposition.) (c) What is the value of SNR at terminals 1-2? (d) What is the value of SNR at terminals 3-4 when filter I is used? when filter II is used?

11.4 Describe, in a general way, how a sampling process can be used to obtain the waveshape of a periodic wave that is much smaller than the noise that is added to the periodic wave. In this process, is it important that the probability density function for the noise voltage be symmetrical about zero? Why?

11.5 What types of measurement problems would warrant the use of a piece of equipment that will perform an autocorrelation on a signal that may contain some information?

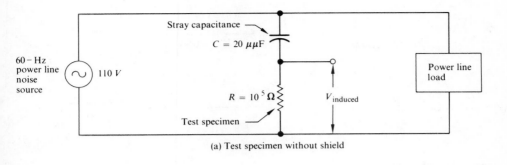

(a) Test specimen without shield

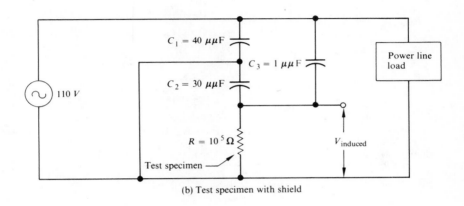

(b) Test specimen with shield

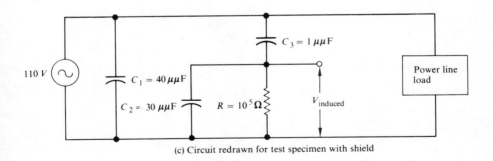

(c) Circuit redrawn for test specimen with shield

Fig. R11.1

11.6   What types of measurement problems would warrant the use of a piece of equipment that will perform a cross-correlation on a signal that may contain some information?

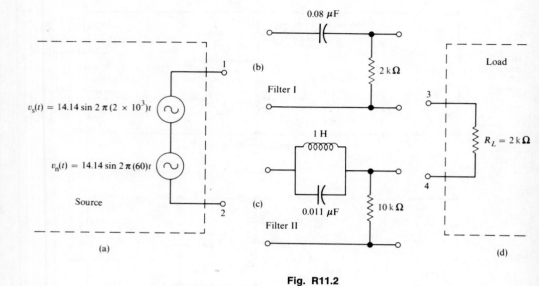

$v_s(t) = 14.14 \sin 2\,\pi\,(2 \times 10^3)t$

$v_n(t) = 14.14 \sin 2\,\pi\,(60)t$

Source

(a)

(b)

0.08 μF

Filter I

2 kΩ

(c)

1 H

0.011 μF

10 kΩ

Filter II

Load

$R_L = 2\,k\Omega$

(d)

Fig. R11.2

12
useful
circuits
and operations

12.1 OBJECTIVES

There are many useful electrical circuits that can help expand the range of things that a scientist can do. The scientist's job may involve much more than a simple measurement of signal current or voltage. The final results of the experiment may require that several operations be performed on the measurement data. The signal may have to be multiplied by a constant or integrated with respect to time. The average value of the signal may be needed. There may be a need to turn on a buzzer or start a recorder whenever the signal level rises above a critical value. All of these operations can be performed by readily available standard circuits.

There may be other situations in which it is important that the timing of various events be controlled automatically. For example, when a light is to be used as a stimulus to an animal and measurements are to be made of the time between the instant that the light goes on and the instant there is a response by the animal, a timing circuit must be set up that will control both the light and the response-time-measuring device. The situation may be more complex in that a specific sequence of different stimuli is to be administered and the animal's response to this combination of conditions is to be studied. Electronic or electromechanical devices are available for these tasks.

Many different kinds of experiments can be imagined that will require the use of a variety of electrical devices and apparatus. Some of the useful circuits and operations that have not been introduced in earlier chapters will be presented in this chapter. The emphasis in our discussion will be to discover what can be done with the circuits rather than detailed circuit analyses of the building blocks. Many examples will be given to show how the building blocks can be used.

The basic operations to be investigated are: multiplication by a constant, summation, integration, differentiation, filtering, generation of pulses, and counting.

12.2 THE OPERATIONAL AMPLIFIER

The *operational amplifier* is a basic building block which can be used to perform a wide variety of functions. These functions will be described in succeeding sections of this chapter. The operational amplifier has the following characteristics:

1. The amplification A_v is very high, with an approximate range of -10^3 to -10^7 (the minus sign indicating 180° phase shift).

2. The input impedance Z_{in} is very high, with an approximate range of 10^5 to 10^{12} Ω.

3. The phase shift is 180° over the useful frequency range.

The signal portion of the operational amplifier is shown in Fig. 12.1. The power supply connections are not included in this figure. The minus sign in the triangular symbol representing the amplifier indicates that any signal applied to this terminal will be inverted at the output, as shown in Fig. 12.1(b).

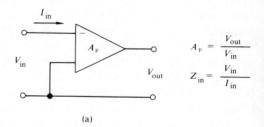

$$A_v = \frac{V_{out}}{V_{in}}$$

$$Z_{in} = \frac{V_{in}}{I_{in}}$$

(a)

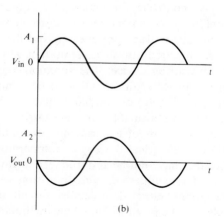

(b)

Fig. 12.1. Operational-amplifier relationships.

When making use of an operational amplifier in a particular problem, three questions come to mind and the answers to them will affect the design of the experiment.

1. What is the maximum attainable output signal voltage V_{out}?
2. What is the maximum usable input signal voltage V_{in}?
3. What is the maximum input current I_{in} required from the circuit providing the input signal?

The power supply voltages for the amplifier will usually give a clue to the answers to these questions. Most operational amplifiers require two power supplies connected to the ground reference point such that one power input voltage is positive and the other power input voltage is negative with respect to the ground reference point. Usually the maximum positive swing of the output signal voltage is approximately equal to the positive power supply voltage, and the maximum negative swing of the output signal voltage is equal to the negative power supply voltage. If the power supplies are $+10$ V and -10 V, the output voltage may range between $+10$ V and -10 V; that is, have a peak-to-peak range of 20 V.

The maximum usable input signal voltage V_{in} depends on the voltage amplification A_v and the maximum output signal voltage. Assuming that the voltage amplification for the operational amplifier is -10^6, if the peak-to-peak output voltage swing is 20 V, as indicated above, the peak-to-peak input voltage swing will be V_{out}/A_v or $20/10^6 = 20$ μV. This is a relatively small voltage, which results from the high value of voltage amplification. If the input voltage exceeds this value, the output signal will be distorted.

The maximum input current I_{in} to the amplifier is very small and is determined by the ratio V_{in}/Z_{in}. Assume that the input impedance is 10^6 Ω and the amplifier characteristics are as given above. The peak-to-peak input current will be V_{in}/Z_{in} or $20 \times 10^{-6}/10^6 = 20 \times 10^{-12}$ A or 20 pA. If the input impedance is as low as 10^3 Ω, the peak-to-peak input current will be 20×10^{-9} A or 20 nA. In either case, the current will be very small.

Points to remember

1. The signal voltage at the input to an operational amplifier must be very small, usually in the order of microvolts.

2. The input current to an operational amplifier is very small, usually 1 nA or less.

12.3 MULTIPLICATION BY A CONSTANT

A time-varying wave can be multiplied by a constant with an operational amplifier connected as shown in Fig. 12.2. The input-output relation for this circuit is

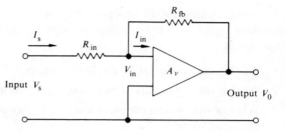

Fig. 12.2. An operational amplifier connected to multiply an incoming signal by a constant.

given by Eq. (12.1):

$$\frac{V_{out}}{V_S} = \frac{1}{\dfrac{R_{in}}{R_{fb}}\left(\dfrac{1}{A_V} - 1\right) + \dfrac{1}{A_V}}, \quad I_{in} << I_S. \tag{12.1}$$

When A_V is much larger than 1 and much greater than R_{fb}/R_{in},

$$\frac{V_{out}}{V_S} = \frac{-R_{fb}}{R_{in}}. \tag{12.2}$$

Equation (12.2) is commonly used to determine the amplification of an operational amplifier connected to be a multiplier. Note that this ratio is valid only
under the assumptions stated above. An important fact is that the amplification
as given by Eq. (12.2) is independent of the amplification of the operational
amplifier, A_V. This means that the operational-amplifier characteristics can change
considerably without affecting the overall performance of the multiplier. The
accuracy of the multiplication depends on the specific values of the R_{fb} and R_{in}
resistors. If these resistor values are affected by aging or temperature fluctuations,
the multiplication factor will also change.

Example 12.1   Multiplication by a factor of ten.   In a particular experiment a
1-V signal is to be multiplied by -10. The current from the signal source to the
multiplier circuit must not exceed 100 μA. Determine the circuit values that must
be used to produce this multiplication.

An operational amplifier can be used to perform this multiplication. Assume
that one is available which has the following characteristics:

$$A_V = -10^6, \quad Z_{in} = 1 \text{ M}\Omega.$$
$$\text{Output voltage range} = \pm 10 \text{ V.}$$

Equation (12.2) shows that the ratio of R_{fb}/R_{in} must be 10 for this example. The
major problem at hand is to determine what values should be chosen for R_{fb} and
R_{in}. Once one of these resistances has been established, the other resistance will
be automatically specified. The input signal current, I_S is the limiting factor in
determining the value of R_{in}. See Fig. 12.3.

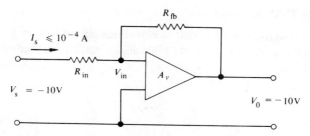

Fig. 12.3. Operational amplifier connection for multiplying the input signal by -10.

Since I_S is the limiting factor, we solve for I_S and then determine R_{in}:

$$I_S = \frac{V_S - V_{in}}{R_{in}}.$$

We have

$$V_{in} = \frac{V_o}{A_V} = \frac{-10}{-10^6} = 10^{-5} \text{ V} \quad \text{when } V_S = 1 \text{ V}.$$

Thus

$$V_{in} << V_S, \quad I_S = \frac{V_S}{R_{in}},$$

and

$$R_{in} = \frac{V_S}{I_S}.$$

It is given in the problem statement that

$$I_S \le 100 \ \mu A.$$

Therefore

$$R_{in} \ge \frac{1 \text{ V}}{100 \times 10^{-6} \text{ A}} \ge 10^4 \ \Omega.$$

If we let $R_{in} = 10^4 \ \Omega$, then R_{fb} must be $10^5 \ \Omega$. If we want to reduce the current flow from the source, we can increase R_{in} which in turn will cause R_{fb} to increase. At this point we will have to refer to the specification sheet for the operational amplifier and determine the maximum allowable resistance that can be used for R_{fb}. The choice of the specific resistor values is also dependent on the availability of precision resistors with these values. The resistors chosen must be stable; that is, able to maintain a fixed resistance value in the environment in which the multiplier is to be used.

12.4   ADDING TWO SIGNALS

An operational amplifier can be used to determine the sum of two or more signal voltages by a simple extension of the multiplier circuit discussed in the previous section (Fig. 12.4).

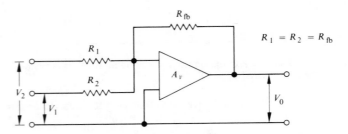

Fig. 12.4.   An operational amplifier used as a summing device.

The output voltage for the circuit shown in Fig. 12.4 is given by Eq. (12.3):

$$V_o = -(V_1 + V_2);$$ (12.3)

the output of the summing circuit is the negative of the sum of the two input voltages. The minimum value of R_1 and therefore R_2 and R_{fb} are determined by the maximum amount of signal current the source can provide. This minimum value of resistance can be calculated in exactly the same way as in Example 12.1.

Example 12.2   A combination of multiplication and summation.   A signal voltage from one source is to be added to a second signal voltage that has been multiplied by a factor of 10. The output voltage amplitude is to be

$$|V_o| = (V_1 + 10\,V_2).$$

Set up a circuit that will produce this result.

   In this example only the amplitude of the sum is needed, so the sign change which usually occurs with an operational amplifier is of no importance. The multiplication and summation can be done with a circuit similar to that shown in Fig. 12.4; it is shown in Fig. 12.5.

Fig. 12.5. Operational amplifier used for multiplication and addition.

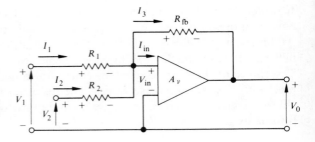

We must determine the appropriate values of the three resistors. Assume that we have an operational amplifier with the same characteristics as given in Example 12.1. The input current I_{in} will be much less than the current I_3, and the output voltage V_o will be much larger than V_{in}. The output voltage equation can be easily obtained in terms of the input voltages. Using Kirchhoff's voltage law, we have

$$V_o - V_{in} + I_3 R_{fb} = 0,$$

$$V_o = -I_3 R_{fb} + V_{in}.$$

Since (refer to example 12.1)

$$V_{in} \cong 0 \text{ V} \quad \text{and} \quad I_3 \cong I_1 + I_2,$$

we have

$$V_o = -I_3 R_{fb} = -(I_1 + I_2) R_{fb}.$$

Similarly,

$$V_1 - V_{in} - I_1 R_1 = 0,$$

$$V_2 - V_{in} - I_2 R_2 = 0,$$

where $V_{in} \ll V_1$ or V_2 (refer to Example 12.1), so that

$$I_1 = \frac{V_1}{R_1}, \quad I_2 = \frac{V_2}{R_2}.$$

Finally,

$$V_o = -\left(\frac{V_1}{R_1} + \frac{V_2}{R_2}\right) R_{fb} = -\left(\frac{R_{fb}}{R_1} V_1 + \frac{R_{fb}}{R_2} V_2\right).$$

Let $R_{fb}/R_1 = 1$ and $R_{fb}/R_2 = 10$. Then

$$V_o = -(V_1 + 10 V_2).$$

From this example we can see that the operations of multiplication and summation can be done simultaneously by means of only one operational amplifier and three appropriately chosen resistors. Once again the signal input current from the sources determines the minimum value of resistors R_1 and R_2 and thus the value of R_{fb}.

Example 12.3   The difference between two signals.   A scientist wants to know the effect of a drug on the response by an animal to periodic flashes of a light of a certain intensity. He wants to note the difference between the responses of two animals, one which has been drugged and the other has not been drugged. How can this difference be displayed on an oscilloscope that has the capability of displaying two signal traces on the screen?

One way of solving this problem is shown in Fig. 12.6. Two operational amplifiers are required to produce the difference between the two input signals. The output of amplifier 1 gives the negative of $s_1(t)$. The second operational amplifier circuit takes the two inputs, $-s_1(t)$ and $s_2(t)$, and produces a sign change to yield an output voltage of $s_1(t) - s_2(t)$. This difference voltage is displayed as trace 1 on the oscilloscope. A light sensor circuit generates a signal every time the light flashes on. This sensor signal provides a time-base reference for the scientist, so he can see when a difference occurs in the responses relative to the light stimulus.

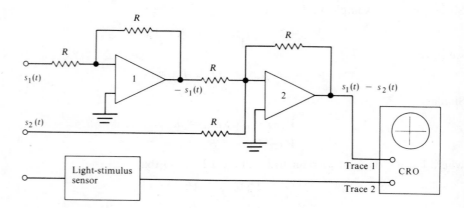

Fig. 12.6. Method taking the difference between two signals and displaying it together with a stimulus-related signal.

If the scientist has a four-trace oscilloscope available, he could show the following traces simultaneously.

1. Trace 1: response of animal 1.
2. Trace 2: response of animal 2.
3. Trace 3: the difference between the responses of animals 1 and 2.
4. Trace 4: response of the light-stimulus sensor.

This problem can also be solved by using an oscilloscope with a differential amplifier input. If this type of oscilloscope is used, the signal from one of the animals must be connected to one of the differential amplifier input terminals on the oscilloscope and the signal from the other animal must be connected to the other input terminal of the differential input amplifier. The oscilloscope will then be set to display the difference between these two input signals. If such an oscilloscope capability is available, the operational-amplifier system shown in Fig. 12.6 will not be needed.

12.5   INTEGRATION

The *integration* of a signal voltage can be accomplished by means of an operational amplifier in a circuit such as shown in Fig. 12.7. The voltage at the output, $v_o(t)$, is given by Eq. (12.4):

$$v_o(t) = \frac{-1}{R_{in}C_{fb}} \int_o^t v_S(t)\ dt. \tag{12.4}$$

If R_{in} and C_{fb} have appropriate values, the term $1/R_{in}C_{fb}$ has units of sec^{-1}. For example, if $R_{in} = 1\ M\Omega$ and $C_{fb} = 1\ \mu F$, the $R_{in}C_{fb} = 1\ \Omega\text{-F} = 1$ sec. *Any product of RC which is 1 Ω-F has a value of 1 sec.*

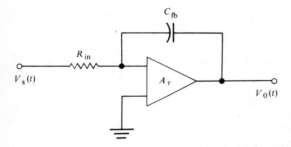

Fig. 12.7. An operational amplifier connected to produce the operation of integration.

There is an upper limit to the output voltage that can be attained by an integrator. This upper limit is determined by the power supply voltages required by the operational amplifier. If the power supply voltage is $+10$ V, then the maximum voltage that can be attained as a result of integration is $+10$ V. Once the output voltage reaches this maximum, the circuit shown in Fig. 12.7 ceases to function as an integrator and a constant maximum voltage will be maintained.

The lower limit of the value of R_{in} is dependent on the maximum amount of current that can be drawn from the signal source. We recall that the input current is $I_S \cong V_S/R_{in}$. The upper limit on the value of R_{in} is determined by the product $R_{in}C_{fb}$ and is dependent on the value of $v_o(t)$ that is desired for a particular integration.

Example 12.4   Integration of a time-varying voltage.   A chemical experiment is to be performed in which the product of the strength of the chemical reaction and the reaction time is to be determined. It is possible to obtain a sensor which will produce a voltage proportional to the strength of the chemical reaction. How is a voltage proportional to this strength-time product to be provided?

This problem statement does not include all of the facts necessary to design the circuit. However, we do know that an integrator circuit is needed. We can make some assumptions which will show what limits we will have to consider when designing such a circuit with an operational amplifier. Let $R_{in}C_{fb} = 1$ sec, the maximum allowable output voltage be 10 V, and assume that the input voltage from the sensor is as shown in Fig. 12.8(a).

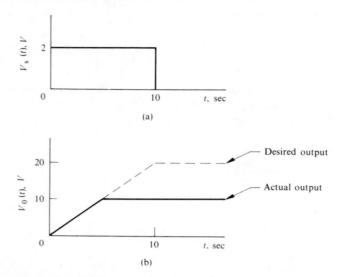

Fig. 12.8. Waveforms for Example 12.4.

The product of the sensor voltage $v_S(t)$ and time is given by the integral of the $v_S(t)$ curve. $v_o(t)$ should be a linearly increasing voltage that rises to 20 V and remains constant thereafter. However, the maximum allowable output voltage is only 10 V, so that the output voltage will rise linearly as desired until it reaches 10 V, after which it will stay constant at 10 V, as shown in Fig. 12.8(b). This is not the desired result.

The operational amplifier integrator circuit must therefore be modified. The variables R_{in} and C_{fb} can be changed to prevent the output voltage from exceeding the 10-V limit. The output voltage can be scaled down by increasing the $R_{in}C_{fb}$ product. Let $R_{in} = 2$ MΩ and $C_{fb} = 2$ μF. Then $R_{in}C_{fb} = 4$ Ω-F or 4 sec. Equation (12.4) then becomes

$$v_o(t) = \frac{1}{4 \text{ sec}} \int_o^t v_S(t) \, dt,$$

while the area under the $v_S(t)$ curve will be given by

$$\int_o^{10} v_S(t) \, dt = 20 \text{ V-sec.}$$

The voltage at the output will be 20/4 when t is greater than 10 sec. (See Fig. 12.9.) Thus the output voltage is directly proportional to the desired product at all times and is scaled down by a factor of 4. This procedure can be used to

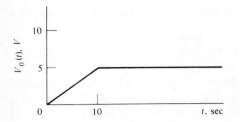

Fig. 12.9. Output voltage for Example 12.4 when a scale-down factor of 4 is used.

prevent the maximum allowable output voltage of the operational amplifier from being exceeded when the actual value of the integration is excessively large.

12.6 DIFFERENTIATION

The rate at which a particular signal varies conveys useful information about the process that produces the signal. This rate is given by the *derivative* of the signal. An operational amplifier can be used to obtain the derivative of a time-varying wave if it is connected as shown in Fig. 12.10.

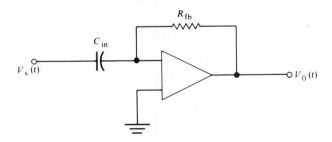

Fig. 12.10. An operational-amplifier circuit which performs differentiation.

The output voltage $v_o(t)$ is related to the derivative of the source voltage $v_S(t)$ by Eq. (12.5):

$$v_o(t) = - R_{fb}C_{in} \frac{dv_S(t)}{dt}. \tag{12.5}$$

The product $R_{fb}C_{in}$ provides a scaling factor in a similar way to that discussed in Example 12.4. If $R_{fb}C_{in} = 1$ sec, the output voltage is equal to the negative of the derivative of the source voltage.

In physical systems which produce signals that change at a relatively slow rate, differentiator circuits will function satisfactorily. If the rate of change of the input signal becomes large, the value of the output voltage given by Eq. (12.5) will exceed the maximum allowable voltage for the operational amplifier and cause distortion in the output signal. High-frequency noise at the input can produce this effect. These factors must be considered when using differentiating circuits in a measurement system.

Example 12.5 Determining the time rate of change of a voltage. A light is to be used to stimulate a rodent. The light intensity is varied to determine how the rate of change of intensity will affect the rodent. An appropriate electrical connection is made to the rodent to pick up the electrical signals as the light intensity is varied. The rodent's response and the derivative of the light intensity are to be displayed by two traces on the screen of an oscilloscope so that a direct comparison can be made. A light-intensity sensor is available to provide a voltage proportional to the light intensity at any instant of time. Show how this can be done.

An operational-amplifier circuit as shown in Fig. 12.10 can be used to obtain the derivative of the voltage provided by the light-intensity sensor. The general circuit diagram for the measurement system is shown in Fig. 12.11.

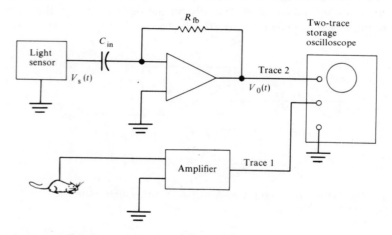

Fig. 12.11. Circuit diagram for Example 12.5.

The signal from the rodent may be too small to be observable on the oscilloscope. If so, an amplifier must be used which will not distort the waveshape of the signal. An operational amplifier with an amplification of 10 or 100 may be satisfactory. The signal will be observed as trace 1. Trace 2 will show the derivative of the light sensor output for appropriate values of C_{in} and R_{fb}. Figure 12.12 will help to give an indication of what value the product $R_{fb}C_{in}$ must have.

The derivative of the sensor voltage takes on three values: 2 V/sec, -2 V/sec, and 0 V/sec. If $R_{fb}C_{in} = 1$ sec, the output voltage $v_o(t)$ will be 2 V, -2 V, or 0. If these are allowable output voltages for the operational amplifier, then the design is satisfactory. It is possible to increase the voltage variation for trace 2 by increasing the product $R_{fb}C_{in}$. For example, we can let $R_{fb} = 1$ MΩ

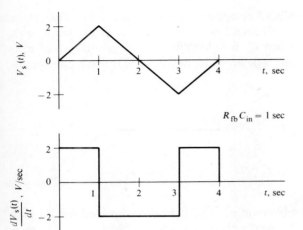

$R_{fb}C_{in} = 1$ sec

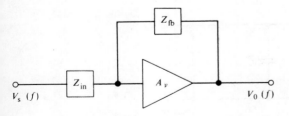

Fig. 12.12. Waveforms for the circuit in Fig. 12.11.

and $C_{in} = 3$ μF. Then $R_{fb}C_{in} = 3$ sec and the voltage input for trace 2 will range from 6 V to −6 V and back to zero.

    A storage oscilloscope can be used to good advantage in this example, because the waveforms shown in Fig. 12.12 each appear only once: $v_s(t)$ is not periodic. The storage oscilloscope will hold these waveforms on the screen so that they can be studied for a period of time. If no storage oscilloscope is available, a camera would have to be used to record the transient waveforms for later study.

12.7 FILTERING

The basic ideas of filtering electrical signals were introduced in Chapter 4, Example 4.3. These ideas can be applied to operational-amplifier filters that are capable of both filtering and amplification. The circuit in Fig. 12.13 shows that impedances are used with the operational amplifiers to produce filter action. As the frequency of the input signal changes, the impedances will change and the overall amplification will change.

Fig. 12.13. Generalized circuit for an operational amplifier used for filtering and amplification.

The output voltage, as a function of frequency, is given by Eq. (12.6).

$$V_o(f) = - \frac{Z_{fb}}{Z_{in}} V_s(f). \qquad (12.6)$$

Let the impedance Z_{fb}, of the feedback components have the characteristics shown in Fig. 12.14. The ratio Z_{fb}/Z_{in} will then have a frequency response curve with the shape shown in Fig. 12.14 when Z_{in} is held constant. If $Z_{in} = 10^3$ Ω, at zero frequency (dc) the output voltage will be $-(10^5/10^3)$ $V_s(0)$; that is, the amplification at dc will be -100.

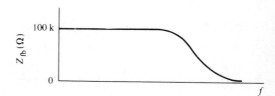

Fig. 12.14. Frequency response characteristic of a particular Z_{fb}.

It may appear that any combination of impedances can be used for Z_{in} and Z_{fb}. This is not true because the feedback component in the circuit, Z_{fb}, may cause a signal to be fed back into the operational amplifier so as to produce oscillations. At the onset of oscillation the circuit will cease to function as a filter. This is a common occurrence. Careful study of the manufacturer's specifications for the operational amplifier may be necessary to prevent oscillations from occurring when using operational amplifiers in filtering circuits.

Example 12.6   Determining the average value of a time-varying voltage.   A scientist wants to determine the average or dc value of a signal voltage when there are noise frequencies present. The source of the signal has an internal resistance (Thevenin resistance) of 10^4 Ω. The experimenter wants to filter out all the noise above approximately 0.1 Hz. He also wants to monitor this average voltage on a chart recorder which has an input resistance of 10^4 Ω. Determine an appropriate filter circuit.

A low-pass filter is needed to filter out all frequencies except those less than 0.1 Hz. This restriction is very stringent. Let us investigate several filters to see what problems must be solved.

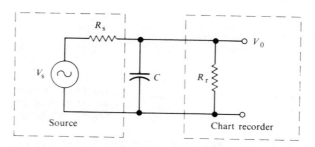

Fig. 12.15. A filter circuit for solution of the problem in Example 12.6.

Figure 12.15 shows the Thevenin equivalent circuit for the source connected to a capacitor and the chart recorder. As the frequency increases, the impedance of the capacitor will decrease, as will the voltage across the chart recorder. Thus filtering action will occur. The output voltage V_o is given by the following equation:

$$V_o = \frac{V_s}{1 + R_s/R_r + j\omega C R_s}.$$

In this example $R_s = 10^4\ \Omega$, $R_r = 10^4\ \Omega$. When $\omega C R_s = 1 + R_s/R_r$,

$$|V_o| = 0.7\ V_s.$$

Assume that

$$|V_o| = 0.7\ V_s \qquad \text{when } f = 0.1\text{ Hz}.$$

Then

$$C = 318\ \mu\text{F}.$$

If this capacitance should have some leakage resistance in parallel with its terminals, the leakage resistance would have the same effect as R_r on the circuit performance. The output voltage at zero frequency is $0.5\ V_s$ for the circuit component values given in this problem.

Consider a second solution. An operation amplifier can be used to provide amplification together with filtering action if the circuit shown in Fig. 12.16 is used. The chart recorder input resistance R_r will have essentially no effect on the

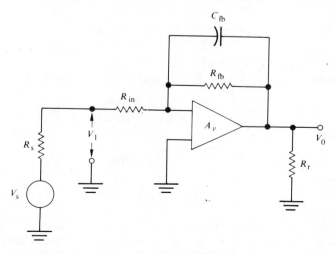

Fig. 12.16. An operational amplifier used in a filter-amplifier circuit.

performance of the operational-amplifier circuit. The output voltage V_o is given by Eq. (12.6):

$$V_o = - \frac{Z_{fb}}{R_{in}} V_1, \tag{12.6}$$

where

$$Z_{fb} = \frac{R_{fb}}{1 + j\omega C_{fb} R_{fb}}, \qquad V_1 \cong \frac{R_{in}}{R_s + R_{in}} V_s.$$

Assume that $V_o/V_1 = -10$ at 0 Hz and that the amplitude of this ratio decreases to -7 at 0.1 Hz. With these conditions in mind, we can determine appropriate values for R_{in}, R_{fb}, and C_{fb}.

Choice for R_{in}. The equation above indicates that V_1 will approach the value of V_s when R_{in} is much greater than R_s. Let us assume that $R_{in} = 10\ R_s$ is sufficiently large. Then $R_{in} = 10^5\ \Omega$.

Choice for R_{fb}. Using the assumption that an amplification of -10 is needed at 0 Hz, we find that the equation for Z_{fb} indicates that $Z_{fb} = R_{fb}$, so that $R_{fb} = 10\ R_{in} = 10^6\ \Omega$.

Determine C_{fb}. Using the condition that $|V_o| = 7V_1$ when $f = 0.1$ Hz, we get the following equation.

$$|V_o| = \frac{|R_{fb}/(1 + j\omega C_{fb}R_{fb})|}{R_{in}} V_1, \qquad \frac{|R_{fb}/(1 + j\omega C_{fb}R_{fb})|}{R_{in}} = 7.$$

Substituting the appropriate component values into the equation yields

$$\frac{1}{1 + j2\pi \times 10^5\ C_{fb}} = 0.7.$$

Solving for C_{fb}, we get $C_{fb} = 1.6\ \mu\text{F}$.

The general expression for the output voltage V_o is given below:

$$V_o \cong \left(\frac{-R_{fb}}{R_{in}(1 + j\omega C_{fb}R_{fb})} \right) \left(\frac{R_{in}}{R_s + R_{in}} \right) V_s$$

$$\cong \frac{-V_s}{(1/R_{fb} + j\omega C_{fb})\ (R_s + R_{in})}.$$

When $f = 0$ Hz

$$V_o \cong -9\ V_s.$$

The filtering action will be the same as in the first solution, but the output voltage will have a different sign and be approximately 18 times larger than the output obtained with the filter in Fig. 12.15. Also a much smaller capacitor is required in this amplifier circuit. The price paid for this increase in output is the requirement of the operational amplifier and its power supplies.

There are many different filter characteristics that can be obtained with operational amplifiers. Many manufacturers provide application information sheets describing specific filter circuits that can be built with their operational amplifiers. It is important to refer to these sheets to determine what precautions must be taken to prevent unwanted oscillations from occurring.

Points to remember

Operational amplifiers may be used in circuits that can perform

1. multiplication of an input signal by a constant,
2. addition of signals,
3. integration of signals,
4. differentiation of signals,
5. filtering of signals.

Unwanted oscillations may occur in operational-amplifier circuits unless precautions recommended by the amplifier manufacturer are followed.

Most analog computers have operational amplifiers that are set up to be used exactly as described in this section. No power supply voltages or extra components are required. However, the operational amplifiers that are purchased as piece parts require additional components in order to make them functional. These parts may include resistors and/or capacitors and dc power supplies. The manufacturers will supply information sheets for their particular amplifiers which indicate how they should be set up to perform the desired operations. They will also help with many of the practical problems that commonly occur in using operational amplifiers.

12.8 GENERATION OF PULSES

A *pulse* can be considered a variation in amplitude of a quantity whose value is normally constant. It is characterized by a rise and a decay within a finite duration. There are several basic pulse shapes that are relatively easy to generate and can be used for a variety of purposes in measurement systems. The pulses may be used to control a stimulus-producing device. They may be used as part of a system to determine the length of the time interval between the onset and the termination of a response. The pulse rate may depend on the magnitude of the response being measured. For example, the temperature of a specific portion of a human body during a period of exercise may be the response, and the data may have to be telemetered to a data-collection point far from the location of exercise; here the measured pulse rate represents a specific body temperature.

The nature of the application will determine the specific pulse waveshapes that will be needed. Some of the easily generated standard waveshapes are shown in Fig. 12.17.

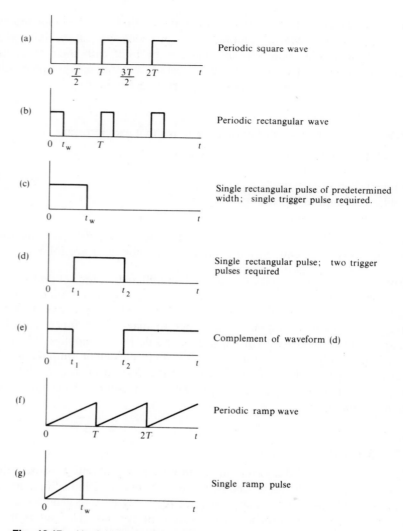

Fig. 12.17. Useful pulse waveshapes.

The waves shown in parts (a), (b), (c), (d), and (e) can be produced by multivibrator circuits.

Waveform	Generating circuit
Periodic square wave (a)	Symmetrical astable multivibrator
Periodic rectangular wave (b)	Nonsymmetrical astable multivibrator
Single rectangular pulse (c)	One-shot multivibrator
Rectangular step wave (d) (e)	Bistable multivibrator

Symmetrical astable multivibrator. Symmetrical astable multivibrators are "free running," which means that they generate the waveform shown in Fig. 12.17(a) whenever their power supply is energized. No external triggering signal is required to cause a symmetrical astable multivibrator to produce the square-wave output voltage.

Nonsymmetrical multivibrator. Nonsymmetrical astable multivibrators are also free running and will generate rectangular square waves whenever the power supply is energized. There may be a control to vary the symmetry t_w of the wave-shape.

One-shot multivibrator. A one-shot multivibrator must have a "trigger" signal voltage to cause the circuit to produce a single rectangular output pulse. The trigger signal does not affect the width t_w of the output rectangular pulse. The output pulse width is determined by the components in the one-shot multivibrator and is controllable.

Bistable multivibrator. A bistable multivibrator is a circuit that has two stable states in which it can operate. The output voltage can have either a high value or a low value. The change from one state to the other takes place almost instantaneously. The output of a bistable multivibrator is shown in Fig. 12.17(d). When the first trigger voltage is applied at t_1, the output becomes positive, when the second trigger voltage is applied at t_2, the output becomes zero. Most bistable multivibrators have two output points so that the waveform shown in Fig. 12.17(e) can be obtained simultaneously with that in Fig. 12.17(d).

The waves shown in Fig. 12.17 are all positive. It is possible to offset these waves by means of an operational amplifier summing circuit, as shown in Fig. 12.18. Note that the output wave is the inverted sum of the two input voltages. A second operational amplifier can be used as a second inverter if needed.

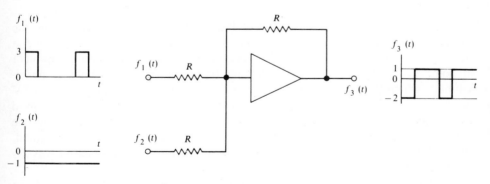

Fig. 12.18.   Summing circuit for offsetting pulse waves.

Example 12.7   Generation of a special sawtooth pulse.   A biologist wants to know how the auditory system of a small animal will respond to different frequencies. Specifically, he wants to determine the response to a sound that starts at 1 kHz and increases linearly to 10 kHz and then stops. He has a sound source that will generate a sinusoidal wave. As the input voltage to this source is varied, the frequency of the sine wave will vary linearly; for example, when the input voltage is 1 V the output frequency is 1 kHz, and when the input voltage is doubled, the output frequency is also doubled. The peak value of the output sine wave is constant regardless of the frequency of the wave. Determine a system of basic building blocks that will provide an appropriate input voltage to this sinusoidal wave source.

The following solution will serve as a good example of how multivibrators and operational amplifiers can be used as building blocks in a measurement system. This problem calls for the generation of an input signal that is a linearly increasing voltage, as shown in Fig. 12.19. This wave can be produced by taking the sum of a rectangular pulse and a ramp-shaped pulse as shown in Fig. 12.17(c) and (g). The rectangular pulse can be produced by a one-shot multivibrator, but the ramp pulse is more difficult to produce by means of the building blocks thus far discussed. A ramp pulse can be produced by integrating a rectangular pulse and adding a rectangular step voltage to the output of the integrator at the appropriate time. Careful study of Fig. 12.20 will show how this can be accomplished.

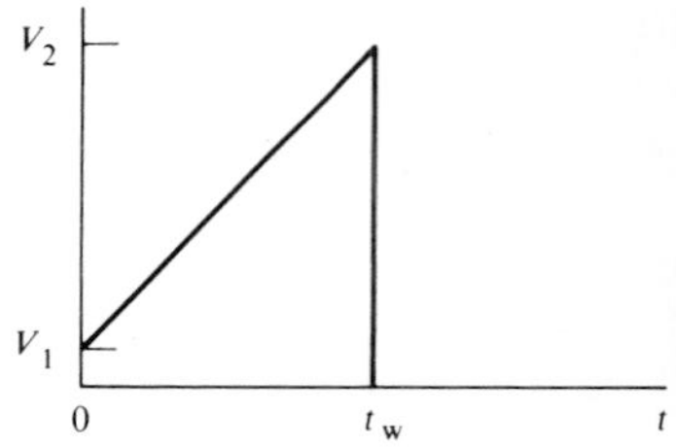

Fig. 12.19.   Input waveform required by the sinusoidal sound source of Example 12.7.

The waveforms at various parts of the circuit are given to show how the ramp pulse is produced. The one-shot multivibrator is used to produce a rectangular wave $f_1(t)$ at point 1. The integrator circuit produces the ramp $f_2(t)$ at point 2. The output of the one-shot multivibrator operates a bistable multivibrator, which has 0 V at point 3 when its input voltage is negative and -10 V at point 3 when its input is zero. The second operational-amplifier circuit is used as a summing circuit to produce the ramp wave at point 4. Provisions must be made to reset the integrator to zero before each ramp wave is to be generated. When the wave at point 1 is added to the wave at point 4, the required wave is produced at point 5.

Let us consider the specific voltage and time requirements shown and see how the various component values can be determined. First, we note the specifications.

Specifications for the output waveform (Fig. 12.19)

$$V_1 = 1 \text{ V}, \quad V_2 = 10 \text{ V}, \quad t_w = 10 \text{ sec.}$$

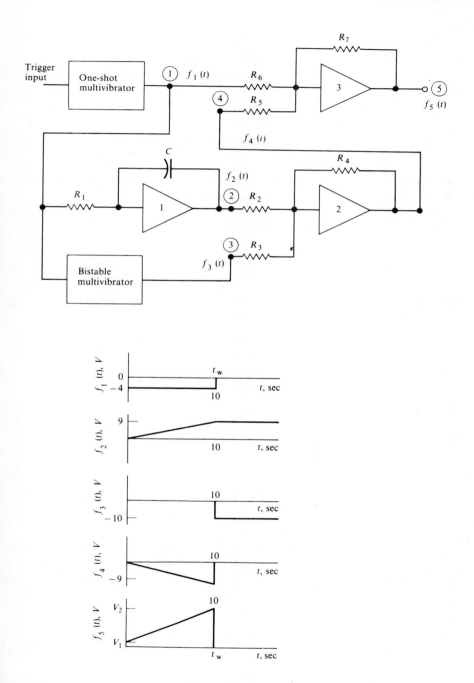

Fig. 12.20. A method of generating the waveform shown in Fig. 12.19.

Specifications for the operational amplifier

Upper limit of output voltage $= +12$ V.
Lower limit of output voltage $= -12$ V.

Specifications for multivibrators.

In the case of a one-shot multivibrator:

Trigger input voltage must be greater than $+1$ V.

Output voltage $= \begin{cases} 0 & \text{when no trigger input voltage has been applied.} \\ -4 & \text{V for a period of 10 sec after the application of} \\ & \text{trigger input voltage.} \end{cases}$

In the case of a bistable multivibrator:

Input voltages $=$ 0 or -4 V.
Output voltage $= \begin{cases} 0 & \text{when input voltage is } -4 \text{ V.} \\ -10 & \text{V when input voltage is 0.} \end{cases}$

The specifications for the multivibrators may not be exactly as we would like them to be, but we will assume that these are what we have to work with.

Design of the integrator. We must determine the values of R_1 and C. We recall the method discussed in Section 12.4. By Eq. (12.4) we get

$$f_2(t) = \frac{-1}{R_1 C} \int_o^t f_1(t) \, dt.$$

The area under the waveform of $f_1(t)$ is -40 V sec. At 10 sec the voltage wave is to be $+9$ V:

$$f_2(10) = 9 \text{ V} = \frac{1}{R_1 C} (40 \text{ V sec})$$

$$R_1 C = \frac{40}{9} \text{ sec.}$$

We let $R_1 = 1$ MΩ. Then $C = 4.45$ μF.

Design of summing circuit 2. The ramp wave at point 2 has the correct shape and voltages from 0 to 10 sec. The output voltage of the bistable multivibrator is -10 V at 10 sec instead of the -9 V required to cancel out the integrator output. This difference can be corrected by appropriate choices of R_2, R_3, and R_4. By Eq. (12.2) we get

$$V_{\text{out}} = \frac{-R_{\text{fb}}}{R_{\text{in}}} V_{\text{in}}, \tag{12.2}$$

$$9 = \frac{-R_4}{R_3} (-10 \text{ V}).$$

Let $R_4 = 1$ MΩ. Then

$$R_3 = \frac{10 \times 10^6}{9} = 1.11 \text{ MΩ.}$$

Since the ramp wave has the correct amplitude, the summing circuit should multiply $f_2(t)$ by -1. Again using Eq. (12.2), we obtain $R_2 = R_4 = 1$ MΩ.

Design of summing circuit 3. The rectangular voltage at point 1 is too large; it must be reduced by summing circuit 3. By Eq. (12.2) we can determine the ratio R_7/R_6:

$$1 \text{ V} = \frac{R_7}{R_6} (-4 \text{ V}).$$

Let $R_7 = 1$ MΩ. Then

$$R_6 = 4 \text{ MΩ.}$$

The ramp voltage does not need to be modified. Therefore, according to Eq. (12.2), $R_5 = R_7 = 1$ MΩ. This completes the design calculations needed to specify the circuit that will produce $f_5(t)$.

12.9 REVIEW QUESTIONS AND PROBLEMS

12.1 A signal of 2 V peak to peak must be amplified by a factor of $+10$. Draw a diagram showing how this can be done with operational amplifiers. Assume that an individual amplifier has an $A_v = -10^5$ in the frequency range of the signal. What values should the resistors have that must be used with the operational amplifiers?

12.2 A signal of 5 V peak to peak must be amplified by a factor of -5. What considerations must be made when picking an operational amplifier to produce this amplification? Draw the circuit diagram for such an amplifier system.

12.3 A signal source has a Thevenin equivalent circuit consisting of an open circuit voltage of 4 V and an internal resistance of 10^5 Ω. This signal source is to be connected to an operational amplifier circuit that has an R_{in} resistance of 10^4 Ω and an R_{fb} resistance of 10^5 Ω. (a) What is the amplification of this operational amplifier circuit? (b) If this source is connected to R_{in}, what will be the voltage that will appear at the output of the operational amplifier?

12.4 A test is to be made to determine the ability of a person to hear a sine-wave signal in the presence of random noise. A sine-wave generator and a random-noise generator are to be used to produce the signal plus noise output. Design an operational amplifier circuit that can be used to sum these two waves together before feeding the combination into an audio power amplifier. Assume that each of the generators has a control to vary the amplitude of its output voltage. Assume each of the generators has a Thevenin equivalent internal resistance of 600 Ω.

12.5   The ramp-shaped voltage wave, $v_R(t)$, shown in Fig. R12.1 is to be added to a variable dc voltage. The ramp generator has no control to vary the peak value of the ramp voltage. We need a means of controlling the amplitude of the ramp voltage so that it ranges from 0 to 4 V peak to peak before it is added to the variable dc voltage. The variable dc voltage is to range from $+4$ V to -4 V. Show an operational amplifier system that can perform all of these operations.

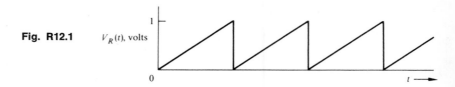

Fig. R12.1 $V_R(t)$, volts

12.6   A small animal is to be stimulated by a ringing bell. An output response from the animal is to be displayed on an oscilloscope screen to see if there is any relationship between the response and the ring of the bell. The suggestion was made that a very narrow positive pulse be displayed on the screen whenever the bell rings. In this way the response on the screen can be timed in relation to the time the bell rings. A pulse generator was found that would produce a very narrow pulse when the bell rings. Set up an operational amplifier circuit that will combine the voltage response from the animal and the narrow pulses. Show how this circuit should be connected to a single channel oscilloscope.

12.7   The area under the curve of voltage as a function of time shown in Fig. R12.2 provides an experimenter with some important information. He has been using a strip chart recorder to plot this voltage curve. Then, he determines the area under the curve. For the waveform shown, design an operational amplifier circuit that will determine this area automatically. Operational amplifiers with an $A_v = -10^6$ and powered by $+10$-V and -10-V dc sources are available. The input resistance of these amplifiers is 10^7 Ω.

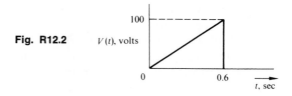

Fig. R12.2 $V(t)$, volts

12.8   Design an operational amplifier integrator that will produce the integral of the $v(t)$ wave shown in Fig. R12.3. Show appropriate component values. Use the same type of operational amplifiers as described in the previous problem.

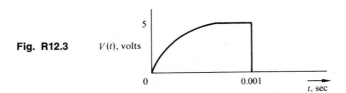

Fig. R12.3 $V(t)$, volts

12.9   The output of the integrator of the previous problem is to be displayed on the screen of a storage oscilloscope along with the $v(t)$ wave. Show a circuit diagram that could be used to do this. Assume the oscilloscope has only one input channel for the y axis.

appendixes

appendices

glossary

Term or word	Page	Definition
ac power	66	The power in an alternating-current circuit; given by the equation ac power = rms voltage × rms current × cosine of the phase angle between the current and the voltage.
ac signal	66	The portion of the alternating-current voltage or current that contains information.
Active transducer	140	A transducer that will produce a voltage in response to a measurand without an excitation by an external source of electrical energy.
Alternating current (ac)	58	An electric current whose instantaneous value and direction change periodically; the term is usually used to refer to a sinusoidally shaped current or voltage wave.
Ammeter	18	A meter used to measure current.
Ampere	6	The unit of current in the International System of Units; abbreviated A.
Amplifier	106	A device that enables an input signal to control the power derived from a source independent of the signal so that the output will bear some relationship to, and be generally greater than, the input signal.
Amplitude-frequency distortion	118	Distortion due to an undesired amplitude-frequency characteristic; the usual desired characteristic is flat over the frequency range of interest (IEEE).

Definitions with IEEE designations are taken from Reference 59.

Term or word	*Page*	*Definition*
Amplitude modulation	130	A process in which the amplitude of a carrier wave is varied in accordance with a modulating wave.
Analog-to-digital conversion system	159	A circuit in which the input is information in analog form (continuous range of values) and whose output is the same information in digital form (discrete set of values arranged in some code form such as a binary-code sequence of 0's and 1's).
Antenna	8	A device for radiating or receiving radio waves (IEEE).
Astable multivibrator	9	A type of oscillator that produces nonsinusoidal waveforms of voltage or current; is free running in that it does not require an input signal to control its operation.
Audio amplifier	7	A device designed to amplify electrical signals that contain frequencies in the range audible to the human ear: approximately 20 Hz to 20 000 Hz.
Autocorrelation	314	A method of comparing a time-varying wave with a time-shifted replica of the wave. For a periodic wave it is defined mathematically to be

$$R(\tau) = \frac{1}{T} \int_0^T f(t)f(t + \tau)\,dt,$$

where $f(t)$ is the time-varying wave, τ is the time-shift variable, $f(t + \tau)$ is the time-varying wave shifted by τ units of time, and T is the period of the wave.

Autotransformer	99	A transformer consisting of one electrically continuous winding with one or more fixed or movable taps that is intended for use in such a manner that part of the winding is common to both primary and secondary circuits (IEEE).
Band-pass filter	302	An electric filter that will let pass a band of frequencies with very little attenuation while severely attenuating frequencies above and below this band.
Band-rejection filter	302	An electrical filter that will severely attenuate a band of frequencies while letting pass frequencies above and below this band with very little attenuation.

Term or word	Page	Definition
Bandwidth	116	A range of frequencies within which performance, with respect to some characteristic, falls within specified limits (IEEE); commonly defined at the points where the response is 3 decibels less than the reference value.
Biotelemetric system	3	A measurement system in which a physiological or physical function is transduced and transmitted through air to a receiver and/or a measurement device.
Biotelemetry	8	The measurement of biological properties from a remote location.
Bistable multivibrator	341	An electrical circuit that will switch from one to the other of two possible stable states whenever an input trigger pulse is applied to the circuit.
Block diagram	3	A diagram representing a circuit or system in which the various parts of the system are not given in detail but are shown in relation to the other parts of the system.
Capacitance	69	That property of a system of conductors and dielectrics which enables the system to store electricity when a voltage exists between the conductors; expressed as the ratio of the electrical charge stored and the voltage across the conductors; basic unit is the farad.
Capacitive reactance	74	The amplitude of the impedance of a capacitor defined by the equation $$X_C = \frac{1}{2\pi f C},$$ where f is the frequency of the sinusoidal wave, C is the value of capacitance; measured in ohms.
Capacitor	57	An electrical component consisting of two conducting materials separated by an insulating material; capable of storing electrical charge.
Cathode-ray oscilloscope	8	An oscilloscope that uses a cathode-ray tube to present the visual display of a fixed or varying voltage.
Cathode-ray tube	200	An electron-beam tube in which the beam can be focused to a small cross section on a luminescent screen and varied in position and intensity to produce a visible pattern (IEEE).

Term or word	*Page*	*Definition*
Circuit	18	A path through which electric current can flow.
Coaxial cable	130	A two-conductor electrical cable with a concentric outer conductor about a central conductor; shown in Fig. 10.7(a).
Complex numbers	247	A number that has a real and an imaginary part such that there are an amplitude and an angle associated with the number.
Composite signal	298	A signal composed of many different parts, for example information signal plus unwanted noise.
Control device	107	A device capable of controlling the flow of electric power from a power source in response to a measurand signal.
Crosscorrelation	317	A method of comparing two different signals by means of Eq. (11.6).
D'Arsonval meter	178	A meter for measuring dc currents; consists of a movable coil with a pointer mounted in a magnetic field set up by a permanent magnet; produces a linear rotation of the pointer as a function of current.
dc power	66	The power in a direct-current circuit; defined by the equation $$\text{dc power} = \text{voltage} \times \text{current}.$$
Deflection factor	203	The ratio of the input signal amplitude to the resultant displacement of the indicating spot on the screen of the cathode-ray tube (IEEE).
Derivative	333	The limit of $\triangle y / \triangle x$ as $\triangle x$ goes to zero for an equation defining y as a function of x.
Differential amplifier	208	An amplifier whose output signal is proportional to the algebraic difference between two input signals (IEEE).
Differentiation	333	The process of finding dy/dx from an equation defining y as a function of x.
Diode	100	An electrical device that has an asymmetric current-vs.-voltage characteristic; tends to be an open circuit when biased with one set of polarities of voltage and a short circuit when biased with the opposite set of voltage polarities.

Term or word	Page	Definition
Diode bridge rectifier	7	A network, consisting of four diodes, that is designed to convert alternating current to current flowing in only one direction; produces full-wave rectification; offers relatively high resistance to current flow in one direction and relatively low resistance to current flow in the other direction.
Direct-coupled system	3	A system in which the various major components are connected with wires.
Direct current (dc)	27	Current that flows in only one direction and is of constant value.
Distortion	118	An undesired change in waveform (IEEE).
Drift, stability	114	Gradual shift or change in the output over a period of time due to change in or aging of circuit components when all other variables are held constant (IEEE).
Drive	16	The delivery of current, voltage, or power to a load.
Ecotelemetry	8	A biotelemetric measurement system used to track animals within their environmental range; the transmitter is usually attached externally to the animal.
Effective value	60	The root-mean-square (rms) value as given by the equation $$\text{Effective value} = \left(\frac{1}{T} \int_{0}^{T} f(t)^2 \, dt \right)^{1/2},$$ where $f(t)$ is a periodic function of time and T is the period of the function. A 1-v rms sinusoidal wave applied to a 1-Ω resistor produces the same heat that 1-v dc will produce in a 1-Ω resistor.
Electric charge	5	A fundamentally assumed concept, like mass, length, and time, required by the existence of experimentally measurable forces; a plus sign indicates that the positive electricity is in excess, a minus sign indicates that the negative electricity is in excess.
Electric current	18	The time rate of change of electric charge passing through a specified area.

Term or word	Page	Definition
Electric field (static)	68	A state of the region in which stationary charged bodies are subject to forces by virtue of their charges (IEEE).
Electron	200	An elementary particle containing the smallest negative electric charge.
Electronic counter	214	An electronic instrument capable of changing from one to the next of a sequence of distinguishable states upon each receipt of an input signal (IEEE); has a digital readout panel to display the numbers.
Electrostatic coupling	284	The interaction of an electric field with an electric circuit involving the induction of a voltage in the circuit by the electric field.
Excitation	138	An external electric voltage and/or current applied to a transducer for its proper operation.
farad	74	The unit of capacitance in the International System of Units (IEEE); abbreviated F.
Filter, electric	121	A filter designed to separate electric waves of different frequencies (IEEE); introduces relatively small insertion loss to waves in one or more frequency bands and relatively large insertion loss to waves of other frequencies.
Flicker noise	287	Noise caused by slow changes in materials used in cathodes and transistors; one form of random noise which becomes noticeable at frequencies below 1 kHz.
Fluctuation noise	286	Noise consisting of random fluctuations.
Free-running multivibrator	9	See astable multivibrator.
Frequency modulation	130	A process in which the instantaneous frequency of a carrier wave is varied in accordance with a modulating wave.
Fuse	98	An electrical circuit-protection device designed to burn out and thus open an electrical path in the presence of excessive current; rated by the currents at which it will burn out and the voltage of the circuit into which it is inserted.
Gage factor	152	The ratio of the relative change in resistance to the relative change in length of a resistive strain gage.

Term or word	Page	Definition
Gaussian curve	289	A bell-shaped curve defined by the equation $$p(x) = \frac{1}{\sigma\sqrt{2\pi}}\, e^{-x^2/2\sigma^2},$$ where σ is a constant called the standard deviation.
henry	80	The unit of inductance in the International System of Units (IEEE); abbreviated H.
hertz	58	A term used to represent cycle per second when describing frequency; 1 hertz equals 1 cycle per second; abbreviated Hz.
High-pass filter	302	An electrical filter that will severely attenuate frequencies from dc up to the lower cutoff frequency while letting pass frequencies above this cutoff frequency with very little attenuation.
Humidity sensor	164	A transducer that will respond to changes in the amount of moisture in the air.
Ideal ac current source	66	An ac source that will deliver a constant peak current to an electrical load regardless of the impedance of the load.
Ideal ac voltage source	66	An ac source that has zero internal impedance and produces a constant peak voltage regardless of the current flow through the source.
Ideal current source	30	A source of power that will deliver a constant current to a circuit regardless of the resistance connected across its terminals.
Ideal voltage source	29	A source of power that will maintain a constant voltage across its terminals regardless of the current flow out of the terminals.
Impedance	16	The impedance of a portion of an electric circuit to a completely specified periodic current and potential difference is the ratio of the effective value of the potential difference between the terminals to the effective value of the current, when there is no source of power in the portion under consideration; commonly said to oppose the flow of current in ac circuits; the basic unit is the ohm.
Induced voltage	77	A voltage produced in a component due to changes in an electric or magnetic field about the component.

Term or word	*Page*	*Definition*
Inductance	79	A property of an electric circuit, or of two neighboring circuits, which determines the voltage induced in one of the circuits by a change of current in either of them; the basic unit is the henry.
Inductive reactance	81	The amplitude of the impedance of an inductor; defined by the equation $$X_L = 2\pi fL,$$ where f is the frequency of the sinusoidal wave and L is the value of inductance; measured in ohms.
Inductor	57	A component that has the property of inductance.
Input resistance	31	The resistance measured between the two terminals that serve as the signal input to a device.
Integration	331	The inverse of differentiation; a process of finding a function of x, $y = f(x)$, from a differential expression dy/dx.
Internal impedance or resistance	16	The impedance or resistance inside a device as distinguished from that connected to the output terminals of the device.
Kirchhoff's current law	232	The sum of currents entering a node in a circuit is equal to zero.
Kirchhoff's voltage law	237	The sum of voltages around a closed loop in a circuit is equal to zero.
Linear potentiometer	154	A resistor made of a material that has uniform resistance along the full length of the resistor; has a movable tap which connects to the resistor and can be positioned mechanically.
Linear resistor	28	A resistor in which the relation between voltage and current does not change as a function of the voltage across the resistor.
Load	14	A part of an electrical circuit across which a signal is applied or a source is connected; may be considered a resistance, an impedance, or a current.
Low-pass filter	302	An electrical filter that will let pass frequencies from zero up to some cutoff frequency with very little attenuation and severely attenuate frequencies above the cutoff frequency.

Term or word	Page	Definition
Magnetic coupling	85	The interaction of a magnetic field with an electrical circuit in which a voltage is induced in the circuit by the magnetic field.
Magnetic field	77	A state produced in a medium, either by current flow in a conductor or by a permanent magnet; observations show that it has both a directional property and a magnitude or strength property; can induce a voltage in a second conductor in the medium when the state changes or when the second conductor moves in prescribed ways relative to the medium.
Magnetic flux	77	The number of lines of force issuing from a magnetic pole; these lines of force indicate a direction from the north pole to the south pole.
Magnetic-tape recorder	8	A recorder in which one or more records are made simultaneously as a function of time on magnetic tape.
Measurand	138	A physical quantity, property, or condition which is being measured.
Megahertz	67	One million hertz or one million cycles per sec; abbreviated MHz.
Microphone	169	A transducer in which variations in the pressure of sound waves are converted into electrical energy.
Microswitch	162	A transducer that will open or close an electrical circuit in response to a very low pressure.
Modulation	130	The process by which some characteristic of a carrier is varied in accordance with a modulating wave (IEEE); the variation of some characteristic of a carrier.
Modulator	130	A device that produces modulation.
Moving-coil meter	178	A D'Arsonval meter.
Multimeter (circuit analyzer)	188	The combination in a single enclosure of a plurality of instruments or instrument circuits for use in measuring two or more electrical quantities in a circuit (IEEE).
Nanovolt	287	10^{-9} volts; abbreviated nV.
Node	237	A point in a circuit where two or more electrical components are connected together.

Term or word	*Page*	*Definition*
Noise, electrical	120	An unwanted voltage or current in an electrical circuit.
Nonsymmetrical astable multivibrator	341	An electrical circuit that will generate a periodic rectangularly shaped wave; the high-voltage and low-voltage time intervals are not equal in length.
Norton equivalent circuit	227	Model of a circuit consisting of a current generator in parallel with an impedance; produces the same voltage and current in a load impedance as that produced by the original circuit connected to the load impedance.
Null detector	148	A device or circuit that is capable of responding to very low current or voltage.
ohm	30	The unit of resistance (and of impedance) in the International System of Units; 1 ohm is the resistance of a conductor such that a constant current of 1 ampere in it produces a voltage of 1 volt between its ends (IEEE); abbreviated Ω.
Ohmmeter	139	A direct-reading instrument for measuring electrical resistance.
Ohm's law	30	Voltage equals current times resistance; $V = IR$.
One-shot multivibrator	341	An electrical circuit that will generate one rectangularly shaped pulse whenever an input trigger pulse is applied to the circuit.
Open circuit	97	An electrical path of almost infinite resistance.
Operational amplifier	324	A dc amplifier that is used in circuits to perform the operations of multiplication, addition, differentiation, and integration; usually has high input impedance and high voltage amplification.
Oscillator	125	A nonrotating device for producing alternating current, the output frequency of which is determined by the characteristics of the device (IEEE); produces oscillations which are the variation, usually with time, of a quantity with respect to a specified reference when the quantity is alternately greater and smaller than the reference.
Oscilloscope	200	An instrument primarily for making visible the instantaneous values of one or more rap-

Term or word	Page	Definition
		idly varying electrical quantities as a function of time or of another electrical or mechanical quantity (IEEE).
Output	138	The electrical quantity produced by a transducer or circuit which is a function of the applied measurand.
Parallel circuit	35	A circuit in which one end of each of the components is connected to one terminal and the other end of each of the components is connected to the other terminal.
Parallel-resonant circuit	247	A circuit consisting of an inductor and a capacitor connected in parallel such that at a particular frequency, called the resonant frequency, the impedance looking into the parallel combination is purely resistive.
Passive transducer	140	A transducer whose electrical characteristic changes with the measurand; does not produce any voltage without excitation.
Periodic wave	58	A wave that is repeated in detail at regular intervals of time.
Phase angle or phase shift	70	Difference between two sinusoidal quantities which have the same period; the fractional part of the period through which the independent variable must be assumed to be advanced with respect to only one of the quantities in order that similar values of the fundamental components of the two quantities shall coincide.
Photoconductor	156	A resistor whose value changes significantly as a function of the light intensity illuminating it.
Photovoltaic cell	164	A transducer that will produce a voltage in response to the light intensity illuminating it.
Physiotelemetry	8	A biotelemetric measurement system used to record physiological changes or activities within an animal or plant; the transmitter is usually implanted in the organism.
Piezoelectric crystal	169	A crystalline dielectric transducer which becomes electrically polarized when it is mechanically strained.
Potential	5	A scalar quantity in which energy is involved as a function of position or condition; sometimes used to mean voltage.

Term or word	Page	Definition
Potential difference	5	An electromotive force between two points that will cause an electric current to flow if a conductive path exists between these two points.
Potentiometer	6	A resistor that has three terminals, one on each end and a movable tap which connects to the resistor and can be positioned mechanically; also a term used for a circuit that measures voltage.
Power	66	The time rate at which energy is used; for a dc circuit, $P = $ voltage $\times$ current; for an ac circuit, $P = $ voltage $\times$ current $\times$ cosine of the angle between the current and the voltage; rms values of voltage and current are used.
Power-density spectrum	288	Watts/Hz as a function of frequency for an electrical signal or noise.
Power source	3	A source of electrical energy; may be an ac or a dc source.
Power supply	30	A device capable of delivering power to an electric circuit; not considered a signal-delivering device; a dc power supply is a device for converting available electric service energy into direct-current energy at a voltage suitable for electronic components; a dc regulated power supply is one whose output voltage is automatically controlled to remain within specified limits for specified variations in supply voltage and load current.
Primary side	82	The side of a transformer that is connected to a source of power.
Probability density function	289	A function from which it is possible to determine the probability that a variable will fall within a given range of values; the total area under the curve of this function is always equal to 1.
Pulse	129	A variation in amplitude of a quantity whose value is normally constant.
Random noise	278	A noise that is not predictable; may be produced by electrical phenomena over which man has little or no control; can be described statistically in terms of probability density functions but cannot be described deterministically in terms of specific waveforms.

Term or word	Page	Definition
Receiver	8	A device that accepts an incoming signal, radio waves, or voltage from wired circuits, and converts it into an intelligible form.
Rectification	103	The process by which electric energy is transferred from an alternating-current circuit to a direct-current circuit (IEEE).
Rectifier	100	A device which produces rectification.
Resistance	16	A scalar property of an electrical circuit which determines for a given current the rate at which electric energy is converted into heat; is commonly said to oppose the flow of current; basic unit is the ohm.
Resistor	27	A circuit element or component that has the property of resistance.
rms or root-mean-square value	60	Value of a periodic function given by the equation $$F_{rms} = \sqrt{\frac{1}{T}\int_0^T f(t)^2\, dt,}$$ where T is the period of the function.
root-mean-square	60	See rms.
Schematic diagram	3	A diagram that shows, by means of graphic symbols, the electrical connections and functions of a particular circuit arrangement.
Secondary side	82	The side of a transformer from which power is taken to drive an electrical load.
Sensitivity	138	The ratio of the change in a transducer output to the change in the value of the measurand.
Series circuit	18	A circuit consisting of circuit elements connected end to end so that current flowing in the circuit must pass through every element.
Series-resonant circuit	247	A circuit consisting of an inductor and a capacitor connected in series such that at a particular frequency, called the resonant frequency, the impedance looking into the series combination is purely resistive.
Short circuit	97	An electrical path of almost zero resistance through which current can flow.
Shot noise	287	Noise caused by random motion of charged carriers which results in discontinuous current; one form of random noise.

Term or word	Page	Definition
Shunt	62	An electrical component connected in parallel with another component such that the same voltage is applied to both components.
Signal	3	A visual, audible, electrical, or other indication of information.
Signal-to-noise ratio (SNR)	280	The ratio of the strength of a desired signal to the strength of noise; may be given in terms of rms values of signal and noise currents or voltages or in terms of signal and noise powers.
Sine wave	60	A wave that varies in a manner described by the mathematical sine function.
Source	3	A device that can supply energy to another device.
Speaker	8	A device that converts electrical waves to acoustic waves.
Step-down transformer	83	A transformer in which the voltage at the secondary side is lower than the voltage applied at the primary side.
Step-up transformer	83	A transformer in which the voltage at the secondary side is higher than the voltage applied at the primary side.
Stimuli	4	The things that incite activity in the specimen or device.
Storage oscilloscope	203	An oscilloscope that has the capability of retaining the image of a waveform on the screen of a cathode-ray tube.
Strain gage	151	A transducer used to measure the deformation of a material that has been acted upon by a force.
Strip-chart recorder	8	A device that makes a permanent record of varying signals, usually voltages, on a strip of paper.
Symmetrical astable multivibrator	341	An electrical circuit that will generate a periodic square wave, with equal high-voltage and low-voltage time intervals.
Test organism	3	The organism being tested in some way or on which measurements are being made.
Thermal or Johnson noise	286	Noise caused by thermal agitation of free electrons in a conduction medium; one form of random noise with a very broad band (up to 10^{13} Hz).

Term or word	*Page*	*Definition*
Thermistor	159	A resistor whose value changes significantly as a function of temperature.
Thermocouple	154	A transducer consisting of a junction of two dissimilar conductors; will produce a very small voltage when the junction is heated.
Thermopile	167	A group of thermocouples assembled so as to act jointly as a source of electrical energy.
Thevenin equivalent circuit	227	Model of a circuit consisting of a voltage generator connected in series with an impedance; produces the same voltage and current in a load impedance as the original circuit connected to the load impedance.
Threshold value	138	The smallest change in the measurand that will result in a measurable change in the transducer output.
Time constant	158	The value of T in an exponential response term $A \exp(-t/_T)$ (IEEE).
Transducer	3	A device which provides a usable output in response to a specified physical quantity, property, or condition which is measured.
Transfer function	121	A mathematical, graphical, or tabular statement of the influence which a system or element has on a signal or action compared at input and at output terminals.
Transformer	6	An electrical device without continuously moving parts which by electromagnetic induction transforms electrical energy from one or more circuits to one or more other circuits at the same frequency, usually with different voltage and current.
Transistor	107	A solid-state device that is capable of controlling the flow of power from a source such that it can be used as a switch or as a control device in an amplifier.
Transmitter	8	A device or apparatus for transmitting signals by means of electric currents or electromagnetic waves.
Vacuum tube	107	Usually refers to an evacuated electron tube having a hot source of electrons that can flow to an electrode; capable of controlling the flow of power from a source such that it can be used as a switch or as a control device in an amplifier.

Term or word	*Page*	*Definition*
Vacuum tube voltmeter (VTVM)	188	A voltmeter with vacuum tubes in its circuits; usually has a high input resistance of 1 $M\Omega$ or more.
volt	6	The unit of voltage or potential difference in the International System of Units; The volt is the voltage between two points of a conducting wire carrying a constant current of 1 ampere, when the power dissipated between these points is one watt (IEEE); abbreviated V.
Voltage	5	The difference in electrical potential between two points; the basic unit is the volt.
Voltage divider	6	A circuit consisting of a series connection of components with appropriate fixed taps or a moving connection such that it can make available a portion of the total voltage; if the voltage divider is composed of a single resistor with a moving tap, it is called a potentiometer.
Voltage source model	228	A Thevenin equivalent circuit.
Voltmeter	14	A meter that is used to measure voltage.
watt	84	A unit of electric power; 1 watt equals 1 volt $\times$ 1 ampere, assuming dc values of voltage and current or rms values of voltage and current when the phase angle is zero.
Wave analyzer	186	An electrical instrument for measuring the amplitude and frequency of the various components of a complex current or voltage wave (IEEE).
Waveform	58	A graphical presentation of the variation of a quantity as a function of time.
Wheatstone bridge	147	A circuit used to measure resistance or impedance.
White noise	288	Noise that has a flat power density spectrum for all frequencies; the power per hertz is the same for all frequencies.
X-Y recorder	193	A device which makes a permanent record on paper of one varying signal with respect to another varying signal; the signals are usually voltages.

2
list of symbols

Component	Circuit symbol	Letter symbol
Air-core transformer		
Ammeter	I	I
Capacitor	C	C
Ideal current source	I_g	I_g or I_s
Ideal voltage source	dc ac	V_g or V_s
Inductor		L
Iron-core transformer		
Resistor		R
Short circuit		

Component	Circuit symbol	Letter symbol
Tapped resistor or potentiometer		R
Variable resistor		R
Variable capacitor		C
Voltmeter		V

The subscripts used with the letter symbols are as closely related to the name for the particular circuit element or component as possible. Some of the commonly used subscripts are listed below.

Symbol	Meaning
$i_g(t)$	Instantaneous current generator output as a function of time
$i_s(t)$	Instantaneous current source output as a function of time
$v_g(t)$	Instantaneous voltage generator output as a function of time
$v_n(t)$	Noise voltage generator; specified by giving power density spectrum for the noise source
$v_s(t)$	Instantaneous voltage source output as a function of time
I_{cr}	Current flow into a chart recorder
I_g	Current generator output
I_i	The ith branch current in a circuit
I_{in}	Input current
I_s	Ideal current source output or source current or sum of currents at a particular point in a circuit
I_{vm}	Current flow into a voltmeter
R_{cr}	Input resistance to a chart recorder
R_{eq}	Equivalent resistance of a combination of resistors: series, parallel, or series-parallel combinations
R_i	The ith resistor in a group of n resistors or the internal resistance of a device
R_{int}	Internal resistance of a device
R_{ij}	Resistance between points i and j in a circuit
R_{Tp}	Total resistance across a parallel combination of resistors
R_{Ts}	Total resistance of a series combination of resistors
R_{vm}	Input resistance to a voltmeter
R_{12}	Resistance between points 1 and 2 in a circuit
V_b	Battery voltage or ideal voltage source output
V_{ij}	Voltage between point i and point j in a circuit

Symbol	Meaning
V_s	Ideal voltage source output or source voltage or sum of voltages in a series circuit
V_{12}	Voltage between point 1 and point 2 in a circuit
Z_i	The ith impedance in a circuit
Z_{in}	Input impedance of a circuit.

The following symbols relate to the numerical values.

Symbol	Meaning
$\cong$	Approximately equal to
$>>$	Much greater than
$<<$	Much less than
G	Giga or times 10^9
GHz	Gigahertz or 10^9 hertz
k	Kilo or times 10^3
kV	Kilovolts or 10^3 volts
m	Milli or times 10^{-3}
mA	Milliampere or 10^{-3} ampere
mV	Millivolt or 10^{-3} volt
M	Mega or times 10^6
MHz	Megahertz or 10^6 hertz
μ	Micro or times 10^{-6}
μF	Microfarad or 10^{-6} farad
n	Nano or times 10^{-9}
nsec	Nanosecond or 10^{-9} second
p	Pico or 10^{-12}
pF	Picofarad or 10^{-12} farad
Σ	Take the algebraic sum of the terms that follow.

3
list of useful equations

The following equations are widely used in the analysis of elementary electrical circuits. They are gathered here for handy reference. The equation numbers are given, so the reader may refer to the points in the text where they first appear and thus refresh his memory as to their applicability in a particular problem.

Equation	Equation Number	Page
Ohm's law: $V = IR$	(3.0)	33

Total resistance of a series of n resistors:

$$R_{Ts} = \sum_{i=1}^{n} R_i$$

(3.1)　　34

Total resistance of two resistors in parallel:

$$R_{Tp} = \frac{R_1 R_2}{R_1 + R_2}$$

(3.21)　　38

Total current in a parallel circuit of n branches:

$$I_T = \sum_{i=1}^{n} I_i$$

(3.26)　　39

Total resistance of n resistors in parallel:

$$R_{Tp} = \frac{1}{\sum_{i=1}^{n} (1/R_i)}$$

(3.27)　　39

Voltage-divider output voltage:

$$V_L = \frac{R_p}{R_1 + R_p} V_b$$

(3.45)　　52

Equation	Equation Number	Page

Total impedance of series of n resistors:

$$Z_{\text{Total}} = \sum_{i=1}^{n} Z_i \qquad\qquad (4.2) \qquad\qquad 59$$

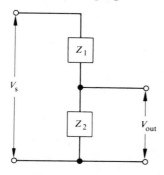

Ohm's law for ac circuits:

$$V = IZ \qquad\qquad (4.5) \qquad\qquad 60$$

Calculating rms value of a sine wave:

rms value = maximum value divided by $\sqrt{2}$ (4.6)   61

maximum or peak value = (rms value) $(\sqrt{2})$ (4.7)   61

Total voltage for a series circuit:

$$V_{\text{Total}} = \sum_{i=1}^{n} V_i \qquad\qquad (4.12) \qquad\qquad 62$$

Output voltage across an impedance voltage divider:

$$V_{\text{out}} = \frac{1}{1 + Z_1/Z_2} V_{\text{s}} \qquad\qquad (4.16) \qquad\qquad 63$$

Total current in a parallel circuit of n branches:

$$I_{\text{Total}} = \sum_{i=1}^{n} I_i \qquad\qquad (4.17) \qquad\qquad 65$$

Equation	Equation Number	Page

Equivalent impedance of n impedances in parallel:

$$Z_{eq} = \dfrac{1}{\displaystyle\sum_{i=1}^{n} (1/Z_i)}$$

(4.19)   65

ac power:

ac power = rms voltage × rms current × cosine of the phase angle

(4.20)   66

dc power:

dc power = voltage × current

(4.21)   66

Defining equation for capacitance:

$$C = \frac{q}{V}$$

(4.22)   69

Defining equation for current:

$$i(t) = \frac{dq}{dt}$$

(4.23)   69

Defining equation for impedance of a capacitor:

$$Z_C = -j\frac{1}{2\pi f C}$$

(4.30)   73

Defining equation for capacitive reactance:

$$X_C = \frac{1}{2\pi f C}$$

(4.31)   74

Induced voltage:

$$V_{ind} = L\frac{di}{dt}$$

(4.33)   79

Impedance of an inductor:

$$Z_L = j2\pi f L$$

(4.35)   80

Inductive reactance:

$$X_L = 2\pi f L$$

(4.36)   81

Transformer voltage and turns ratios:

$$\frac{V_{out}}{V_{in}} = \frac{N_2}{N_1}$$

Transformer impedance and turns ratios:

$$Z_{in} = \left(\frac{N_1}{N_2}\right)^2 Z_{out}$$

Voltage regulation:

$$\text{Voltage regulation} = \frac{V_{no\ load} - V_{rated\ load}}{V_{rated\ load}} \times 100\%.$$

Decibels, voltage:

$$\text{Number of dB} = 20\ \log_{10}\frac{V_2}{V_1}.$$

Decibels, power:

$$\text{Number of dB} = 10\ \log_{10}\frac{P_2}{P_1}.$$

Distortion factor:

$$\text{Distortion factor} = \left(\frac{\text{Sum of the squares of amplitudes of all harmonics}}{\text{Square of amplitude of the fundamental frequency}}\right)^{1/2}.$$

Transfer function:

$$\text{Transfer function} = \frac{\text{Output signal voltage as a function of frequency}}{\text{Input signal voltage as a function of frequency}}.$$

Determining the shunt resistance for ammeters
constructed with microammeters or milliammeters:

$$R_{sh} = \frac{I_m R_m}{I - I_m}$$

Equation	Equation Number	Page

where I_m = full-scale meter current, I = maximum current to be measured, R_m = resistance of meter movement.

Determining the series resistance for voltmeters constructed with milliammeters:

$$R_{ser} = \frac{V}{I_m} - R_m, \qquad\qquad (7.2) \qquad\qquad 181$$

where V = full-scale voltage to be measured, I_m = full-scale meter current, R_m = resistance of meter movement.

Kirchhoff's voltage law: The sum of the voltages   232
around a closed loop is equal to zero or

$$\sum_{i=1}^{n} V_i = 0,$$

where n = number of components in series around the loop.

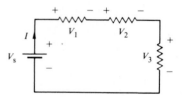

Kirchhoff's current law: The sum of all the cur-   237
rents entering a node is equal to zero, assuming
that all currents at the node enter the node, or

$$\sum_{i=1}^{n} I_i = 0,$$

where n = number of parallel branches at the node.

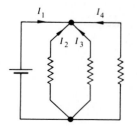

$$I_1 + I_2 + I_3 + I_4 = 0$$

Equation   Equation Number   Page

or

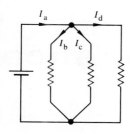

$$I_a - I_b - I_c - I_d = 0$$

4
references

PART A

The references that are relevant to each chapter are listed after the chapter number according to their list numbers in Part B of this appendix.

Chapter	Reference Numbers
1	4,5,6,7,9,11,16,17,24,27,30,31,32,38,40,46,52,56
3	2,3,28,38
4	2,28,38
5	2,23,28,45
6	1,12,13,14,15,25,26,33,35,36,37,39,41,48,49,53,54
7	8,18,22,23,28,42,43,44,45,47,50,51,55
8	4,7,27,46,57
9	2,3,28,38
10	2,10,19,34
11	2,10,20,34
12	2,28,29,41

PART B

1. Ambroziak, A., *Semiconductor Photoelectric Devices*. Gordon and Breach Science Publishers, New York, 1970.
2. Benedict, R. R., *Electronics for Scientists and Engineers*. Prentice-Hall, Englewood Cliffs, N. J., 1967. (This book is intended for the nonspecialist with no prior knowledge of the subject. The approach is analytical and quantitative. It includes material on transducers, noise, data systems, as well as electronic instruments, amplifiers and components.)

3. Brophy, J. J., *Basic Electronics for Scientists*. McGraw-Hill, New York, 1966. (Written to provide the undergraduate science major with a basic understanding of electronic devices and circuits.)
4. Caceres, C. A., *Biomedical Telemetry*. Academic Press, New York, 1965.
5. Cooper, W. D., *Electronic Instrumentation and Measurement Techniques*. Prentice-Hall, Englewood Cliffs, N. J., 1970.
6. Cornsweet, T. N., *The Design of Electric Circuits in the Behavioral Sciences*. Wiley, New York, 1963.
7. Craighead, F. C., Jr., *et al.*, "Bio-telemetry," *Proceedings of the Interdisciplinary Conference* (L. E. Slater, Ed.) Pergamon Press, New York, 1963.
8. Dewhurst, B. J., *Physical Instrumentation in Medicine and Biology*. Pergamon Press, New York, 1966.
9. Edwards, D. F., *Electronic Measurement Technique*. Transatlantic Arts, Levittown, N. Y., 1971.
10. Ficchi, R. F., *Electrical Interference*. Hayden, New York, 1964. (The purpose of this book is to provide the tools and techniques to enable the engineer to minimize interference in electronic equipment and systems. Topics include shielding, filtering, cables, and grounding, among others. Has an extensive bibliography.)
11. Geddes, L. A., and L. E. Baker, *Principles of Applied Biomedical Instrumentation*. Wiley, New York, 1968.
12. Geddes, L. A., "Interface design for bioelectrode systems," *IEEE Spectrum,* 1972, **9**(10):41-48. (Proper specification of input impedances for recorders is the key to design of distortion-free measurement systems. This article describes electrocardiographic electrodes, electroencephalographic electrodes, floating electrodes, and needle electrodes. It also discusses the electrical models of bioelectric electrodes to serve as a working guide to aid in specifying the input impedance needed for a recorder used when measuring bioelectric potentials.)
13. Giles, A F., *Electronic Sensing Devices*. Newnes, London, 1966. (The book aims at providing assistance to those engaged in developing or applying industrial sensing devices. Includes solid-state, electrolytic, gaseous ion, capacitive, and magnetic-induction sensors as well as electronic sensors for physical quantities and for chemistry.)
14. Harvey, G. F. (Ed.), *ISA Transducer Compendium,* Second Edition, Part I. IFI/Plenum, New York, 1969. (Detailed listing of specific transducers manufactured for measurement of pressure, level, and flow.)
15. Harvey, G. F. (Ed.), *ISA Transducer Compendium,* Second Edition, Part 2. Instrument Society of America, Pittsburgh, 1970. (Detailed listing of specific transducers manufactured for measurement of sound, force and torque, motion and dimension.)
16. Kashin, P., and H. G. Wakeley, "An insect 'bitometer'," *Nature,* 1965, **208**:462-464.
17. Kavanau, J. L., and K. S. Norris, "Behavior studies by capacitance sensing," *Science,* 1961, **134**:730-732.
18. Kidwell, W. M., *Electrical Instruments and Measurements*. McGraw-Hill, New York, 1969.
19. Lathi, B. P., *Communication Systems*. Wiley, New York, 1968. (Discusses modulation systems and noise, among other communications-related topics.)

20. Lathi, B. P., *An Introduction to Random Signals and Communication Theory*. International Textbook Company, Scranton, Pa., 1968. (Very technical discussion of autocorrelation, cross-correlation, and optimum filtering. Gives the elements of probability theory.)

21. Lee, Y. W., *Statistical Theory of Communication*. Wiley, New York, 1960. (Very thorough and technical discussion of autocorrelation, cross-correlation, and sampling techniques, in addition to other topics.)

22. Lenk, J. D., *Handbook of Oscilloscopes: Theory and Application*. Prentice-Hall, Englewood Cliffs, N. J., 1968. (The book can be used to supplement the operating instructions of any oscilloscope. Includes oscilloscope basics, cameras, measuring voltage and current; measuring time, frequency, and phase; measuring impedance, strain, pressure, and noise, among other topics.)

23. Lenk, J. D., *Handbook of Electronic Test Equipment*. Prentice-Hall, Englewood Cliffs, N. J., 1971. (Describes the purpose and operating principles related to test equipment. Includes analog meters, digital and differential meters, bridge-type test equipment, signal generators, electronic counters, oscilloscopes and recorders, amplifiers, probes and transducers, among other topics.)

24. Lenk, J. D., and A. Marcus, *Measurements for Technicians*. Prentice-Hall, Englewood Cliffs, N. J., 1971.

25. Levins, S., "Stress and behavior," *Scientific American*, 1971, **224**(1):26-31. ("Startle" response is measured by placing a rat in a cage with a movable floor and exposing it to a sudden loud noise. The rat tenses or jumps, and the resulting movement of the floor is transduced into movement of a pen on a recording paper.)

26. Lippold, O., "Physiological tremor," *Scientific American*, 1971, **224**(3):65-73. (The subject's forefinger interrupts a beam of parallel light falling on a ground-glass slit. Behind the slit is a photodetector, the output of which is amplified and fed into a small fixed-program averaging computer.)

27. MacKay, R. S., *Biomedical Telemetry*. Wiley, New York, 1970. (Includes electronics, modulation, plastics, and other materials, pressure-sensing and transmission, temperature-sensing and transmission, bioelectric and chemical electrode potentials, sensors and transmitters for other variables, frequency and antenna selection, receivers and demodulators, calibration and response control, among other topics.)

28. Malmstadt, H. V., and C. G. Enke, *Electronics for Scientists*. Benjamin, New York, 1963. (Introduction to basic electrical measuring instruments, amplifying devices, measurements, servo systems, operational amplifiers, electronic switching and timing circuits, among other topics. Includes a short review of elementary electrical circuit theory. Experiments.)

29. Malmstadt, H. V., and C. G. Enke, *Digital Electronics for Scientists*. Benjamin, New York, 1969. (Introduction to the digital circuits, the concepts and the systems that are basic to the new instrumentation-computation revolution. Assumes little or no background in digital electronics or other electronics. Includes switching devices, logic gates, flip-flops and multivibrators, counters, registers, readout and digital and analog-digital instruments and systems, among other topics. Experiments.)

30. McClelland, W. J., "An electronic apparatus for recording movement in small animals," *J. Exp. Anal. Behav.*, 1965, **8**(4):215-218.
31. McLean, D. L., and M. G. Kinsey, "A technique for electronically recording aphid feeding and salivation," *Nature*, 1964, **202**:1358-1359.
32. McLean, D. L., and W. A. Weigt, "An electronic measuring system to record aphid salivation and ingestion," *Ann. Ent. Soc. Amer.*, 1969, **61**:180-185.
33. Menaker, M., "Nonvisual light reception," *Scientific American*, 1972, **226**(3):22-29. [Microswitches used under perches (one near water and one near food) to record activity by means of a recorder.]
34. Morrison, Ralph, *Grounding and Shielding Techniques in Instrumentation*. Wiley, New York, 1967. (Discussion of noise sources and noise problems. Offers techniques for avoiding noise pickup. Uses electrostatics and mutual capacitance as the bases and gives general rules for shielding signal paths and grounding signal lines.)
35. Neubert, H. K. P., *Instrument Transducers: An Introduction to Their Performance and Design*. Clarendon Press, Oxford, England, 1963.
36. Norton, H. N., *Handbook of Transducers for Electronic Measuring Systems*. Prentice-Hall, Englewood Cliffs, N. J., 1969. (Very complete discussion of transducers, is application oriented. Will be useful to users of transducers and those responsible for selecting and purchasing transducers. Definitions of terms.)
37. Noton, D., and L. Stark, "Eye movements and visual perception," *Scientific American*, 1971, **224**(6):34-43. (The subject viewed pictures displayed on a rear-projection screen by a random-access slide projector. Diffuse infrared light was shined on his eyes; his eye movements were recorded by photocells, mounted on a spectacle frame that detected reflections of the infrared light from the eyeball. Eye movements were displayed on oscilloscope and also recorded on tape.)
38. Offner, F. F., *Electronics for Biologists*. McGraw-Hill, New York, 1967. (Introduces fundamentals of electronics and the principles of some of the instruments employed in the biological sciences. The purpose of the book is to permit the reader to intelligently select, use, and understand the limitations of equipment which he will usually obtain from commercial sources. It includes electrophysiological electronic practice, transducers, electrodes and stimulations, among other topics.)
39. Oliver, F. J., *Practical Instrumentation Transducers*. Hayden, New York, 1971. (A comprehensive book that discusses a wide variety of transducers and some associated circuitry. Its primary purpose is to serve as a guide to transducer selection and application by control systems and instrumentation engineers.)
40. Powell, J. A., H. Esch, and G. B. Craig, Jr., "Electronic recording of mosquito activity," *Ent. Exp. and Appl.*, 1966, **9**:385-394.
41. Prensky, S. D., *Electronic Instrumentation*. Prentice-Hall, Englewood Cliffs, N. J., 1971. [Discusses comparison measurement methods (potentiometer and bridge types), transducers, analog computers, among other topics. Assumes knowledge of basic electronics.]
42. Prensky, S. D., *Advanced Electronic Instruments and Their Use*. Hayden, New York, 1970.
43. Ragosine, V. E., "Magnetic recording," *Scientific American*, 1969, **221**(5):71-82.

44. Roth, C. H., *Use of the Oscilloscope: A Programmed Text*. Prentice-Hall, Englewood Cliffs, N. J., 1970.

45. Schuster, D. H., *Basic Electronic Test Equipment: A Programmed Introduction*. McGraw-Hill, New York, 1968. (A programmed introduction to the theory and use of basic electronic test equipment. Three basic types of test equipment are covered: meters, signal generators, and oscilloscopes.)

46. Slater, L. E., "Biotelemetry," *Bioscience*, 1965, **15**:79-120.

47. Squires, T. L., *Beginner's Guide to Electronics*. Philosophical Library, New York. 1967.

48. Stacy, R. W., *Biological and Medical Electronics*. McGraw-Hill, New York, 1960. (Written as an introductory book. Discusses theory of measurement, detecting and sensing elements, recording and readout devices, complete instrumentation schemes, trouble-shooting instruments and computers as laboratory instruments, among other topics.)

49. Summer, S. E., *Electronic Sensing Controls*. Chilton, Philadelphia, 1969. (Presents the fundamentals of a large class of industrial electronics equipment. Includes material that would be of interest to many biologists. Discusses sensors and transducers, photoelectric controls, temperature controls, among other topics. Not highly technical or theoretical.)

50. Thomas, H. E., and C. A. Clark, *Handbook of Electronic Instruments and Measurement Techniques*. Prentice-Hall, Englewood Cliffs, N. J., 1967.

51. Tiedmann, A. T., *Elements of Electrical Measurements*. Allyn and Bacon, Boston, 1967. (Book is designed to introduce to the reader some of the basic aspects of electrical measurements. Not written for the specialist but does require an understanding of electric-circuit theory. Includes cathode-ray oscilloscopes, indicating instruments, balance methods of measurement, analog computer, among other topics.)

52. Vurek, G. G., *Proceedings of the Annual Conference on Engineering in Medicine and Biology*, Conference Commemorating the Nineteenth Anniversary of the Conference on Medicine and Biology, 1966.

53. Wedlock, B. D., and J. K. Roberge, *Electronic Components and Measurements*. Prentice-Hall, Englewood Cliffs, N. J., 1969. (Introduction to basic electrical concepts used in measurements. Introduction to basic measuring instruments and their operation. Very little mathematical development.)

54. Wolff, H. S., *Biomedical Engineering*. McGraw-Hill, New York, 1970. (A nontechnical introduction to the general area of bioengineering with strong emphasis on biomedical engineering. Introduces types of measurements to be done and ways of doing them, including kinds of transducers and instruments used. Discusses hospital automation and prosthetic devices, among other topics.)

55. Yanof, H. M., *Biomedical Electronics*. F. A. Davis, Philadelphia, 1965.

56. Zucker, M., and W. E. Howard, "A transistorized body capacitance relay for eco-behavioral studies," *Anim. Behav.*, 1968, **16**(1):65-66.

57. *The A.R.R.L. Antenna Book*. American Radio League, West Hartford, Conn., 1960.

The following dictionaries are useful references on the definitions of technical terms that appear in books and articles related to electrical phenomena and measurements.

58. Carter, H., *Dictionary of Electronics*. Hart, New York, 1963.
59. *IEEE Standard Dictionary of Electrical and Electronics Terms*. The Institute of Electrical and Electronics Engineers, Wiley-Interscience, New York, 1972.
60. *IRE Dictionary of Electronics Terms and Symbols*. The Institute of Radio Engineers, New York, 1961.

5
list of examples

6
list of
basic electrical units and
multiplier abbreviations

Term	Unit	Symbol for Unit	Multiplier	Symbol	Value
Capacitance	farad	F	Pico	p	10^{-9}
Current	ampere	A	Micro	μ	10^{-6}
Inductance	henry	H	Milli	m	10^{-3}
Resistance	ohm	Ω	Kilo	k	10^3
Voltage	volt	V	Mega	M	10^6
Power	watt	W	Giga	G	10^9

7
color code used on carbon-composition resistors

Color	Value
Black	0
Brown	1
Red	2
Orange	3
Yellow	4
Green	5
Blue	6
Violet	7
Gray	8
White	9
Gold	$\pm 5\%$ tolerance
Silver	$\pm 10\%$ tolerance

Most significant digit ────▶ ①
Next most significant digit ────▶ ②
Power of 10 multiplier exponent ────▶ ③
Percent tolerance ────▶ ④

Example Assume that color band 1 is red, color band 2 is green, color band 3 is orange, and color band 4 is gold. Resistance $= 25 \times 10^3 \Omega \pm 5\%$.

8
answers
to selected review
questions and problems

3.6   (a) 12.5 V, 50 V.

     (b) 100 V.

3.11 (a) $\Delta V_{R_1} = 3.08$ V.

     (b) $\Delta V_{R_1} = 4$ V.

3.12 $I_s = 0.237$ mA, $V_{12} = 0.527$ V.

3.13 $I_a = 0.667$ mA.

3.14 (a) circuit a : $R_1 = 3$ kΩ,
           circuit b : $R_1 = 100$ Ω.

     (b) circuit a : $R_1 = 4.28$ kΩ,
           circuit b : $R_1 = 80$ Ω.

3.15 Proposal I $\Delta I_s = 0.147$ mA.
     Proposal II $\Delta I_s = 0.081$ mA.

4.1 $V_{rms} = 5.3$ V, $f = 1.43$ Hz.

4.2 $I_{peak} = 5.66$ mA.

4.10 $P = 1057$ W.

4.25 (a) Checkpoints

R_2, Ω	500	800	1k	1.2k	1.5k
P, W	0.0222	0.0247	0.025	0.0248	0.024

     (b) $R_2 = R_1$.

4.26 $R_2 = R_1$.

4.27 $N_1/N_2 = 4.47$.

5.6   Use transformer with $N_1/N_2 = 1.83$.

5.19 (a) $P_{out}/P_{in} = 1000$.

(b) $V_{out}/V_{in} = 3.316$.

5.21 $V_{out}/V_{in} = 0.708$ or $P_{out}/P_{in} = 0.501$.

5.26 When $V_{s_{in}} = 0.1A$, $SNR_{out} = 3.33$ and there will be noise of significant amplitude.

6.3   When the light is 0.4 lumens, the voltage across the device is 47 V.
When the light is 0.1 lumens, the voltage across the device is 158 V.

6.4   Connect the light-sensitive resistor in series with a 20-V dc power supply and a load resistor. When the light is off, the current is almost zero and the voltage across the light-sensitive resistor is almost 20 V. This is the maximum allowable voltage across the light-sensitive resistor. The load resistance can range from 4.8 kΩ to 5.73 kΩ and produce a maximum variation of about 6.8 V. Lower or higher values of load resistance produce a smaller output voltage variation.

6.5 $100 \, \Omega \leqslant R_2 \leqslant 1000 \, \Omega$.

6.6   Maximum $\Delta V = 15.8$ V.

6.7   (a) $\Delta V_o = 0.267 \, V_{battery}$.

(b) $\Delta V_o = 0.25 \, V_{battery}$.

6.8   Assuming $V_{R_1} = 0.3$ V and battery current is 10 mA : $R_1 = 30 \, \Omega$, $R_2 = 570 \, \Omega$, $P_{R_1} = 3$ mW.

6.9   0.43 V.

7.1   (a) $8.7 \, V \leqslant V \leqslant 9.3 \, V$.

(b) $2.1 \, V \leqslant V \leqslant 2.7 \, V$.

(c) 3.22% for 9 V reading;
11.1% for 2.4 V reading.

7.2   Connect a 2-Ω, ¼-W resistor in parallel with a milliammeter. Impossible to obtain ±5% tolerance at low end of the scale.

7.3   Connect a 3980-Ω, ¼-W resistor in series with a milliammeter.

7.4   Connect a 1480-Ω, ¼-W resistor in series with a 1.5-V battery and the milliammeter.

Scale calibration:

R_T, Ω	500	600	700	800	900	1000
I, mA	0.75	0.714	0.682	0.652	0.625	0.60

7.5 23.5%.

7.6 Chart recorder "loads down" the circuit by voltage divider action.

9.1 $V_{int} = 18$ V, $R_{int} = 1200$ Ω, $V_{12} = 8.18$ V.

9.2 Checkpoints:

R_L, k Ω	0.5	1	1.5	2	2.5	3
V_{12}, V	5.29	8.18	10.0	11.25	12.16	12.86

9.3 No unique solution. If $R_L = 250$ Ω, $I_{ps} = 0.1$ A.
Build a voltage divider with a 60-Ω and a 47.6-Ω resistor. Connect R_L across the 47.6-Ω resistor. Then 3.5 V $< V_{R_L} < 4.15$ V when 100 $\Omega < R_L$ < 400 Ω.

9.9 Assume clockwise currents in each loop.
$I_1 R_1 + I_1 R_2 + I_1 R_3 - I_2 R_3 + V_s = 0.$
$I_2 R_3 - I_1 R_3 + I_2 R_4 + I_2 R_5 - I_3 R_5 - V_s = 0.$
$I_3 R_5 - I_2 R_5 + I_3 R_6 = 0.$

9.10 $P_{R_3} = 0.521$ W.

9.11 For 100-W operation, use 35.9-Ω, 90-W resistor in series with heater. For 200-W operation, use a 13.7-Ω, 70-W resistor.

9.12 (a) 30.8 V, (b) 2.31 A, (c) 227 W, (d) 15.4 V.

9.13 $V_{int} = 57.14$ V, $R_{int} = 17.14$ Ω.

9.15 Assume all currents leave node 1.

$$\frac{V_{12} - V_s}{R_1} + \frac{V_{12}}{R_2} + \frac{V_{12}}{R_3 + R_4} = 0.$$

9.16 23.2 mA, 1.61 W.

9.17 Assume all currents leave nodes 1 and 3.

$$\frac{V_{14}}{R_1} + \frac{V_{14} - V_s}{R_2} + \frac{V_{14} - V_{34}}{R_3} = 0.$$

$$\frac{V_{34} - V_s}{R_4} + \frac{V_{34} - V_{14}}{R_3} + \frac{V_{34}}{R_5} = 0.$$

9.18 10.52 W.

9.19 37.84 V.

9.20 $V_s = 7.13$ V, $I_s = 1.53$ mA.

9.21 $\Delta V_{12} = 1.08$ V, $\Delta P_{R_0} = 0.237$ mW.

9.22 7.24 mA.

9.23 (a) 8.26 W   (b) 90.9 mA

 (c) 95.2 mA when $R_x = 50\ \Omega$
  76.9 mA when $R_x = 300\ \Omega$

9.24 $R_x\ \Omega$ I_{R_n}, mA   Direction of current flow
  500   1.02   right to left.
  1000   0.413   right to left.
  2000   0.3   left to right.

9.25 $|Z|$ θ degrees
 (a)   5   53.1
 (b)   35.36   45
 (c)   36.06   −33.69
 (d)   42.06   −28.39
 (e)   9.49   −18.43
 (f) 120.1   2.38
 (g) 117.15   50.19
 (h)   7.81   −39.8
 (i)   23.6   −53.6
 (j)   37.74   −32.0

9.26 (a) $9.06 + j\ 4.23$
 (b) $22.63 - j\ 22.63$
 (c) $11.64 + j\ 43.47$
 (d) $6.06 - j\ 3.5$
 (e) $50.0\ + j\ 86.6$
 (f) $294.0\ - j\ 89.8$
 (g) $66.2\ + j124.5$
 (h) $72.1\ - j\ 48.6$
 (i) $8.42 - j\ 11.18$
 (j) $12.27 + j\ 25.17$

9.27 Checkpoints

f, Hz	100	500	1000	50 000
Z, Ω	$-j1592$	$-j318$	$-j159.2$	$-j3.18$

9.28 Checkpoints

f, Hz	100	500	1000	50 000
Z, Ω	$-j79\ 600$	$-j15\ 920$	$-j7960$	159.2

9.29 Checkpoints

f, Hz	100	500	1000	50 000
X_L, Ω	628.3	3142	6283	314 200

9.30 $20 + j30\ \Omega$, $36\ \angle 56.3°\ \Omega$.

9.31 $100\ \Omega$

9.33 1591 Hz, 70.7 V.

9.35 Checkpoints

f, Hz	800	1200	1591	2000	2500
$|V_R|$, V	39.4	61.37	70.7	64.27	51.68

9.37 $10^3\ \Omega$

9.39 Checkpoints

f, Hz	3000	3200	3558	3700	4000
$|V_R|$, V	10.47	7.12	0	2.76	7.73

9.40 The $0.04 \mu F$ capacitor reduces the noise by a factor of 8.13 relative to the signal voltage.

9.41 Checkpoints

f, Hz	10	50	100	300	1000
$|V_{34}/V_{12}|$	0.995	0.893	0.705	0.315	0.099

9.42 Checkpoints

f, Hz	10	50	100	300	1000
$|V_o/V_s|$	0.962	0.698	0.444	0.163	0.049

9.43 $V_{12} = 50\ \angle 59.9°$.

10.4 1mV.

10.5 (a) 0.5 mV, (c) 7.5 mV.

11.1 Circuit a : 0.754 mV.
 Circuit c : 0.0377 mV.

11.3 (a) Filter I, (c) $SNR_{34} = 23.6$ with Filter I
 $SNR_{34} = 0.0998$ with Filter II.

12.1 No unique answer.

12.3 $A_v = -10$, $V_{out} = -3.64$ V.

12.7 No unique answer.

12.8 $R_{in}\ C_{fb} = 5 \times 10^{-4}$.

index

Index

index